Infectious Diseases and Microbiology

Emergency and Intensive Care Medicine

Nova Medicine & Health
New York

Infectious Diseases and Microbiology

Critical Care and COVID-19
Salim Surani (Editor)
Syed Anjum Khan (Editor)
Reena Shah (Editor)
2023. ISBN: 979-8-88697-940-4 (Hardcover)
2023. ISBN: 979-8-88697-969-5 (eBook)

Infectious Diseases: From Prevention to Control
Yvette S. Brewer (Editor)
2023. ISBN: 979-8-88697-657-1 (Hardcover)
2023. ISBN: 979-8-88697-664-9 (eBook)

More information about this series can be found at
https://novapublishers.com/product-category/series/infectious-diseases-and-microbiology/

Emergency and Intensive Care Medicine

Environmental Emergencies and Injuries in Nature
Murat Yücel, MD (Editor)
Murat Güzel, MD (Editor)
İbrahim İkizceli, MD (Editor)
2022. ISBN: 978-1-68507-833-1 (Hardcover)
2022. ISBN: 978-1-68507-917-8 (eBook)

Multidisciplinary Approach to Trauma
Mehmet Cenk Turgut, MD (Editor)
Asli Turgut, MD (Editor)
2022. ISBN: 978-1-68507-761-7 (Hardcover)
2022. ISBN: 978-1-68507-915-4 (eBook)

More information about this series can be found at
https://novapublishers.com/shop/peritonitis-causes-diagnosis-and-treatment/

Salim Surani
Syed Anjum Khan
and Reena Shah
Editors

Histoplasmosis

From Diagnosis to Treatment

nova
Medicine & Health
New York

Library of Congress Cataloging-in-Publication Data

Names: Surani, Salim, editor. | Khan, Syed Anjum, editor. | Shah, Reena (Physician), editor.
Title: Histoplasmosis: from diagnosis to treatment / Salim Surani, editor, Clinical Professor, University of Houston, Houston, TX, USA, Syed Anjum Khan, editor, Assistant Professor of Medicine, Mayo Clinic, Mankato, MN, USA, Reena Shah, editor, Associate Professor and Chief of Medicine, Aga Khan University, Nairobi, Kenya.
Description: New York : Nova Science Publishers, [2023] | Series: Emergency and intensive care medicine | Includes bibliographical references and index. |
Identifiers: LCCN 2023041587 (print) | LCCN 2023041588 (ebook) | ISBN 9798891131293 (hardcover) | ISBN 9798891132283 (adobe pdf)
Subjects: LCSH: Histoplasmosis. | Histoplasmosis--Diagnosis. | Histoplasmosis--Treatment.
Classification: LCC RC147.H7 H574 2023 (print) | LCC RC147.H7 (ebook) | DDC 616.2/4--dc23/eng/20231002
LC record available at https://lccn.loc.gov/2023041587
LC ebook record available at https://lccn.loc.gov/2023041588

Published by Nova Science Publishers, Inc. † New York

Contents

Preface

This book is an attempt to demystify Histoplasma infection and enhance your knowledge about this recluse fungus. The Pharaoh's curse, which led to the deaths of several team members involved in the discovery of Tutankhamun's tomb in 1922, is believed to be caused by Histoplasma infection. Although some still attribute the deaths to the curse, microbiologists believe Histoplasma capsulatum, a thermal fungus commonly found in the ground, as the likely culprit.

Histoplasma infection is a global phenomenon, with more than 500,000 cases reported annually in the United States alone. The fungus is prevalent in Ohio and the Mississippi River valley, where residents have a high positivity rate. Infection occurs when spores found in bird and bat droppings are inhaled. Airborne transmission is common during activities such as demolition, landscaping, and farming. Although most people are asymptomatic, immunocompromised individuals can suffer life-threatening infections that affect various parts of the body.

In disseminated histoplasmosis, the fungus can invade the liver, spleen, pancreas, intestine, and other organs, leading to fever, weight loss, anorexia, coughing, vomiting, diarrhea, abdominal pain, and, in some cases, tuberculosis-like symptoms. Patients can also develop multi-system involvement, including meningitis, pneumonia, pericarditis, and adrenal insufficiency. Our goal is to shed light on this elusive organism and the life-threatening complications it can cause if untreated especially in immunocompromised individual.

In this book you will learn from chapters on global prevalence of the disease, its diagnosis, histopathology, and radiology findings; systemic involvement, differential diagnosis, histoplasma and pregnancy, hemophagocytic syndrome and many other interesting aspects of the disease.

We assure you that the time spent in reviewing the content will be invaluable.

Salim Surani, MD
Syed Anjum Khan, MD
Reena Shah, MD

Chapter 1

The Global Prevalence of Histoplasmosis

Ladan Panahi[1,*]
Niraj Patel[1]
Jessica Kaestner[1]
Ella Lorng[1]
Roxana Merino[1]
Jessica Milligan[1]
Ricco Rizo[1]
Augusta Udeani[1]
Salim Surani[2]
and Laura Vasquez[1]
[1]Department of Pharmacy Practice,
Texas A&M Rangel School of Pharmacy, Texas, USA
[2]Department of Medicine & Pharmacology,
Texas A&M University, Mayo Clinic, Rochester, Minnesota, USA

Abstract

This chapter provides a topic update on the global prevalence of Histoplasmosis. Recent years have seen an expansion of Histoplasma geographic distribution due to climate change, environmental disruption, and host factors. This chapter examines the recent shifts and expansions in the prevalence of some of these endemic fungi. It is hypothesized that these changes are due to human migration, agricultural practices,

* Corresponding Author's Email: panahi@tamu.edu.

In: Histoplasmosis
Editors: Salim Surani, Syed Anjum Khan and Reena Shah
ISBN: 979-8-89113-129-3

occupational exposures, deforestation, soil movement, and climate change. Although organ transplantation has advanced, these emerging insights enhance our understanding of Histoplasmosis, particularly in those with a higher risk of infection and severity of the disease. This review discusses epidemiologic beliefs about the disease, its geographic distribution, prevalence, and burden in the United States and the world.

Keywords: histoplasmosis, solid organ transplantation, infection, endemic mycoses, immunocompromised, prevalence, epidemiology

Introduction

Histoplasmosis, first described by Samuel T. Darling in the early 20th century, is a fungal infection caused by a diverse group of fungi [1]. There are three identified varieties of Histoplasma [2]. The two well-defined organisms of histoplasmosis in humans are *Histoplasma capsulatum* and *Histoplasma* duboisii [3]. *Histoplasma capsulatum* is an endemic fungal pathogen that can cause histoplasmosis, a fungal infection caused by the inhalation of Histoplasma species [4, 5] Compared to *H. capsulatum*, *H. duboisii* primarily causes skin and soft tissue infections and hardly involves the lungs [6].

Typically found in bird or bat feces, it is commonly centered around the Mississippi and Ohio River Valley in the United States.1 In the environment of the midwestern states, Histoplasma species exist as mold but are then converted to yeast at body temperature within a human host [2].

These fungi can cause disease in healthy and immunocompromised patients [1] These fungi are termed endemic mycoses due to their common occurrence in specific geographic ranges and cause morbidity and mortality in HIV/AIDS and immunocompromised patients [6]. Among these species, there are differences in geographical distribution, clinical presentation, diagnostic approach, and therapeutic interventions [1].

Clinical Presentation

One of the most common sites for infection in all cases of blastomycosis is the lungs, with pneumonia being the most common manifestation [4]. Most infections are caused by inhaling the microconidia in the environment [2]. Other dissemination sites include the bone marrow, lymph nodes, spleen, liver,

GI tract, skin, and the central nervous system (CNS) [2]. Depending on the host immune state, clinical manifestations can occur after a 3 to 17-day incubation period [5]. Some of these manifestations are presented as asymptomatic, acute/chronic pulmonary, and life-long infections [5]. Although *H. capsulatum* is mainly asymptomatic, patients exposed to a greater infection can develop symptomatic pulmonary infections requiring hospitalization [7]. Aside from pulmonary symptoms, other symptoms such as fever, night sweats, and weight loss occurred progressively or in a waxing-waning manner [8]. Fever and shortness of breath are the most common clinical manifestations, followed by diarrhea, cough, diaphoresis, and headache [9]. Other symptoms may include malaise, cough, dyspnea, hepatosplenomegaly, and other gastrointestinal symptoms [2]. Presentation specific to CNS histoplasmosis includes headaches, altered mental status, and focal neurological deficits [2]. These symptoms may last up to three weeks [9]. In about 5% of the cases, rheumatologic, cardiac, and cutaneous manifestations showed signs of arthritis, pericarditis, erythema nodosum and erythema multiforme occurring as a systemic response, not as part of the dissemination [8].

Diagnosis

Due to the highly variable clinical manifestations, diagnosing histoplasmosis can be extremely challenging [2]. The selection of a diagnostic tool will depend on the symptomology, the patient's immune status, and the epidemiological context [3]. Diagnosis of Histoplasmosis is confirmed with culture or histopathology, along with other tests such as a urine antigen test or a Histoplasma serological test [4, 9]. The identification of yeast via culture growth of mold at incubated room temperature is the gold standard for diagnosis [8]. Blood and tissue cultures may take 4 to 6 weeks to show growth, which can slow down treatment [2, 8]. Cytology and histopathology, by contrast, can lead to faster diagnosis but sensitivity and specificity are lower [8]. Therefore, positive blood cultures and radiology imaging may also help identify the presence of histoplasmosis and disseminated infection [4].

The urine serum antigen test helps diagnose histoplasmosis rapidly and can be helpful in longitudinal assessment [1]. The urine antigen test is a very sensitive diagnostic test and can still be present in the body after treatment is complete [4]. It has been shown that the urine antigen test may have a positive result for a period even after treatment for histoplasmosis, notably in solid organ transplant patients [4]. Serum testing may be more helpful on chronic pulmonary histoplasmosis patients than on immunosuppressed patients [1].

Antigen detection is a valuable tool that provides noninvasive evidence of disseminated histoplasmosis [8]. Due to the culture identification and serologic testing problems in transplant recipients and immunocompromised patients, antigen testing has become the primary diagnostic tool for histoplasmosis [2]. Urine testing is considered more sensitive than serum antigen testing, potentially due to the increased antigen concentration in urine, with some data suggesting enhanced sensitivity with combined testing [2]. Antigen testing may also be performed on other body fluids, including bronchoalveolar lavage (BAL), CSF, and pleural fluid, though result interpretation is less established [2]. In recent studies, developing a qualitative lateral flow assay (LFA) has led to faster histoplasmosis antigen detection in the urine, which can provide results within 40 minutes without needing special equipment [2]. However, the FDA has not approved any assays for human histoplasmosis detection to date [2].

Computed tomography (CT) or magnetic resonance imaging (MRI) in CNS disease often reveals mass lesions, meningeal enhancement, and/or infarcts though also findings may be expected [2]. Mediastinal granuloma can often be identified by CT imaging, showing the patchy distribution of contents [8]. The most common abnormalities revealed on a chest CT scan were multiple nodular lesions, and diffuse bilateral infiltrates [9]. Additional common radiologic abnormalities include intra-thoracic and abdominal lymphadenopathy and hepatosplenomegaly [2]. Positron emission tomography (PET) is often used as part of this workup, but PET radionuclide uptake is increased similarly in both malignancy and infection [8].

Typical laboratory findings include pancytopenia, transaminitis, hyperbilirubinemia, elevated inflammatory markers (e.g., erythrocyte sedimentation rate, C-reactive protein, and ferritin), and hypercalcemia [2]. Blood work can help diagnose severe histoplasmosis if there are elevated alkaline phosphate, lactate dehydrogenase, and ferritin levels and the presence of hepatosplenomegaly or mediastinal/hilar adenopathy on radiological imaging [8].

Biopsies can often be conducted in the liver, lung, lymph nodes, bone marrow, and skin [2]. Granuloma formation can also be seen in the biopsies; however, it is less consistent in immunocompromised patients [2]. A noninvasive procedure can also be conducted to diagnose by using a fine needle to aspirate the specimen in the tissues [2]. Polymerase chain reaction (PCR) testing offers high sensitivity, specificity, and fast turnaround. Still, it is not comparable to the sensitivity and specificity reported in the literature when using methods such as culture, antigen testing, serology, and clinical criteria [8]. There is a large variety of PCR testing that can be considered, but the high cost isn't ideal for routine use [2].

Histoplasmosis is endemic in much of the world [6]. In many parts of the world, histoplasmosis is not diagnosed as often due to the unavailability of tests or clinician awareness, which often leads to the misdiagnosis of histoplasmosis [6].

Treatment

Histoplasmosis treatment involves two drug classes of antifungal agents: triazoles and polyenes. Triazoles inhibit the biosynthesis of an essential component of the fungal cell membrane, ergosterol [3]. Itraconazole (ITZ), voriconazole, and posaconazole, which are part of the triazole drug class, are thought to be able to destroy Histoplasma. Still, fluconazole is believed only to inhibit the growth of the fungus [3]. Amphotericin B (AmB), like other polyenes, forms a complex with ergosterol in the fungal plasma membrane, leading to disruption in the cell membrane and cell death (Aráuz, 2021). Furthermore, the foundation of histoplasmosis therapy has always been amphotericin B and/or itraconazole, with intravenous AmB being preferred for severe infections [2]. Liposomal AmB is the favored formulation versus traditional deoxycholate because of reduced toxicity to the kidneys and the higher rate of survival when used in HIV patients and disseminated histoplasmosis [2]. (Aráuz, 2021). The American Society of Transplantation guidelines suggests that oral ITZ therapy should be given after one to two weeks of AmB administration when clinical stabilization is apparent [2]. Longer courses of AmB therapy are recommended in patients with central nervous system (CNS) disorders [2]. ITZ monotherapy can be used in cases of mild or moderate disease [2]. Generally, antifungal therapy should last at least 12 months, regardless of disease severity [2]. For patients needing continuous immunosuppression or after a relapse, indefinite therapy may be an option, especially with CNS involvement [2]. Echinocandin use is not supported because of insufficient data, but fluconazole has been used in place of ITZ in case of intolerance [2].

Other antifungal or FDA-approved drugs with different indications exist as alternative medications and may help manage Histoplasma [2]. For instance, encochleated amphotericin B deoxycholate is a newly developing polyene formulation that uses a novel lipid nanocrystal for oral administration [2]. Tetrazoles are developing azoles that will help avoid drug interactions because of their greater selectivity for fungal Cyp51 [2]. Among these drugs, VT-1598 was granted orphan drug status for treating coccidioidomycosis [2]. Other novel drugs related to Histoplasma are olorofim, fosmanogepix, and nikkomycin Z [2].

Corticosteroids are suggested in patients with acute distress syndrome in addition to fungal antifungal therapy [8]. Antifungal treatment for many cases of acute histoplasmosis can last 12 weeks when dissemination is not present [8]. Patients with chronic pulmonary histoplasmosis must get treated to avoid the degradation of lung tissues [8]. Treatment helps decrease the rate of deaths, the disappearance of fungus in sputum, and the decrease in pulmonary infiltrates in two-thirds of cases [8].

Prognosis

Healthcare providers need to be conscious of the possibility of a histoplasmosis and blastomycosis infection after a transplant; because the infection may be inactive and not present any particular symptoms, this could retard diagnosis and increase the chances of death [4]. The onset of infection in non-immunocompromised people is frequently caused by breathing in fungal conidia, which can either be undetectable or present deadly symptoms [4]. In solid organ transplant recipients (SOTRs), histoplasmosis can be due to a primary respiratory infection, the rising of a dormant infection, or an asymptomatic infection that progressed into an apparent illness during the use of immunosuppressants [4]. SOTRs have a higher tendency to serious infections that spread outside the lungs due to a decrease in their immune function, leading to increased morbidity and mortality [2]. The clinical presentation extends from being self-limiting to a deadly disease, and complications may involve pulmonary nodules, erythema nodosum, pericarditis, mediastinal lymphadenitis, granulomas, fibrosis, and presumed ocular histoplasmosis syndrome [10]. The evidence of the relationship between presumed ocular histoplasmosis syndrome (POHS) and histoplasmosis is not unanimous. This complication should not be neglected because it accounts for approximately 40% of histoplasmosis codes in insurance claims data, meaning that it possibly plays a significant role in *Histoplasma* infection [10]. In a patient with early and asymptomatic mediastinal granuloma (MG), chest pain may indicate upcoming complications [8]. These complications involve attachment to nearby structures, and fistulization, with subsequent drainage of semiliquid, purulent-appearing contents to adjacent structures, including bronchi, lung parenchyma, esophagus, or surgical tracts following a mediastinoscopy [8].

According to the Food and Drug Administration (FDA), delay in treating histoplasmosis increases the risk of a life-threatening or fatal outcome [11]. Patients should be educated about what types of environment *H. capsulatum* resides in, activities to avoid, and symptoms to watch for that require medical attention [11].

Epidemiology

Infections by *H capsulatum* are primarily caused by bird and bat excrement found in damp soil being inhaled during events such as cave expeditions or construction [3]. Activities such as demolition, construction, renovation, and cleaning pest or chicken water removal can lead to disruption and inhalation of aerosolized microconidia [3]. In Indiana, out of a pool of 590 people, there were 189 confirmed cases of histoplasmosis. At the same time, 308 were likely cases, and 93 met the Council of State and Territorial Epidemiologists (CSTE) case definition, but because of a lack of data, they couldn't be categorized [5]. Histoplasmosis infections most likely occur in southern and central parts of the US and may be affected by higher temperatures [10]. Recently, the Northern states of Minnesota, Wisconsin, and Michigan are now highly endemic for histoplasmosis. Insufficient data on asymptomatic histoplasmosis with symptoms prevents the ability to determine its prevalence [10]. The incidence of histoplasmosis is 6.1 cases per 100,000 people with 90% lifetime exposure to *Histoplasma capsulatum* [8]. The risk of progressive disseminated Histoplasmosis (PDH) increases in the immunocompromised, such as HIV/AIDS patients, the young and elderly, organ transplant recipients, or patients getting TNF-α inhibitors [8].

Since bat droppings can be used as herbal remedies, they can increase the chance of getting histoplasmosis [6]. Histoplasmosis has been attributed to donor transference of *H. capsulatum*, unlike blastomycosis [4]. In soil saturated with greater nitrogen content, Histoplasma is found in higher concentrations since there is typically more bird and bat excrement in such soil [2]. Only about one-quarter of people with periodic histoplasmosis remember being exposed to bird and bat excrement, even though they are involved in over three-quarters of histoplasmosis outbreaks [10].

Histoplasmosis infection can affect transplant recipients either from the organ donor, infection reactivation, or from environmental exposure [2]. Cuellar et al., reported an incidence of *H. capsulatum* infection was 2.9 cases out of 1,000 transplantations in organ transplant recipients [9]. Unanticipated histoplasmosis in lung transplant recipients was 18 out of 1000 transplants, with most patients experiencing lung parenchyma and involvement with their lymph nodes [9].

Histoplasmosis Prevalence in the United States

Less than 1000 cases of histoplasmosis are detected annually in 12 states via surveillance, with a lack of surveillance data in the remaining states [5]. Histoplasmosis affects a much more extensive range than previously reported spreading to the Central and Eastern United States in states like Michigan, Wisconsin, and Minnesota [10].

Ohio and Mississippi River Valleys

Histoplasmosis is primarily found in the Mississippi and Ohio River Valley regions in the United States [3]. These regions have been known to be highly endemic for histoplasmosis since 1945 [9]. Within these regions, 80% of young adult males tested positive for *H. capsulatum* exposure in seminal studies utilizing skin test antigens [3]. However, besides these highly endemic regions, there are reported cases and outbreaks of histoplasmosis all throughout the United States and even worldwide [3]. For example, histoplasmosis cases in humans and animals have also been documented as far as California, New York, Florida, and Alaska [10].

Global Distribution of Histoplasmosis

Although the central United States has the most significant *Histoplasma capsulatum* prevalence, these infections also occur in other parts of the world [7]. Regions outside the United States are recognized as favorable for *H. capsulatum* based on their climate, humidity, and soil characteristics [3].

These favorable regions typically contain moderate temperatures, many rivers, and high nitrogen content [3].

North America

In North America, St. Lawrence, Mississippi, and Ohio River basins are the highest endemic regions of histoplasmosis, and microfoci appear in the mid-eastern states [1]. In 1983, it was reported that multiple patients had AIDS and progressive disseminated Histoplasmosis [7]. One histoplasmosis report came from Indiana, a hyper-endemic area, and the other reports came from less common regions like Texas and Michigan and even places where it was thought that histoplasmosis wasn't present, like New York and Colorado [7]. Autochthonous cases of histoplasmosis, due to point environmental sources, have been reported in various regions of the United States that have not been considered endemic before [8]. These regions include the Rocky Mountain states, such as Montana and Idaho; the southeast, such as Florida and South Carolina; the northeast, such as New York; and the North Central states, like Minnesota and North Dakota [8]. Outside of the United States, *H. capsulatum* is moderately endemic in Puerto Rico, where it is recognized as a site of outbreaks [8].

Asia

The central area of Myanmar, within Southeast Asia, is one of the endemic regions of histoplasmosis [3]. Histoplasmosis has been present in Asia for many years [6]. Beginning in 1963, within Malaysia, Histoplasmosis was first isolated from the soil [6]. In 1970, in India, Malaysia, Indonesia, Singapore, Thailand, Vietnam, and Japan, 30 possible native cases were reviewed by Rhadhawa [6]. China has also had an increased rate of infections over recent years [7]. From 1990 to 2011, 300 infections were reported, and 75% of those cases were found to occur along the Yangtze River [7]. In Thailand, between 1984 and 2010, a spike in PDH cases linked to the AIDS epidemic reported more than 1,200 cases [7]. In India, cases of progressive disseminated histoplasmosis have increased among HIV-positive and/or diabetic patients, and some believe it might be under-recognized and mistaken for tuberculosis [7]. Other regions of Asia where cases have been reported include Bangladesh, Nepal, Pakistan, and Sri Lanka [8].

Africa

In West Africa, there have been over 400 reported cases of histoplasmosis, with most of them secondary to *Histoplasma duboisii* [1]. In Africa, Histoplasmosis is caused by *H. capsulatum*, found throughout Africa, and H. duboisii, which is found mainly in West African regions such as Nigeria, the Democratic Republic of Congo, Uganda, Tanzania, and Madagascar [6]. In addition to these regions, sporadic cases have appeared in Central and South America, Oceania, and northern sub-Saharan Africa [7]. In a literature review, it was found that from 1972 to 2017, there were 470 published cases of histoplasmosis, with the highest number of cases from West Africa [6]. Most of these cases were reported from Nigeria, where histoplasmosis skin sensitivity studies were performed and results ranged from 4.4% in the urban population to 35% near rural parts, including near bat caves [6].

Northern Hemisphere

Histoplasmosis capsulatum is most commonly found in the central US. Still, small case reports have also come from Brazil and Argentina [7]. Histoplasmosis is widely present in the Americas, with an estimated 32% skin test positivity in Latin America [3]. In Mexico, infection prevalence ranges from 5% to 50% [3]. The level of prevalence varies in different regions due to climate, soil, and factors such as HIV co-infection [3]. South and Central America have high numbers of patients with histoplasmosis, many in persons infected with HIV [7]. Brazil is highly endemic for histoplasmosis in the northern and mid-western states and the south-eastern regions [7]. Latin America, including Brazil, French Guiana, Argentina, Colombia, Venezuela, Guatemala, and Panama, is highly endemic for histoplasmosis. In some parts of Brazil, up to 90% of the population has been exposed to *H. capsulatum,* according to seroepidemiologic studies [7, 8].

Europe

Histoplasmosis is uncommon in Europe and usually only occurs in people who have acquired it from endemic areas. However, there have been some locally acquired cases reported in Italy [8]. A 5-year study in Europe reported 118 instances of histoplasmosis, including locally acquired cases in Germany, Italy, and Turkey [1].

Prevalence in Specialized Populations

Human Immunodeficiency Virus (HIV)/Acquired Immunodeficiency Syndrome (AIDS)

The disease is often seen in advanced HIV or other immunosuppression, typically treated with L-AmB. Weak immune systems can be innate, caused by drugs, or associated with other illnesses such as HIV or cancer. A study in Brazil reported a higher than 40% prevalence in people living with HIV in the Central-Northeast region, compared to 10% in the South [3]. Disseminated histoplasmosis is particularly problematic for those with HIV. It has been under-recognized in India as tuberculosis [7, 10]. Immunocompromised individuals are typically at a higher risk of developing severe histoplasmosis, particularly in disseminated histoplasmosis related to HIV, with a mortality rate of almost 40% in recent studies [10]. Moreover, hospitalizations for histoplasmosis have risen in the US over the past decade, especially among patients with immunocompromising conditions beyond HIV/AIDS [8].

Autoimmune Disorders

Most symptomatic cases are of progressive disseminated histoplasmosis, and the disease has become a concern for people with autoimmune conditions. Patients with confirmed histoplasmosis cases are more likely to have a weakened immune system compared to those with probable cases (41% vs. 26%, 2.0 odds ratio, 1.2-3.2 confidence interval) [5]. An impaired T-cell function can result from innate defects (e.g., Job syndrome, severe combined immunodeficiency syndrome), immunosuppressive medications, or other conditions such as malignancy or HIV [7]. Patients from Latin America and sub-Saharan Africa who immigrated to non-endemic regions in Europe are also at risk for progressive disseminated histoplasmosis due to the reactivation of previous infection and decreased T-cell function [7]. Individuals with autoimmune diseases like rheumatoid arthritis using immunosuppressive drugs are also susceptible to PDH [7]. Immunocompromised patients are at least ten times more likely to develop progressive disseminated histoplasmosis than the general population [8].

Immunosuppressant Use

People with progressive disseminated histoplasmosis are usually experiencing significant problems with their cellular immunity, particularly in those with advanced HIV; however, it is becoming more common in individuals who take immunosuppressant drugs for long-term inflammatory illnesses and organ transplant recipients [3].

Tumor Necrosis Factor Blocker therapy

Histoplasmosis is the most common invasive fungal infection in patients taking TNFα inhibitors [8]. Despite being well-recognized in this population, diagnosis is often delayed, and the infection is associated with a 20% mortality rate [8]. As of 2010, 88 cases of histoplasmosis have been reported among patients using TNF-α inhibitors, most of which were disseminated [7]. In experimental infections, TNF blockade prevented the formation of a protective immune response by inhibiting the activation of macrophages [11]. In a local study, only 0.64% (3 out of 469) adult patients treated with TNF blockers for inflammatory bowel disease from 2000 to early 2009 developed histoplasmosis, a rate similar to that of organ transplant patients before the three outbreaks (0.5%) [11]. For patients about to start TNF-α inhibitors, it is recommended to inform the doctor if they have lived in an area with an increased risk of fungal infections (such as the Ohio and Mississippi River valleys) [10]. Histoplasmosis systemic infection resulting from tumor necrosis factor-α inhibitor therapy necessitates stopping the TNF-α inhibitor during antifungal treatment [1, 11].

Solid Organ Transplant Patients

Histoplasmosis is a rare occurrence in solid-organ transplantation (SOT), despite their increased risk of infection, happening less than 1% of the time, even in areas with high incidence. Only 1 in 10,000 transplants are donor-derived [2, 8]. The incidence of histoplasmosis in solid-organ transplant recipients is estimated to be low, with only a few documented cases, mostly in kidney and liver transplant recipients [9]. There are only isolated reports of histoplasmosis among lung or heart transplant recipients [9]. For ten years (1997-2007), 3572 solid-organ transplantations were performed, and 38 patients were identified with post-transplantation histoplasmosis [9]. Other studies have shown that post-transplant Histoplasmosis and blastomycosis incidence was less than 1% but often resulted in disseminated infection [4]. The accuracy of diagnosing histoplasmosis in immunocompromised patients, especially solid-organ transplant recipients, varies and is generally lower [3]. Histoplasmosis is uncommon in solid organ transplant patients, but severe infection may lead to graft loss or death. Complications are even more pronounced in post-transplant patients who are immunocompromised [2].

The Impact of Travel and Immigration on Histoplasmosis Prevalence

The growing number of reports of histoplasmosis cases is due to increased travel to endemic areas for tourism or work and migration to these areas [7]. Imported cases of histoplasmosis are becoming more common due to increased global connectivity and travel [8]. A systematic review of the literature found that the most common destination for travelers contracting Histoplasmosis was South and Central America (57%), followed by North America (21%), and the most common risk factor was exposure to bat guano or spelunking (61%) [8]. However, many exposures to histoplasmosis are not travel-related and occur near the home rather than from traveling, despite nearly a quarter of patients reporting travel in the month before symptom onset [5]. Histoplasmosis cases have been reported in HIV-positive and HIV-negative patients and among individuals who have traveled to Malaysia [7]. Patients who are immunocompromised should be advised to avoid activities like visiting caves during travel to decrease their risk of histoplasmosis [3].

Conclusion

Endemic mycoses cause considerable morbidity and mortality in immunocompetent and immunocompromised individuals worldwide and each has its own changing regions of endemicity. Diagnosis is often missed or delayed, especially outside of endemic areas, due to a lack of knowledge about the pathogen which is due to a lack of data on its geographic distribution. Disease surveillance and wider public health reporting are needed to detect locally acquired cases and track changes in distribution. Additionally, environmental and epidemiological studies are necessary to accurately estimate the incidences and geographic distribution of these fungi worldwide. Histoplasmosis, although an uncommon infection in the SOT population, has significant clinical implications. Given its clinical manifestations and expanding worldwide distribution, it should increasingly be suspected in the appropriate clinical context. Laboratory testing and antifungal drug options are growing, and with diligent monitoring and post-transplant antifungal prophylaxis, serious infection can largely be avoided in those at the highest risk.

References

[1] Thompson G R 3rd, Le T, Chindamporn A, Kauffman C A, Alastruey-Izquierdo A, Ampel N M, Andes D R, Armstrong-James D, Ayanlowo O, Baddley J W, Barker B M, Lopes Bezerra L, Buitrago M J, Chamani-Tabriz L, Chan J F W, Chayakulkeeree M, Cornely O A, Cunwei C, Gangneux J P, Govender N P, Hagen F, Hedayati M T, Hohl T M, Jouvion G, Kenyon C, Kibbler C C, Klimko N, Kong D C M, Krause R, Lee Lee L, Meintjes G, Miceli M H, Rath P M, Spec A, Queiroz-Telles F, Variava E, Verweij P E, Schwartz I S, Pasqualotto A C. Global guideline for the diagnosis and management of the endemic mycoses: An initiative of the European Confederation of Medical Mycology in cooperation with the International Society for Human and Animal Mycology. *The Lancet Infectious Diseases*. 2021; 21(12):e364-e374.

[2] Saullo J L, Miller R A. Updates on Histoplasmosis in Solid Organ Transplantation. *Current Fungal Infection Reports*. 2022:1-14.

[3] Arauz A B, Papineni P. Histoplasmosis. *Infect. Dis. Clin. North Am.* Jun 2021; 35(2):471-491. doi:10.1016/j.idc.2021.03.011.

[4] Grim S A, Proia L, Miller R, Alhyraba M, Costas-Chavarri A, Oberholzer J, Clark N M. *A multicenter study of histoplasmosis and blastomycosis after solid organ transplantation*. Wiley Online Library; 2012.

[5] Benedict K, McCracken S, Signs K, Ireland M, Amburgey V, Serrano J A, Christophe N, Gibbons-Burgener S, Hallyburton S, Warren K A, Keyser Metobo A, Odom R, Groenewold M R, Jackson B R. *Enhanced surveillance for histoplasmosis*—9 states, 2018–2019. Oxford University Press US; 2020:ofaa343.

[6] Ashraf N, Kubat R C, Poplin V, Adenis A A, Denning D W, Wright L, McCotter O, Schwartz I S, Jackson B R, Chiller T, Bahr N C. Re-drawing the maps for endemic mycoses. *Mycopathologia*. 2020;185:843-865.

[7] Bahr N C, Antinori S, Wheat L J, Sarosi G A. Histoplasmosis infections worldwide: thinking outside of the Ohio River valley. *Current tropical medicine reports*. 2015; 2:70-80.

[8] Azar M M, Loyd J L, Relich R F, Wheat L J, Hage C A. *Current concepts in the epidemiology, diagnosis, and management of histoplasmosis syndromes*. Thieme Medical Publishers; 2020:013-030.

[9] Cuellar-Rodriguez J, Avery R K, Lard M, Budev M, Gordon S M, Shrestha N K, van Duin D, Oethinger M, Mawhorter S D. Histoplasmosis in solid organ transplant recipients: 10 years of experience at a large transplant center in an endemic area. *Clinical Infectious Diseases*. 2009;49(5):710-716.

[10] Benedict K, Toda M, Jackson B R. *Revising conventional wisdom about histoplasmosis in the United States*. Oxford University Press US; 2021:ofab306.

[11] Hage C A, Bowyer S, Tarvin S E, Helper D, Kleiman M B, Wheat L J. Recognition, diagnosis, and treatment of histoplasmosis complicating tumor necrosis factor blocker therapy. *Clinical Infectious Diseases*. 2010;50(1):85-92.

Chapter 2

The Incidences and Prevalence of Histoplasmosis

Maryam Ahmed[1]
Zara Borkowski[2]
Sneha Reddy[3]
Reena Shah[4]
and Salim Surani[4,5,*], MD

[1] Department of Medicine, Punjab Medical College, Faisalabad, Pakistan
[2]Premedicine department, Incarnate Word Academy, Corpus Christi, Texas, USA
[3]Premedicine Department, University of Texas, Austin, Texas, USA
[4]Department of Medicine, Aga Khan University, Nairobi, Kenya
[5]Department of Medicine & Pharmacology, Texas A&M University, Texas, USA

Abstract

Histoplasmosis Capsulatum causes Histoplasmosis, and the infection is acquired through inhalation of airborne spores from contaminated soil or bird or bat droppings. The disease can spread to systemic organs and lead to hospitalization in severe cases. The disease is globally distributed, although some regions are hyper-endemic while others are considered non-endemic regions. The incidence and prevalence of histoplasmosis vary depending on the geographical location. The incidence ranges between 0.1 to 1 case per 100,000 people annually in temperate climates and between 10 and 100 cases per 100,000 in the humid tropics, and more than 100 cases per 100,000 people among the groups that are areas considered to be high risk. Global annual prevalence is estimated at 100,000, and about 50% of the world lives in endemic areas. In American

---

[*] Corresponding Author's Email: srsurani@hotmail.com.

In: Histoplasmosis
Editors: Salim Surani, Syed Anjum Khan and Reena Shah
ISBN: 979-8-89113-129-3

continents, the disease is endemic in Ohio and Mississippi River valleys, the Great Lakes, and Central and South America. In the USA, the incidence is approximately 2.5 cases per 100,000 population and about 3.8 cases per population of 100,000 people in Minnesota. In Canada, the incidence is estimated 0.14 cases per 100,000 people. In Africa, the disease is more prevalent in West, South, and East Africa, and the positivity rate of the disease is between 0 to 35%. Europe is considered a non-endemic region, although few cases are reported in Spain, France, Italy, and Germany. In comparison to these European countries, the disease is more prevalent in Asia, China, India, and Thailand. Factors influencing Incidence and Prevalence include immunosuppressants, especially HIV/AIDS, age, and environmental factors.

Keywords: histoplasmosis, incidence, prevalence, HIV/AIDS, environmental factors, fungal infection, histoplasma capsulatum

Introduction

Histoplasmosis is a fungal infection caused by the inhalation of the spores of the fungus Histoplasma Capsulatum [1]. The infection is acquired by inhaling airborne spores from contaminated soil or bird or bat droppings. The fungus spores are found in soil and areas with high bird or bat droppings [2]. The symptoms of histoplasmosis vary depending on the severity of the infection. The most common symptom is a fever, occasionally accompanied by chills, sweat, headaches, muscle aches, and fatigue. Other symptoms include coughing, chest pain, shortness of breath, and weight loss. In severe cases, the infection can spread to other organs, including the brain, and can be fatal. Histoplasmosis is treated with anti-fungal medications. In extreme cases, hospitalization may be necessary [3].

Prevalence and Incidence of Histoplasmosis

Different studies showed varying incidence and prevalence rates worldwide in various continents and countries. This review looks at the incidence and prevalence rates as captured and documented by various global authors. This review highlights the knowledge gaps regarding the epidemiological aspects of histoplasmosis.

Global Incidence and Prevalence of Histoplasmosis

Histoplasmosis is currently among the most prevalent systemic infections in the world [1]. The outbreaks frequently occur due to activities that disturb the soil, particularly samples containing bird or bat droppings [1]. Another article further says that each continent has experienced a histoplasmosis outbreak, and about 50% of the world's population lives in endemic areas [4]. This endemic area includes West Africa (Zimbabwe, Congo), Australia, South America, Southeast Asia (Malaysia, Taiwan, India, Taiwan), South Africa, Europe, and Central and North America. On the other hand, another article indicates that the global incidence of histoplasmosis varies widely, from 2 to 300 cases per 100,000 population [4]. The global prevalence of disseminated histoplasmosis is approximately 100,000 [5, 6].

Incidence and Prevalence of Histoplasmosis in America

Another article also notes that histoplasmosis occurs worldwide and is endemic in many areas, including the American continent [7]. Also, it concluded that the disease is highly prevalent in South America and the US, especially around Ohio and the Mississippi River Valley [7].

About 80% of young adults who reside in Mississippi Valley and Ohio Valley have been infected by H. Capsulatum at least once in their lifetime [3]. Further, about 250,000 have been infected with the disease in the USA and clinical symptoms are evident in only 5% of the population infected. Another study by Paige A Armstrong noted that in the United States, the annual incidence is approximately 2.5 cases per 100,000 population. They argue that histoplasmosis disease is not readily identifiable; thus, the incidence and prevalence data are hard to find. An article by Fayyaz J also agrees with CDC that at one point in their life, about 60 to 90% of those residing in the Mississippi River valley and Ohio were infected by Histoplasma. The disease incidence among the elderly 65 years and above who reside in the USA is 3.4 cases per 100,000 [8, 9].

According to the Minnesota Department of Health, the incidence of histoplasmosis was 3.8 cases per 100,000 people (214 cases in a population of about 5.6 million people). 62% of those infected were males, 93% were whites, 37% were immunocompromised, and 49% of those infected by the disease were hospitalized [10].

Linder KA, Kauffman CA note that despite the disease being reported globally, many cases have been reported in Latin and North America. They indicated that Histoplasma microfoci are connected to the cases in Florida, mid-Atlantic coastal states as well as the rural areas of New York. An article notes that this mycosis, the most common in the USA, is majorly distributed in the Southeastern and the Midwest regions. The study further indicates that there have been about 1000 outbreaks from 1938 to 2013 in Puerto Rico and in 26 states of the USA. During the outbreaks, there were about 3000 reported cases. The article defines an outbreak as more than two cases [11].

A review has similar findings to the study by Benedict K, Mody RK cases were approximately 2850. There were two reported outbreaks [12]. About 28% of the outbreaks reported 3 to 5 cases, 17% of the outbreaks reported 6 to 9 cases, 18% of the outbreaks reported more than 30 cases, 16% of the outbreaks reported 2 cases, 11% of the outbreaks had 6 to 9 cases, and 10% of the outbreaks had 20 to 29 cases [12]. Benedict K, Mody RK further found out that males accounted for 60% of the cases during the outbreaks that occurred in 26 states, as also reported [12]. In their review, additionally found out that most of the cases (28%) were reported in Indiana, 15% reported in Ohio, Iowa reported 8%, Michigan reported 6% of the cases, Illinois reported 6%, Nebraska reported 5% and Arkansas reported 5% of the cases [12].

Brazil is one endemic country, and a systematic review found that histoplasmosis had been reported all over Brazil. Still, most cases had been reported in Brazil's Northeastern, Midwest, central-West, and Southeastern regions [13]. They reviewed 207 studies between 1939-2018. The authors found that 78.3% of the cases reported were males, while females accounted for 21.7% of the remaining cases. The male-to-female ratio was about 4:1 [13]. Most incidences were reported in individuals in their 4th and 5th decades of life. The mortality rate was 33.1% [13].

Canada has a high disease prevalence in the Quebec and Ontario regions [14]. There is a high prevalence among males (71%), and the incidence was approximately 0.14 cases per 100,000 people [14]. Another study reported that the incidence of the disease was 0.8 cases per 100,000 between 1990 to 2015, the prevalence among males was at 80%, and the prevalence among those in the 5th decade of their lives was at 29.7% [15].

Incidence and Prevalence of Histoplasmosis in Africa

A review explains that some microfoci of Histoplasma are found in various African regions, including West, South and East Africa [11]. However, the ideal incidence of the disease is difficult to arrive at in Africa due to the unavailability of testing in the better part of Africa. According to Rahim MA, Zaman S et al., it has been challenging to find data on the prevalence, mortalities, incidence and morbidity of Histoplasma since it's not a notifiable disease. Despite that, that the disease is prevalent in Madagascar, West Africa, as well as Central Africa [7]. Most prevalent species in Africa are Hcd (African histoplasmosis) and Hcc. Despite the limited data about the incidence of the disease in Africa, some reported and documented cases have been reported [7].

The disease cases have been reported in at least 32 countries. Cases of Hcc have been noticed to be more prevalent in North and South Africa, while cases of Hcd have been majorly reported in Western, Eastern and Central Africa. However, only Morocco and Egypt were the only countries in Northern Africa that reported cases of Hcc [7]. A portion of Hcc cases reported in S. Africa have been E. africanus, while several Hcc microfoci have been reported in Kenya, DRC, Senegal, Benin and Ivory Coast [7]. The review revealed 470 cases were reported from 32 countries, 52.5% of the cases were Hcd, and 39.6% were Hcc [7]. Nigeria had the highest prevalence in Africa at 26.4% [7].

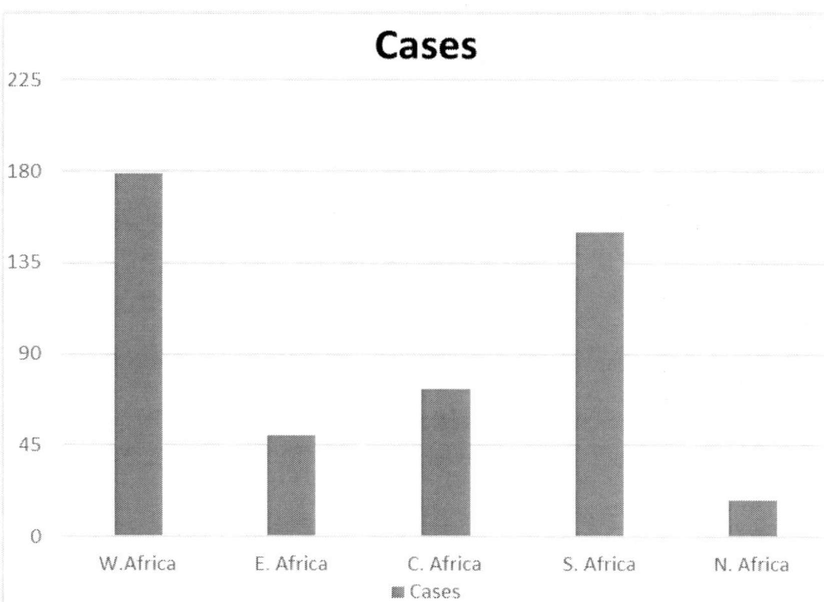

Figure 1. Distribution of Reported Histoplasmosis Cases in Africa from 1952 to 2017.

A study notes that the cases of histoplasmosis have increased in Africa since the advent of HIV/AIDS [16]. The study notes that about 470 cases were reported in Africa between 2017 and 1952. The study additionally noted that 38.1% of the cases were reported in West Africa, and about 32% were reported in South Africa. The article says that the positivity rate of the disease is between 0 to 35% in Africa [16]. further notes that there is little data on the incidence of histoplasmosis in Africa, especially sub-Saharan Africa, despite the burden of HIV in the region. According to the study, 35% of cases diagnosed in Nigeria were reported among those living in rural areas. The distribution of cases in Africa is shown in Figure 1 [16].

Incidence and Prevalence of Histoplasmosis in Europe

A review notes that there have been reported cases of the disease in different parts of Europe, especially Spain, France, Italy and Germany.[11] Many cases reported in Europe were common among those who migrated from endemic areas in Africa. The study by Rahim MA, et al., contrasts with that of Linder KA, Kauffman CA since it indicates that there are very rare cases of the disease in Europe except for a few cases in Italy. According to a systemic review, about 133 articles were published between 2020 and 2005, and there were about 730 cases of histoplasmosis cases in Israel together with 17 countries in Europe. The males were the most prevalent at 60.4%, as per (17). 89.5% of the cases were prevalent among those living with HIV, and the mortality rate was approximately 32% [17].

Some countries in Europe are considered non-endemic for histoplasmosis. For instance, the prevalence in Spain is 0.31 cases per 100,000 people yearly; most cases are those that have traveled from endemic regions of the world, while the incidence was approximately 0.53 per 100,000 people in Spain [18]. Additionally, there had been a rise in the number of reported cases in Spain, and this is due to immigration. Also, there were about 286 cases of the disease between 2014 and 1997 and of the 286 cases, males were the most prevalent at 67.5% [18].

Incidence and Prevalence of Histoplasmosis in Australia

In Australia, most cases have been reported in Queensland and New South Wales, and rare cases have been reported in the rest of the country [11].

Incidence and Prevalence of Histoplasmosis in Asia

A review of reported cases of histoplasmosis in Asia in 2019 was about 1692. 36.8% of the cases were reported in India, 36.1% in China, 13.8% in Thailand and the rest were distributed in other Asian countries [11]. Other counties, for instance, Qatar, Lebanon, Saudi Arabia, Jordan, Japan and Kuwait, did not have any disease cases [19].

A review illustrates that the disease has also been reported in the Yangtze region in China, and some cases have also been diagnosed in Thailand among those living with HIV [11]. China, one of the world's largest countries and one of the most populated countries, had the highest prevalence of histoplasmosis in Yunnan (27.7%), 15% in Jiangsu and 8.9% in Hunan provinces [20]. Antinori S additionally noted that a survey in Sichuan province among healthy students indicated that the prevalence was between 6% and 35%, and the highest prevalence was recorded in the southern region of that province. Antinori S further showed that disseminated disease cases accounted for 86% of the total reported cases. On the other hand, 52% of those who were positive for H. capsulatum had no underlying condition. A review also adds the Hubei, Yunnan and Chongqing regions of China as areas of high prevalence [20].

Moreover, Antinori S reviewed the prevalence of the disease in India, which is also one of the most populated countries in the world. The review found that the disease is most prevalent in the country's North- eastern and Eastern regions, mainly Assam and Calcutta. The prevalence was found to be about 12.3%. In India, areas in Uttar Pradesh, West Bengal, Delhi, Haryana, Maharashtra, and Rajasthan are considered endemic areas with high incidence and prevalence [21-23].

A mapping of histoplasmosis in S. East Asia. Baket et al., found about 407 cases of the disease in S.E Asia, 57.2% of the cases were reported in Thailand, and 18.6% were reported in Malaysia, 11.7% in Indonesia and 5.1% in Singapore. Other countries reported very few or no cases of the disease [24].

Factors Influencing Incidence and Prevalence of Histoplasmosis

Several factors influence the prevalence and incidence of histoplasmosis. Fayyaz J in his article, expresses that the individual's immune status and environmental exposures are the major factors influencing the incidence and prevalence of histoplasmosis. Immunosuppressed individuals, especially AIDS patients, are the most burdened. Other factors include extreme age [3]. Various factors are discussed and supported by various findings as follows:

HIV/AIDS

According to an article by Scully MC and WHO, there has been a surge in the incidence of histoplasmosis due to the rising population of immunocompromised individuals, specifically HIV patients. The CDC supports this, indicating that histoplasmosis is mainly common among people living with HIV/AIDS globally, especially in areas where the management of HIV through ART has been poor or low. The article cites Latin America as one of the regions where histoplasmosis has been a burden to those living with HIV; about 30.0% of the HIV patients succumb to histoplasmosis [9].

The link between histoplasmosis and AIDS dates back to the 1980s, when most disseminated histoplasmosis cases were reported among those newly diagnosed with HIV. The reports of histoplasmosis in those living with HIV were even reported in areas that previously never reported any cases, such as Trinidad and Thailand. Other areas considered non-endemic also reported histoplasmosis cases among newly diagnosed HIV patients and AIDS led to an increase in the number of histoplasmosis cases reported in Thailand by approximately 1200 [25, 26]. ART patients have shown lower histoplasmosis incidences [26].

Adenis A also agrees that AIDS is a major determinant of the incidence and prevalence of histoplasmosis. Adenis A illustrates that histoplasmosis, an opportunistic disease, causes most AIDS-related mortalities. The study additionally found that the incidence of histoplasmosis increased by 3 folds in HIV patients and led to 45.3% deaths [27].

A study supports the idea that AIDS influences the incidence and prevalence of this disease [28]. The study notes that the incidence of histoplasmosis among those newly diagnosed with HIV is about 8.3%, which was more than double the incidence of those not living with HIV who have been diagnosed with histoplasmosis (3.8%) [28, 29]. The incidence was 4.8% in the HIV patients adhering to ART [28]. The study further notes that the mortality rate caused by histoplasmosis among those newly diagnosed with HIV was 21.2%, while the mortality rate among ART was 18.5%. The mortality increased to 28.6% for those who defaulted to HIV care [28].

Leedy et al., note that the incidence of the disease in those living with HIV is about 4.1 cases per 100 persons or 4100 cases per 100,000 persons, as compared to the average incidence among the general population ranging between 2 and 300 cases per 100,000 people [26].

Other Immunosuppressants

Other immunosuppressors, such as steroid medication and chemotherapies, can lead to cases of histoplasmosis [30].

Age

Age is a factor that influences the incidence of histoplasmosis, and people older than 55 years and humans in infancy are at a high risk of being infected by the disease [30].

Environmental Factors

The environment is a factor that determines the incidence of histoplasmosis. Several studies have unearthed and supported various factors as follows:

A study indicates that the area of residence determines the incidence and prevalence of histoplasmosis. The study found that most of those diagnosed with histoplasmosis (64.8%) lived in rural areas, while 35.2% lived in urban areas [28].

Environmental settings and various human activities are determinants of the incidence and prevalence of the disease [12]. Benedict K et al., found out in their study that the most common settings contributing to histoplasmosis are farms, old buildings and buildings under renovation, chicken coops, caves and campsites. Moreover, Benedict K et al., found out that activities that involved soil disruption contributed to 32% of the outbreaks in the USA, and activities that involved disruption in the accumulation of bats and birds' dropping was related to 40% of the outbreaks. Demolition, together with construction activities, likely contributed to about 25% of the outbreaks. In the USA's outbreaks between 2013 and 1938, birds' and bats' droppings were found in 79% of the outbreak areas [12].

Conclusion

In conclusion, histoplasmosis is a fungal infection caused by H. capsulatum. Despite being distributed globally in all continents, the incidence and prevalence are higher in some regions, such as Latin America, the USA, and some regions in India, China, Africa and South America. On the other hand, other regions like the larger regions of Europe are considered non-endemic areas, and the few cases reported result from immigration. Moreover, more studies have shown that the disease is more prevalent in males. Factors influencing the prevalence and incidence of the disease are immunosuppressants. For instance, AIDS is a major factor. Other factors are age, where infants and elderly people above 55 are at greater risk. Environmental factors such as soil disturbance, demolition and building of structures, living on farms, being in caves, and bats and birds' droppings are determinants of the incidence and prevalence of histoplasmosis.

References

[1] Rodrigues A M, Beale M A, Hagen F, Fisher M C, Terra P P D, de Hoog S, Brilhante R S N, De Aguiar Cordeiro R, De Souza Collares Maia Castelo-Branco D, Rocha M F G, Sidrim J J C & De Camargo Z P. The global epidemiology of emerging Histoplasma species in recent years. *Stud. Mycol.* [Internet]. 2020; 97:100095. Available from: https://doi.org/10.1016/j.simyco.2020.02.001.

[2] Kauffman C A. Histoplasmosis: A clinical and laboratory update. *Clin. Microbiol. Rev.* [Internet]. 2007;20(1):115–32. Available from: https://www.ncbi.nlm.nih.gov/pmc/articles/PMC1797635/pdf/0027-06.pdf.

[3] Fayyaz J. Histoplasmosis [Internet]. *Medscape*. 2020. Available from: https://emedicine.medscape.com/article/299054-overview#a6.

[4] Sami M. Akram J K. Histoplasmosis. *PubMed* [Internet]. 2022; Available from: Sami M. Akram; Janak Koirala.

[5] Bongomin F, Gago S, Oladele R, & Denning D. Global and multi-national prevalence of fungal diseases—estimate precision. *J. Fungi* [Internet]. 2017;49(3):408–9. Available from: https://www.sciencedirect.com/science/article/pii/S016606162030004X#bib1.

[6] Azar M M, Loyd J L, Relich R F, Wheat L J & Hage C A. Current Concepts in the Epidemiology, Diagnosis, and Management of Histoplasmosis Syndromes. Pubmed [Internet]. 2020; Available from: https://pubmed.ncbi.nlm.nih.gov/32000281/.

[7] Rahim M A, Zaman S, Amin M R, Uddin K N, Chowdhury M A J. Histoplasmosis: An emerging or neglected disease in Bangladesh? A systematic review. *Oman Med. J.* [Internet]. 2020;35(1):1–17. Available from: https://www.ncbi.nlm.nih.gov/pmc/articles/PMC5773084/pdf/pntd.0006046.pdf.

[8] Paige A, Armstrong B R J. Multistate Epidemiology of Histoplasmosis, United States, 2011-2014. *PubMed* [Internet]. 2018; Available from: https://pubmed.ncbi.nlm.nih.gov/29460731/.

[9] CDC. How common is histoplasmosis? *CDC* [Internet]. 2020; Available from: https://www.cdc.gov/fungal/diseases/histoplasmosis/statistics.html.

[10] Minnesota Department of Health. *Histoplasmosis*, 2019 [Internet]. Minnesota Department of Hiealth. 2021. Available from: https://www.health.state.mn.us/diseases/reportable/dcn/sum19/histoplasmosis.html.

[11] Linder K A, Kauffman C A. Histoplasmosis : Epidemiology, Diagnosis, and Clinical Manifestations. 2019;120–8. Available from: https://link.springer.com/content/pdf/10.1007/s12281-019-00341-x.pdf.

[12] Benedict K, Mody R K. Epidemiology of histoplasmosis outbreaks, United States, 1938-2013. *Emerg. Infect. Dis.* [Internet]. 2017;22(3):370–8. Available from: https://www.ncbi.nlm.nih.gov/pmc/articles/PMC4766901/pdf/15-1117.pdf.

[13] Almeida M de A, Almeida-Silva F, Guimarães A J, Almeida-Paes R, Zancopé-Oliveira R M. The occurrence of histoplasmosis in Brazil: A systematic review. *Int. J. Infect. Dis.* [Internet]. 2019;86:147–56. Available from: https://doi.org/10.1016/j.ijid.2019.07.009.

[14] Dingle T C. Histoplasmosis acquired in Alberta, Canada: an epidemiological and genomic study. *Lancet* [Internet]. 2021; Available from: https://www.thelancet.com/journals/lanmic/article/PIIS2666-5247(20)30229-9/fulltext#.

[15] Brown E M, McTaggart L R, Dunn D, Pszczolko E, Tsui K G, Morris S K, Stephens D, Kus J V & Richardson S E. Epidemiology and geographic distribution of blastomycosis, histoplasmosis, and coccidioidomycosis, Ontario, Canada, 1990–2015. *Emerg. Infect. Dis.* [Internet]. 2018;24(7):1257–66. Available from: https://www.ncbi.nlm.nih.gov/pmc/articles/PMC6038754/pdf/17-2063.pdf.

[16] Oladele R O, Ayanlowo O O, Richardson M D & Denning D W. Histoplasmosis in Africa: An emerging or a neglected disease? *PubMed* [Internet]. 2018; Available from: https://pubmed.ncbi.nlm.nih.gov/29346384/.

[17] Antinori S, Giacomelli A, Corbellino M, Torre A, Schiuma M, Casalini G, Parravicini C, Milazzo L, Gervasoni C, Ridolfo A L. Histoplasmosis diagnosed in Europe and Israel: A case report and systematic review of the literature from 2005 to 2020. *J. Fungi* [Internet]. 2021;7(6). Available from: https://www.ncbi.nlm.nih.gov/pmc/articles/PMC8231918/pdf/jof-07-00481.pdf.

[18] Molina-Morant D, Sánchez-Montalvá A, Salvador F, Sao-Avilés A, Molina I. Imported endemic mycoses in Spain: Evolution of hospitalized cases, clinical characteristics and correlation with migratory movements, 1997-2014. *PLoS Negl. Trop. Dis.* [Internet]. 2018 Feb 15;12(2): e0006245. Available from: https://doi.org/10.1371/journal.pntd.0006245.

[19] Bongomin F. *Histoplasma and Histoplasmosis* [Internet]. CHAPTER METRICS OVERVIEW. 2020. Available from: https://www.intechopen.com/chapters/72189.

[20] Antinori S. *Editorial Histoplasma capsulatum: More Widespread than Previously Thought*. 2017; 90(6):982–3. Available from: https://com-mendeley-prod-publicsharing-pdfstore.s3.eu-west-1.amazonaws.com/6284-PUBMED/10.4269/ajtmh.14-0175/tropmed_90_982_pdf.pdf?X-Amz-Security-Token=IQoJb3JpZ2

luX2VjEGoaCWV1LXdlc3QtMSJHMEUCIQDg9lo%2FhM2KLR46cHjJPpu9up RYjS1IPX%2FbszoHRoHRyQIgaRT4M5b1Q.

[21] Rozaliyani A and Setianingrum F. The Review of Histoplasmosis Endemicity and Current Status in Asia. CHAPTER METRICS Overv [Internet]. 2020; Available from: https://www.intechopen.com/chapters/72189.

[22] Baker J, Setianingrum F, Wahyuningsih R, Denning D W. Mapping histoplasmosis in Southeast Asia–implications for diagnosis in AIDS. *Emerg. Microbes Infect.* [Internet]. 2019;8(1):1139–45. Available from: https://www.ncbi.nlm.nih.gov/pmc/articles/PMC6711083/pdf/TEMI_8_1644539.pdf.

[23] Scully M C, Baddley J W. Epidemiology of Histoplasmosis. *Curr. Fungal Infect. Rep.* [Internet]. 2018;12(1):51–8. Available from: https://doi.org/10.1007/s12281-018-0309-x.

[24] WHO. *Guidelines for diagnosing and managing disseminated histoplasmosis among people living with HIV.* WHO [Internet]. 2020; Available from: https://www.who.int/publications/i/item/9789240006430.

[25] Bah. N C. Histoplasmosis infections worldwide: thinking outside of the Ohio River valley. *Rev. Del. Col. Am. Cardiol.* [Internet]. 2018;72(23):2964–79. Available from: https://www.ncbi.nlm.nih.gov/pmc/articles/PMC4535725/pdf/nihms680311.pdf.

[26] Adenis A, Nacher M, Hanf M, Vantilcke V, Boukhari R, Blachet D, Demar M, Aznar C, Carme B & Couppie P. HIV-Associated Histoplasmosis Early Mortality and Incidence Trends: From Neglect to Priority. *PLoS Negl. Trop. Dis.* [Internet]. 2014 Aug 21;8(8):e3100. Available from: https://doi.org/10.1371/journal.pntd.0003100.

[27] Medina N, Rodriguez-Tudela J L, Aguirre L, Salazar L R, Gamboa O, Bonilla O, Pérez J C, Arathoon E, Denning D W & Alastruey-Izquierdo A. Incidence of histoplasmosis in a cohort of people with hiv: From estimations to reality. *Microorganisms*. 2021;9(12).

[28] Leedy N, Cari E V, Wheat L J. *HIV-Associated Histoplasmosis: Current Perspectives*. 2020;113–25. Available from: https://www.ncbi.nlm.nih.gov/pmc/articles/PMC7090190/.

[29] Ferreira S da C, Nóbrega F J F, de Araújo R C, de Almeida P H, Villanova M G, Santana R de C, Ramalho L N Z, Martinelli A de L C, Troncon L E de A. Histoplasmosis related to immunosuppression in a patient with crohn's disease: A diagnostic challenge. *Am. J. Case Rep.* [Internet]. 2021;22(1):1–6. Available from: https://www.ncbi.nlm.nih.gov/pmc/articles/PMC8438646/pdf/amjcaserep-22-e925345.pdf.

Chapter 3

Clinical Features of Histoplasmosis

Ayushi Mendiratta[1,*], MD
Piyush Garg[2], MBBS
Rahul Kashyap[3], MD
and Salim Surani[4], MD
[1]PGY1 Resident, Internal Medicine, Parkview health system, Pueblo, Colorado, USA
[2]Department of Medicine, Heart Institute, Medanta- The Medicity, Gurgaon, Haryana, India
[3]Department of Research, Wellspan Health, York, USA
[4]Department of Medicine and Pharmacology, Texas A&M University, Texas, USA

Abstract

Histoplasmosis is a disease of worldwide endemicity with a greater predilection to river valleys. In the United States, it is usually seen in midwestern and central states. It is a dimorphic fungus, and the infection is usually acquired by inhalation of conidia present in the soil. Therefore, any activity related to the soil that might be occupational or any kind of recreational activity may lead to its transmission. Caves and old buildings which have increased amounts of bat guano have a high prevalence of histoplasmosis conidia. Clinically infections are classified into pulmonary and disseminated histoplasmosis and most of the infections are asymptomatic, although severe infection may be seen in individuals with compromised immune systems. The most common symptoms are fever, cough, chest pain, lymphadenopathy and hepatosplenomegaly. In pulmonary histoplasmosis, chest radiography is mainly suggestive of diffuse reticulonodular infiltrates with hilar and mediastinal

* Corresponding Author's Email: amendiratta95@gmail.com.

In: Histoplasmosis
Editors: Salim Surani, Syed Anjum Khan and Reena Shah
ISBN: 979-8-89113-129-3

lymphadenopathy. Majorly the T cells play a role in fighting histoplasmosis and any disease process leading to decreased cellular immunity (e.g., HIV infection) can lead to failure to activate macrophages which ultimately leads to progressive disseminated histoplasmosis. This serious infection may present with multiple organ failure like liver and kidney failure, respiratory distress, shock, etc.

Keywords: histoplasmosis, acute pulmonary histoplasmosis, disseminated histoplasmosis

Introduction

The pathogenic varieties of histoplasmosis are *H. capsulatum* var. *capsulatum* and *H. capsulatum* var. *Duboisii* [1]. Airborne spores of Histoplasma, once inhaled, are deposited in the alveoli. Germination requires an average temperature and is ingested by the pulmonary macrophages. They act as a parasite within them and migrate to mediastinal and hilar lymph nodes, from where they can easily disseminate to various organs via the bloodstream [2].

Cellular immunity develops after approximately a couple of weeks, and macrophages clear the infection in an immunocompetent host. Initially, necrosis develops at the site of infection, and years later, calcified granulomas develop. Immunocompromised hosts are at a high risk of disseminated infections [3].

Clinical Manifestations

Clinical features develop only in a small number of exposed individuals and are classified into Pulmonary Histoplasmosis and Disseminated Histoplasmosis as shown in Table 1.

Table 1. Pulmonary and Disseminated Histoplasmosis Clinical Features

Pulmonary Histoplasmosis	• Acute pulmonary histoplasmosis • Chronic cavitary pulmonary histoplasmosis.
Disseminated Histoplasmosis	• Acute disseminated histoplasmosis • Chronic progressive disseminated histoplasmosis.

Pulmonary Histoplasmosis

Acute Pulmonary Histoplasmosis

It is usually a self-limited condition. The clinical presentation involves symptoms like headache, malaise, and fever. Symptoms indicating a pulmonary infection: Chest congestion, dyspnea, and cough, usually dry [4].

In the immunocompetent population, the infection is cleared off by itself, but fatigue patients may be fatigued for a longer period of time. It usually involves one or two lobes of the lungs and is radiologically evident as patchy lobular pneumonia with hilar and mediastinal lymphadenopathy [5, 6].

Although in patients exposed to a large inoculum of this fungus, like from cleaning an attic or chicken coop, it can lead to an acute severe infection [4, 7]. It is marked by sudden onset fever with sudden onset fever with chills, dyspnea, and chest pain. This can progress to acute respiratory distress syndrome. Physical examination findings are significant for rales throughout the lungs. Chest X-ray shows diffuse reticulonodular infiltrates. With or without lymphadenopathy [8, 9]. This acute severe infection can also occur in an immunocompromised host due to suppressed cell-mediated immunity.

Extrapulmonary Manifestations: Occurs in almost 5% of infected individuals.

- Skin involvement: Erythema nodosum and multiforme are thought to be due to a hypersensitivity response to the antigen [10].
- Rheumatologic manifestations: Polyarticular symmetrical arthritis, which are transient in nature and responds to NSAIDs [11].

Chronic Cavitary Pulmonary Histoplasmosis

This is usually seen in older patients with underlying lung pathology, usually emphysema. Due to the infection, the emphysematous bullae become thickened, followed by necrosis and fibrosis. This is commonly seen in the apical and apical posterior portions of the lung [12]. Necrosis continues to increase the size of the cavity and can involve the entire lobe of the lung (also known as the "marching cavity"). Lymphadenopathy is uncommon, but calcified nodes may be seen on chest x-rays [6]. Pleural involvement may occur in the form of thickening, but effusion is rarely seen [4].

Clinical presentation is similar to the tuberculosis reactivation, i.e., fever, night sweats, fatigue, weight loss, anorexia, and sometimes mild hemoptysis. If left untreated, the course of illness is progressive and can lead to deterioration in lung condition, ultimately leading to death [13].

Complications of Pulmonary Histoplasmosis

Granulomatous Mediastinitis

The usual course of lymph node involvement in histoplasmosis is enlargement followed by a decrease in size and calcification. But sometimes, there is a massive increase in the size of lymph nodes, which coalesce together. The nodes involved are hilar, subcarinal, and paratracheal. Caseating necrosis occurs in these lymph nodes from the center of which the yeast can sometimes be isolated with the help of tissue biopsy.

The patients are usually asymptomatic, and the lymph nodes are an incidental finding on x-ray. Symptoms may be present because of the pressure effect of the lymph nodes over the mediastinal structures like superior vena cava (SVC), esophagus, and bronchi presenting as chest pain, cough, dyspnea, dysphagia or SVC syndrome (face/neck swelling, distended neck veins, cough, dyspnea, orthopnea, upper extremity swelling, distended chest vein collaterals, and conjunctival suffusion) [6, 14]. Ultimately the condition resolves by calcification of these lymph nodes.

Sometimes these calcified lymph nodes erode the bronchus, and broncholithiasis develops. Features of obstruction and inflammation develop, leading to features of cough and focal wheeze.

Fibrosing Mediastinitis

It is a rare but lethal complication of pulmonary histoplasmosis. It was earlier thought to be evolving from granulomatous mediastinitis, but there is no relevant data suggesting the relationship between these two [15]. It is thought to be due to excessive fibrosis around the infected lymph nodes leading to compression of mediastinal structures [15, 16]. Biopsy shows mature collagen formation. Involvement of pulmonary arteries and SVC leading to right heart failure and SVC syndrome, respectively. Chest x-rays are suggestive of mediastinal widening.

Pericarditis and Pleural Effusion

Due to host immune response, patients develop pericarditis along with exudative, hemorrhagic, culture-negative pleural effusion in the background of pneumonia and mediastinal lymphadenopathy [17-19]. Pericarditis presents as chest pain and dyspnea and the mainstay of symptom management is nonsteroidal anti-inflammatory drugs [17]. Corticosteroids are sometimes used to lower the immune response of the host.

Disseminated Histoplasmosis

Pathogenesis

During infection, cytokines like Interleukin [12] and Interferon gamma trigger macrophages, which lead to the spread of the organism to the adjacent lymph nodes via lymphatics and, from there it spreads hematogenously via activated macrophages to the reticuloendothelial system [20]. Failure to activate macrophages due to reduced cell-mediated immunity leads to disseminated infection.

Reinfection and Reactivation

Sometimes the infection is controlled in the form of controlled foci of fungus-like tuberculosis, which can reactivate years later [21, 22]. The patient population at risk for uncontrolled disseminated histoplasmosis are those with reduced cell-mediated immunity who live in endemic areas.

Risk Factors

Drugs

Many cases have been reported to the FDA Adverse Events Reporting systems after the use of corticosteroids, tumor necrosis factor antagonists (Etanercept or Infliximab), Methotrexate [23]. Screening has been recommended before starting a patient on a TNF inhibitor. Patients who are at high risk are usually those who belong to the endemic areas, i.e., United States (particularly Midwestern and Central states), Mexico, Central, and South America, Africa, and Asia with a history of working in old buildings, caves, cleaning chicken coops, etc. High-risk patients, patients with a history of histoplasmosis within the last two years or symptoms of histoplasmosis, are the ones who undergo a chest X-ray before starting the treatment [24, 25].

Post-Transplant Patients

There are three ways in which solid organ transplant patients can develop histoplasmosis- new infection by inhalation of conidia, reactivation of old infection, or transmission of infection from the infected donor [25]. Both living and deceased donors are thus tested for the infection before transplantation.

Patients with AIDS or Hematological Malignancies

AIDS patients are at a high risk of primary infection in endemic areas or reactivation when CD4 count < 150 cells/μL [25]. However, this risk has decreased in the United States due to effective antiretroviral therapy [26].

Pathology

In patients with histoplasmosis, infiltration of tissues is usually seen with macrophages (i.e., histiocytosis) and not neutrophils, lymphocytes, and plasma cells [27].

Tissue response is of three types in disseminated histoplasmosis:

- Diffuse histiocytosis
- Focal histiocytosis
- Tuberculoid granuloma.

Clinical Features

Disseminated histoplasmosis occurs in two classical forms depending on the time frame of the infection- Acute and chronic. Clinical manifestations depend on the host's immune status as well as fungal load [27]. Involvement of one extrapulmonary site (e.g., GI or CNS) is also classified as disseminated disease [28]. In severely immunocompromised hosts, the infection usually spreads to multiple organs and thus constitutes progressive disseminated histoplasmosis.

Acute Infection

They are usually seen in severely immunocompromised hosts. Systemic signs of infection include fever, chills, anorexia, weight loss, lymphadenopathy, or hepatosplenomegaly. Mucosal ulceration can also occur in the form of superficial and deep ulceration with heaped-up borders. Severe disease can also present sepsis, like a picture with disseminated intravascular coagulation, hypotension, acute kidney injury, or acute respiratory distress syndrome [29].

Chronic Infection

It is generally seen in older individuals and is also known as chronic progressive disseminated histoplasmosis. The usual presentation is hepatosplenomegaly with pancytopenia along with adrenal gland involvement.

Patients with disseminated disease can sometimes present with signs and symptoms predominant to the particular organ involvement [28].

Unique features due to specific system involvement are as follows.

Gastrointestinal

GI histoplasmosis is a rare entity mostly presenting as severe diarrhea with malabsorption and tenesmus, anorexia, abdominal pain, and tenderness [30]. It can also involve the colon and cause ulcerations, strictures, and perforations [30]. Another complication that can occur is protein-losing enteropathy due to malabsorption leading to hypogammaglobulinemia. The disease usually mimics many other GI pathologies like Inflammatory bowel disease, GI tuberculosis, GI carcinomas, and lymphomas.

Pathologic Forms of GI Histoplasmosis:

1. Subclinical form: macrophages in the form of clusters in lamina propria.
2. Fungus-containing macrophages form plaques and polyps
3. Inflammatory symptoms (pain abdomen, bleeding) due to tissue necrosis and ulcerations (single or continuous mucosal ulcers, deep bleeding ulcers, or friable necrotic masses)
4. Localized bowel thickening [30-32].

Adrenal Glands

This is another rare sequela of disseminated histoplasmosis. It sometimes presents as signs and symptoms of adrenal insufficiency, such as orthostatic hypotension, nausea, and vomiting [33]. CT scan is usually suggestive of bilateral adrenal enlargement. This adrenal mass has peripheral enhancement and central hypodensity due to necrosis or hemorrhage [33]. This particular characteristic of the scan narrows the differential of the disease to histoplasmosis and tuberculosis, and thus histopathological and cytological analysis can help confirm the diagnosis.

Genitourinary

The GU tract is rarely involved in disseminated histoplasmosis or maybe remains underdiagnosed due to lack of symptoms. Urinary tract involvement usually causes bladder ulceration and immune complex-mediated glomerulonephritis in the mesangium [34]. Testicles are infrequently involved and usually present as epididymo-orchitis, which, just like other disseminated histoplasmosis, mimics other granulomatous infections like testicular tuberculosis and in any immunosuppressed case, should be considered as an important differential, especially in the endemic areas [35].

Osteoarticular Infection

In primary acute infection, polyarthritis or arthralgias involving knees, ankles, wrists, or small joints of the hand in 6% of reported cases which may occur due to initial sensitization to Histoplasma antigen, as noted in a study in Indianapolis in 1978 [36]. It can cause septic monoarthritis of joints and rarely, osteomyelitis [37]. In a study by Berbari et al., few cases of culture-negative prosthetic joint infections on prolonged incubation grew Histoplasma [38]. It can also cause inflammation of tendons and carpal tunnel syndrome and can be seen in immunocompetent hosts as well in the absence of disseminated disease presenting as focal inflammation of the tendons [39].

CNS Infection

Infection usually occurs in about 5-10% of the infected individuals and is due to hematogenous dissemination to the brain or meninges. Meningitis occurs due to infection of the basilar meninges and can lead to communicating hydrocephalus. It can cause brain and spinal cord mass lesions, like brain abscess, neoplasm, or encephalitis. Brain lesions on MRI appear as multiple rings enhancing lesions on Magnetic Resonance Imaging [40].

Endocarditis

Heart valve involvement is rare in histoplasmosis and is usually difficult to diagnose due to consistently negative blood cultures [41]. The diagnosis is delayed by an average of nine months because of this [42]. It can involve native or prosthetic valves. Timely diagnosis and management are crucial since the infection is uniformly fatal. Patients present with fever, fatigue, and weight loss. Sometimes they have signs and symptoms of heart failure like shortness of breath, edema, or neurological features like altered mental status. In some patients, vegetation may embolize vessels of the cerebrum, causing stroke, extremities causing acute limb ischemia, or major organs like the spleen, kidneys, etc., causing infarcts [43].

Skin Involvement

This is commonly seen in patients with advanced HIV, and lesions includes dermatitis, nodules, plaques, and abscesses but rarely can also cause cellulitis, panniculitis, necrotic vasculitis, and exfoliative erythroderma [44]. Skin biopsy showing infiltration of macrophages with *H. capsulatum* is the mainstay in diagnosis [45].

Others

Peritonitis [46, Pancreatitis, Cholecystitis [47], Panniculitis [48], Mastitis [49], Chorioretinitis [50], Hypercalcemia (due to increased calcitriol production by activated macrophages) [51], Hemophagocytic lymphohistiocytosis [52], Thrombotic microangiopathy [53].

Histoplasmosis during COVID-19

SARS-CoV-2 is the causative agent of the coronavirus infection, which leads to a variety of clinical features ranging from cough and fever to acute respiratory distress syndrome (ARDS).

Pulmonary histoplasmosis also shows FDG avidity in PET/CT, both in the primary pulmonary infection and the mediastinal and hilar lymph nodes. FDG-PET/CT is a noninvasive tool capable of early detection and assessment of disease involvement [54]. Computed Tomography (CT) findings of the chest during the infection show multiple areas of ground-glass/linear opacities and consolidations. The areas most affected were peripheral regions of the lower lobe of both lungs [55].

The immunosuppressive state during COVID-19 infection may increase the susceptibility to invasive fungal infections like Pneumocystis jirovecii, cryptococcosis, histoplasmosis, Coccidioides, etc.

Taylor et al., [56] reported a case of [50] years of a male patient who was admitted due to Covid-19 pneumonia, and a CT scan showed a right upper lung lobe mass. The bronchoalveolar lavage, biopsy of the lung, bone marrow biopsy, and Histoplasma urine antigen test confirmed the patient with disseminated histoplasmosis. It is reported that there was an increase in the incidence of histoplasmosis co-infected with the COVID-19 pandemic. Macedo et al., [57] reported two cases of pulmonary histoplasmosis after COVID infection. The patient was treated with Itraconazole [58]. Mild infection is treated by Itraconazole. Moderate and severe infection is treated by Amphotericin B.

In AIDS patients, COVID-19 has not increased susceptibility to opportunistic infections, like histoplasmosis, coccidioidomycosis, etc. Some case reports report the occurrence of histoplasmosis in the context of COVID-19.

The patient neither developed a severe infection nor was admitted to the ICU, probably because of the low CD4 count, which might have prevented him from developing cytokine storm and immune reconstitution syndrome [59].

Conclusion

Histoplasmosis is caused by a dimorphic fungus called histoplasma capsulatum. It is highly prevalent in the United States and occurs because of inhalation of fungal spores. It commonly affects the lungs, and the infections are mostly asymptomatic. In some cases, it may cause acute pulmonary histoplasmosis, or a more serious form of infection called disseminated histoplasmosis.

Acute pulmonary histoplasmosis usually manifests as high-grade fever, cough, chest pain and is radiologically identified with diffuse reticulonodular infiltrates. COVID-19 may also increase the susceptibility to fungal infections. In patients who are immunosuppressed with decreased cellular immunity, histoplasmosis causes an aggressive form of the disease called disseminated histoplasmosis which involves multiple organ systems like liver, kidney, CNS, gastrointestinal system, etc.

References

[1] Kauffman, C. A. 2003. Histoplasmosis, p. 285-298. In W. E. Dismukes, P. G. Pappas, and J. D. Sobel (ed.), *Clinical mycology*. Oxford University Press, New York, NY.

[2] Conces, D. J. *Histoplasmosis. Semin Roentgenol.* 1996;31:14-27.

[3] Wheat, J. Histoplasmosis. Experience during outbreaks in Indianapolis and review of the literature. *Medicine.* 1997;76:339-54.

[4] Goodwin, R. A., Jr., J. E. Loyd, and R. M. des Prez. 1981. Histoplasmosis in normal hosts. *Medicine* (Baltimore) 60:231-266. [PubMed] [Google Scholar].

[5] Gurney, J. W., and D. J. Conces, Jr. 1996. Pulmonary histoplasmosis. *Radiology* 199:297-306. [PubMed] [Google Scholar].

[6] Wheat, L. J., D. Conces, S. D. Allen, D. Blue-Hnidy, and J. Loyd. 2004. Pulmonary histoplasmosis syndromes: recognition, diagnosis, and management. *Semin. Respir. Crit. Care Med.* 25:129-144. [PubMed] [Google Scholar].

[7] Wheat, L. J., and C. A. Kauffman. 2003. Histoplasmosis. *Infect. Dis. Clin. N. Am.* 17:1-19. [PubMed] [Google Scholar].

[8] Kataria, Y. P., P. B. Campbell, and B. T. Burlingham. 1981. Acute pulmonary histoplasmosis presenting as adult respiratory distress syndrome: Effect of therapy on clinical and laboratory features. *South. Med. J.* 74:534-537. [PubMed] [Google Scholar].

[9] Wynne, J. W., and G. N. Olsen. 1974. Acute histoplasmosis presenting as the adult respiratory distress syndrome. *Chest* 66:158-161. [PubMed] [Google Scholar].

[10] Ozols, I. I., and L. J. Wheat. 1981. Erythema nodosum in an epidemic of histoplasmosis in Indianapolis, Indiana. *Arch. Dermatol.* 117:709-712. [PubMed] [Google Scholar].

[11] Rosenthal, J., K. D. Brandt, L. J. Wheat, and T. G. Slama. 1983. Rheumatologic manifestations of histoplasmosis in the recent Indianapolis epidemic. *Arthritis Rheum.* 26:1065-1070. [PubMed] [Google Scholar].

[12] Goodwin, R. A., Jr., F. T. Owens, J. D. Snell, W. W. Hubbard, R. D. Buchanan, R. T. Terry, and R. M. des Prez. 1976. Chronic pulmonary histoplasmosis. *Medicine* (Baltimore) 55:413-452. [PubMed] [Google Scholar].

[13] Furcolow, M. L. 1963. Comparison of treated and untreated severe histoplasmosis. *JAMA* 183:121-127. [Google Scholar] [Ref list].

[14] Parish, J. M., Rosenow E. C., III. Mediastinal granuloma and mediastinal fibrosis. *Semin Respir Crit Care Med* 2002;23:135–143.

[15] Davis, A., D. Pierson, and J. E. Loyd. 2001. Mediastinal fibrosis. *Semin. Respir. Infect.* 16:119-130. [PubMed] [Google Scholar] [Ref list].

[16] Goodwin, R. A., Jr., J. A. Nickell, and R. M. des Prez. 1972. Mediastinal fibrosis complicating healed primary histoplasmosis and tuberculosis. *Medicine* (Baltimore) 51:227-246. [PubMed] [Google Scholar] [Ref list].

[17] Picardi, J. L., C. A. Kauffman, J. Schwarz, J. C. Holmes, J. P. Phair, and N. O. Fowler. 1976. Pericarditis caused by Histoplasma capsulatum. *Am. J. Cardiol.* 37:82-88. [PubMed] [Google Scholar] [Ref list].

[18] Young, E. J., B. Vainrub, and D. M. Musher. 1978. Pericarditis due to histoplasmosis. *JAMA* 240:1750-1751. [PubMed] [Google Scholar] [Ref list].

[19] Schwarz, J., M. D. Schaen, and J. L. Picardi. 1976. Complications of the arrested primary histoplasmic complex. *JAMA* 236:1157-1161. [PubMed] [Google Scholar] [Ref list].

[20] Deepe, G. S. Jr., Bullock W. E. Histoplasmosis: a granulomatous inflammatory response. In: *Basic Principles and Clinical Correlates,* Gallin J. I., Goldstein I. M., Snyderman R. (Eds), Raven, New York 1988. p. 733.

[21] Deepe, G. S. Jr. 1988. Protective immunity in murine histoplasmosis: functional comparison of adoptively transferred T-cell clones and splenic T cells. *Infect. Immun.* 56:2350-2355. [PMC free article] [PubMed] [Google Scholar] [Ref list].

[22] Newman, S. L. 2001. Cell-mediated immunity to Histoplasma capsulatum. *Semin. Respir. Infect.* 16:102-108. [PubMed] [Google Scholar] [Ref list].

[23] US Food and Drug Administration. *MedWatch.* http://www.fda.gov/Drugs/DrugSafety/PostmarketDrugSafetyInformationforPatientsandProviders/ucm124185.htm (Accessed on October 06, 2011).

[24] Chadi, A. Hage 1, Suzanne Bowyer, Stacey E. Tarvin, Debra Helper, Martin B. Kleiman, L. *Joseph Wheat: Recognition, diagnosis, and treatment of histoplasmosis complicating tumor necrosis factor blocker therapy.*

[25] Limaye, A. P., Connolly P. A., Sagar M., Fritsche T. R., Cookson B. T., Wheat L. J., Stamm W. E., *N Engl J Med.* 2000;343(16):1163: Transmission of Histoplasma capsulatum by organ transplantation.

[26] Hajjeh, R. A., Pappas P. G., Henderson H., Lancaster D., Bamberger D. M., Skahan K. J., Phelan M. A., Cloud G., Holloway M., Kauffman C. A., Wheat L. J., National

Institute of Allergy and Infectious Diseases Mycoses Study Group. Multicenter case-control study of risk factors for histoplasmosis in human immunodeficiency virus-infected persons. *Clin Infect Dis* 2001; 32:1215.

[27] Goodwin, R. A., Jr., J. L. Shapiro, G. H. Thurman, S. S. Thurman, and R. M. des Prez. 1980. Disseminated histoplasmosis: clinical and pathological correlations. *Medicine* (Baltimore) 59:1-33. [PubMed] [Google Scholar] [Ref list].

[28] Franklin, D. A., Lindsey Larson, Adriana M Rauseo, Sasinuch Rutjanawech, Michael Joshua Hendrix, William G Powderly, *Andrej Spec: A comparison of presentations and outcomes of histoplasmosis across patients with varying immune status.*

[29] Gutierrez, M. E., A. Canton, N. Sosa, E. Puga, and L. Talavera. 2005. Disseminated histoplasmosis in patients with AIDS in Panama: a review of 104 cases. *Clin. Infect. Dis.* 40:1199-1202. [PubMed] [Google Scholar] [Ref list].

[30] Kahi, C. J., Wheat L. J., Allen S. D., Sarosi G. A. Gastrointestinal histoplasmosis. *Am J Gastroenterol.* 2005;100:220–231. [PubMed] [Google Scholar] [Ref list].

[31] Lamps, L. W., C. P. Molina, A. B. West, R. C. Haggit, and M. A. Scott. 2000. The pathological spectrum of gastrointestinal and hepatic histoplasmosis. *Am. J. Clin. Pathol.* 113:64-72. [PubMed] [Google Scholar] [Ref list].

[32] Kok, J., Chen S. C., Anderson L., Berglund L., Sleiman S., Moss A., Bourke M., Fulcher D., Gilroy N. Protein-losing enteropathy and hypogammaglobulinemia as first manifestations of disseminated histoplasmosis coincident with Nocardia infection. *J Med Microbiol.* 2010;59:610–613. [PubMed] [Google Scholar] [Ref list].

[33] Mukherjee, J. J., Villa M. L., Tan L., Lee K. O. Bilateral adrenal masses due to histoplasmosis. *J Clin Endocrinol Metabol.* 2005;90:6725–6726. [PubMed] [Google Scholar] [Ref list].

[34] Bullock, W. E., R. P. Artz, D. Bhathena, and H. S. K. Tung. 1979. Histoplasmosis: association with circulating immune complexes, eosinophilia, and mesangiopathic glomerulonephritis. *Arch. Intern. Med.* 139:700-702. [PubMed] [Google Scholar] [Ref list].

[35] Valberto, S., Gynara Rezende Gonzalez do Valle Barbosa, B. Bruna Miranda, B. Rafael H. Bastos, B. and Alessandro C. Pasqualotto, *Epididymo-orchitis caused by Histoplasma capsulatum.*

[36] Darouiche, R. O., R. M. Cadle, G. J. Zenon, M. F. Weinert, R. J. Hamill, and M. D. Lidsky. 1992. Articular histoplasmosis. *J. Rheumatol.* 19:1991-1993. [PubMed] [Google Scholar] [Ref list].

[37] Rosenthal, J., Brandt K. D., Wheat L. J., Slama T. G. Rheumatologic manifestations of histoplasmosis in the recent Indianapolis endemic. *Arthritis Rheum.* 1983;26:1065–70. doi: https://doi.org/10.1002/art.1780260902. [PubMed] [CrossRef] [Google Scholar] [Ref list].

[38] Hadi, E. Berbari, M. S., Pooja Gurram, M. B. B. S., Maryam Mahmood, M. B. Ch. B., Paul J. Deziel, P. A. C., Randall C. Walker, M. D., and Raymund R. *Razonable, Prosthetic Joint Infections Due to Histoplasma capsulatum: A Report of 3 Cases.*

[39] Strayer, D. S., M. B. Gutwein, D. Herbold, and R. Bresalier. 1981. Histoplasmosis presenting as the carpal tunnel syndrome. *Am. J. Surg.* 141:286-288. [PubMed] [Google Scholar] [Ref list].

[40] Wheat, L. J., B. E. Batteiger, and B. Sathapatayavongs. 1990. Histoplasma capsulatum infections of the central nervous system: a clinical review. *Medicine* (Baltimore) 69:244-260. [PubMed] [Google Scholar] [Ref list].

[41] McLeod, R., Remington J. S. Fungal endocarditis. In: Rahimtoola S. H., editor. *Infective endocarditis*. New York: Grune and Stratton; 1977. p. 211–90.

[42] Blair, T., Raymond L. Histoplasma endocarditis. *Chest* 1981; 70:620.

[43] Riddell, J., IV, Carol A. Kauffman, Jeannina A. Smith, Maha Assi, Sky Blue, Martha I. Buitrago, Stan Deresinski, Patty W. Wright, Douglas A. Drevets, Steven A. Norris, Holenarasipur R. Vikram, Paul J. Carson, Paschalis Vergidis, John Carpenter, Steven M. Seidenfeld, and L. Joseph Wheat. *Multicenter Case Series with Review of Current Diagnostic Techniques and Treatment: Histoplasma capsulatum Endocarditis*.

[44] Cunha, V. S., Zampese M. S., Aquino V. R., Cestari T. F., Goldani L. Z., *Clin Exp Dermatol.* 2007;32(3):250: Mucocutaneous manifestations of disseminated histoplasmosis in patients with acquired immunodeficiency syndrome: particular aspects in a Latin-American population.

[45] Cohen, P. R. 1, D. E. Bank, D. N. Silvers, M. E. *Grossman: Cutaneous lesions of disseminated histoplasmosis in human immunodeficiency virus-infected patients.*

[46] Reddy, P. A., Brasher C. A., Christianson C., Gorelick D. F. Peritonitis due to histoplasmosis. *Ann Intern Med* 1969; 72:79.

[47] Patrick, C. C., Flynn P. M., Henwick S., Pui C. H. Disseminated histoplasmosis presenting as a cystic duct obstruction. *Pediatr Infect Dis J* 1992; 11:593.

[48] Pottage, J. C. Jr., Trenholme G. M., Aronson I. K., Harris A. A. Panniculitis associated with histoplasmosis and alpha 1-antitrypsin deficiency. *Am J Med* 1983; 75:150.

[49] Osborne, B. M. Granulomatous mastitis caused by histoplasma and mimicking inflammatory breast carcinoma. *Hum Pathol* 1989; 20:47.

[50] Macher, A., Rodrigues M. M., Kaplan W., Pistole M. C., McKittrick A., Lawrinson W. E., Reichert C. M. Disseminated bilateral chorioretinitis due to Histoplasma capsulatum in a patient with the acquired immunodeficiency syndrome. *Ophthalmology* 1985; 92:1159.

[51] Walker, J. V., Baran D., Yakub N., Freeman R. B. Histoplasmosis with hypercalcemia, renal failure, and papillary necrosis. Confusion with sarcoidosis. *JAMA* 1977; 237:1350.

[52] Townsend, J. L., Shanbhag S., Hancock J., Bowman K., Nijhawan A. E. Histoplasmosis-Induced Hemophagocytic Syndrome: A Case Series and Review of the Literature. *Open Forum Infect Dis* 2015; 2:ofv055.

[53] Dwyre D. M., Bell A. M., Siechen K., Sethi S., Raife T. J. Disseminated histoplasmosis presenting as thrombotic microangiopathy. *Transfusion* 2006; 46:1221.

[54] Eibschutz, L. S., Rabiee, B., Asadollahi, S., Gupta, A., Assadi, M., Alavi, A., & Gholamrezanezhad, A. (2022). FDG-PET/CT of COVID-19 and Other Lung

Infections. *Seminars in nuclear medicine,* 52(1), 61–70. (https://doi.org/10.1053/j.semnuclmed.2021.06.017).

[55] Stasiak, C. E. S., Nigri, D. H., Cardoso, F. R., Mattos, R. S. A. R., Gonçalves Martins, P. A., Carvalho, A. R. S., Altino de Almeida, S., Rodrigues, R. S., & Rosado-de-Castro, P. H. (2021). Case Report: Incidental Finding of COVID-19 Infection after Positron Emission Tomography/CT Imaging in a Patient with a Diagnosis of Histoplasmosis and Recurring Fever. *The American journal of tropical medicine and hygiene,* 104(5), 1651–1654. https://doi.org/10.4269/ajtmh.20-0952.

[56] Taylor, M., Ghodasara, A., Ismail, A., Gauhar, U., & El-Kersh, K. (2021). Disseminated Histoplasmosis in an Immunocompetent Patient After COVID-19 Pneumonia. *Cureus*, 13(8), e17269. https://doi.org/10.7759/cureus.17269.

[57] de Macedo, P. M., Freitas, A. D., Bártholo, T. P., Bernardes-Engemann, A. R., Almeida, M. A., Almeida-Silva, F., Zancopé-Oliveira, R. M., & Almeida-Paes, R. (2021). Acute Pulmonary Histoplasmosis Following COVID-19: Novel Laboratorial Methods Aiding Diagnosis. *Journal of fungi* (Basel, Switzerland), 7(5), 346. https://doi.org/10.3390/jof7050346.

[58] Casalini, G., Giacomelli, A., Ridolfo, A., Gervasoni, C., & Antinori, S. (2021). Invasive Fungal Infections Complicating COVID-19: A Narrative Review. *Journal of fungi* (Basel, Switzerland), 7(11), 921. https://doi.org/10.3390/jof7110921.

[59] Basso, R. P., Poester, V. R., Benelli, J. L., Stevens, D. A., Zogbi, H. E., Vasconcellos, I., Pasqualotto, A. C., & Xavier, M. O. (2021). COVID-19-Associated Histoplasmosis in an AIDS Patient. *Mycopathologia,* 186(1), 109–112. https://doi.org/10.1007/s11046-020-00505-1.

Chapter 4

Advances in the Diagnosis of Histoplasmosis: An Update into the Laboratory Diagnosis of *Histoplasma capsulatum*

M. A. Toscanini[1,2]
C. Rodriguez Laboccetta[1,2]
A. Videla Garrido[2]
V. Briceño Fernández[1,2]
K. Hermida Alava[2]
A. Etchecopaz[2]
C. A. Iovannitti[2]
A. D. Nusblat[1]
and M. L. Cuestas[2,*]

[1]Department of Microbiology, Faculty of Medicine, Universidad de Buenos Aires, CONICET, Instituto de Nanobiotecnología (NANOBIOTEC), Cátedra de Biotecnología, Facultad de Farmacia y Bioquímica, Buenos Aires, Argentina
[2]Department of Microbiology, Faculty of Medicine, Universidad de Buenos Aires, CONICET, Instituto de Investigaciones en Microbiología y Parasitología Médica (IMPaM), Departamento de Microbiología, Facultad de Medicina, Buenos Aires, Argentina

Abstract

Histoplasmosis is a life-threatening systemic infection caused by the thermally dimorphic fungal pathogen *Histoplasma capsulatum*, whose

---

* Corresponding Author's E-mail: marilucuestas@gmail.com.

In: Histoplasmosis
Editors: Salim Surani, Syed Anjum Khan and Reena Shah
ISBN: 979-8-89113-129-3

natural reservoirs are thought to be soil enriched with bird excreta and bat guano. Infection is most frequently diagnosed in the Americas, but it has been reported worldwide. Among immunocompetent individuals, histoplasmosis is mostly asymptomatic and spontaneously self-limited. However, in patients with an acquired or congenital T cellular immunity deficiency, histoplasmosis is responsible for an important morbidity and mortality. In HIV infected patients, its extrapulmonary or disseminated form, known as progressive disseminated histoplasmosis (PDH) became an AIDS-defining illness, especially in Latin America, where an estimated 15,000 new infections and 9,000 deaths occur among people living with HIV (PLHIV).

Histoplasmosis diagnosis is still challenging and limited in many countries. Symptoms of PDH are often nonspecific, and among PLHIV, they may be similar to those of other diseases, especially tuberculosis, complicating diagnosis and treatment. As PDH is associated with high mortality rates due to late diagnosis rapid detection of histoplasmosis and specific treatment are needed. In this regard, some progress has been recently achieved, such as the publication of World Health Organization (WHO)/Pan American Health Organization guidelines for diagnosis and management of PDH among PLHIV and the inclusion of *Histoplasma* antigen testing in the WHO list of Essential Diagnostics.

Conventional laboratory methods used for diagnosis of histoplasmosis, such as culture and histopathology, pose many challenges, including the need for complex laboratory infrastructure and staff with mycology training, a turnaround time of up to several weeks, and limited sensitivity. Diagnosis using serologic methods is further complicated by a low antibody test sensitivity when performed in immunocompromised individuals. Several molecular "in-house" tests were also developed and showed promising results but none of these tests are commercially available, and their standardization and validation are still pending. Detection of urine *Histoplasma* antigen has been described as the best option to diagnose PDH due to its high sensitivity. However, cross-reactivity with other related fungi is common. Moreover, this assay is expensive and only performed in a few laboratories. Novel protein antigen candidates have been recently identified and produced by DNA-recombinant techniques in order to obtain standardized and specific reagents for the diagnosis of histoplasmosis, in contraposition to the unspecific antigens or crude extracts used. This chapter describes the currently available diagnostic assays, highlighting their strengths and limitations, and reports the latest approaches to achieve reliable and rapid diagnostic tests for histoplasmosis.

Keywords: histoplasmosis, *Histoplasma capsulatum*, diagnosis, culture, histopathology, antibody detection assays, antigen detection assays, molecular assays

Introduction

Histoplasmosis is a deep pulmonary/systemic mycosis caused by the thermally dimorphic ascomycete fungus *Histoplasma capsulatum*. This respiratory pathogen was first described as a protozoan parasite in Panamá (Ancon, Canal Zone) in 1906 by the pathologist Samuel T. Darling who found it after examining smears from the lungs, spleen and bone marrow in a fatal case that appeared to be disseminated tuberculosis. He proposed the name of *Histoplasma capsulate* owing to its residence within "histiocytes" or macrophages, and the observation that these intracellular organisms appeared to have capsules. [1]

Over the next decades it became evident that *H. capsulatum* is a saprobiotic fungus with no capsule, whose environmental reservoir is nitrogen/phosphate (often bird excreta and bat guano) enriched soils, and that histoplasmosis is primarily a pulmonary disease that may secondarily spread to other organs, especially those of the reticuloendothelial system. [2-4]

As a saprophyte in soil, it is mycelial, but it becomes a budding yeast as a parasite in susceptible hosts. These morphological phases can be reproduced reversibly *in vitro* by shifting the temperature from 25°C at which it is mycelial, to 37°C when it becomes a budding yeast. The process of mycelial-to-yeast conversion is of particular interest since it is triggered by an increase in temperature, and it leads to conversion to a virulent form. [5]

Histoplasmosis is highly endemic in the Americas, where the fungus tends to cause the highest disease burden, but is also distributed in Africa [6-7], India [8], Australia [9], China [10], Southeastern Asia [11] and some regions of Europe [12-13]

According to the clinical manifestations, morphologies and geographical occurrence, three different varieties of *Histoplasma* have been historically recognized: *H. capsulatum* var. *capsulatum*, which is a globally dispersed New World human pathogen responsible for pulmonary and systemic (i.e., classical) histoplasmosis [14]; *H. capsulatum* var. *duboisii*, a human pathogen confined to Central and West Africa, causing African histoplasmosis, whose principal features are skin or bone lesions [15, 16]; and *H. capsulatum* var. *farciminosum*, an Old World animal pathogen, responsible for epizootic lymphangitis in equines. [17] Phylogenetic analyses based on genome sequence variation of four protein-coding genes defined at least eight clades within seven phylogenetic species that display distinct geographical distribution: (i) North American class 1 clade (NAm 1); (ii) North American class 2 clade (NAm 2); (iii) Latin American group A clade (LAm A); (iv) Latin American group B clade (LAm B); (v) Australian clade; (vi) Netherlands (Indonesian?) clade; (vii) Eurasian clade and (viii) African clade. [18, 19] With the exception of the Eurasian clade, which originated from the LAm A clade, the remaining clades are considered phylogenetic species. Kasuga et al. (2003) [18] also described seven multilocus genotypes, named lineages that do not belong to any of the eight clades described and they are also distant from each other (i.e., H140, H81, H66, H69, H153, H167 and EH315). [18]

A further revision of the phylogenetic distribution and population structure carried out by Teixeira et al. proposed that the *Histoplasm*a species complex comprises at least six new phylogenetic species: LAm A1, LAm A2, LAm B1, LAm B2 (corresponding to LAm B clade, Kasuga et al. 2003), RJ (which corresponds to the LAm A clade described by Kasuga et al. [18] and BAC-1 (a bat-associated species-specific clade). [20.]

Recently, Sepúlveda et al. [21] proposed a taxonomic rearrangement of the genus, based on whole genome data from 30 isolates embebbed in five of the groups proposed by Kasuga et al. [18] and showed that the *Histoplasma* genus is composed of at least four species that are genetically isolated and rarely interbreed: *H. capsulatum sensu stricto* when referring to the Panamanian lineage (H81), *Histoplasma mississippiense* sp. nov. (formerly known as NAm 1), *Histoplasma ohiense* sp. nov. (formerly known as NAm 2) and *Histoplasma suramericanum* sp. nov. (formerly known as LAm A). [21]

From here on, we refer to classical histoplasmosis caused by *H. capsulatum* var. *capsulatum* as *H. capsulatum* for simplicity.

Infection with H. capsulatum begins in the lungs by inhaling aerosolized microconidia and mycelial fragments after disruption of the contaminated soils followed by a rapid conversion to yeast that can persist in host tissues causing histoplasmosis (Figure 1). Yeast cells evade phagocytic killing, multiply within alveolar macrophages and use phagocytic cells as vehicles to spread to multiple organs of the reticuloendothelial system (i.e., spleen, liver, lymph nodes, bone marrow). In the vast majority of human cases, inhalation of these fungal propagules leads to a primary pulmonary infection that is unapparent, subclinical or completely benign and self-limited. The remaining human cases can develop acute severe pulmonary disease, chronic progressive lung disease, chronic systemic or disseminated disease, or an acute fulminating systemic or disseminated disease. [3] Involvement of the central nervous system (CNS) either as one manifestation of disseminated infection or as an isolated focal infection might also occur. [3] Chronic meningitis is the most common presentation of histoplasmosis in CNS, due to hematogenous dissemination to meninges, but brain abscesses were also described.

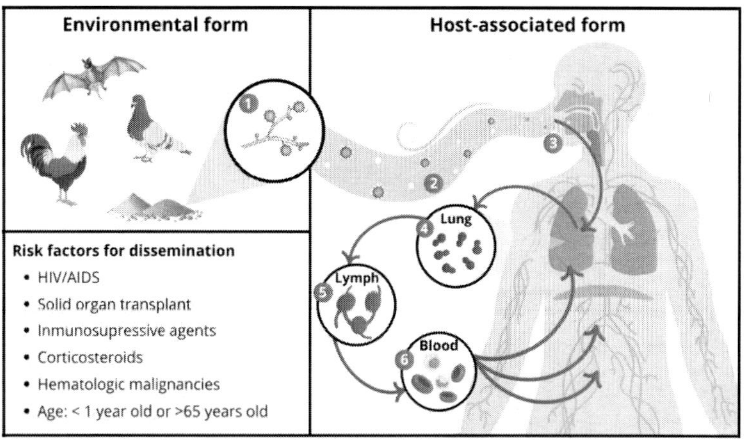

Figure 1. Biology of histoplasmosis.

Hematogenous dissemination from the lungs via infected macrophages is thought to occur even in asymptomatic infections, during the pre-immune phase. [3] It should be noted that neutrophils are unable to destroy the organism and macrophages can ingest but cannot destroy the fungus. Indeed, it is the T-cell-mediated immune response that serves to control the infection and enhances the antifungal response of phagocytes. [14]

Whereas polymorphonuclear and dendritic cells inhibit fungal growth, the organism replicates within macrophages prior to cellular activation. Cytokines such as IL-12, IL-6, and IL-23 are produced during the innate response and are involved in the polarization of naïve T cells. Th1 cells, characterized by IFN-γ, are the predominant T cell population during infection. A smaller population of Th17 population emerges, but only plays a minor role in resolving infection. In addition to IFN-γ, other Th1 cytokines including TNF-α, IL-1β, and GM-CSF activate macrophages to prevent intracellular growth, by producing -for instance- nitric oxide and limiting the amount of iron, copper and zinc accessible to *H. capsulatum.* [22, 23]

In the environment, *H. capsulatum* exists as a mold and its natural reservoirs are soils enriched with bird excreta and bat guano as a mold, whose hyphae produce macroconidia and microconidia. [1] After disruption of the contaminated soils, aerosolized microconidia and mycelial fragments [2] are inhaled by a susceptible host, beginning the infection in the lungs [3] followed by a rapid conversion to oval, budding yeasts due to the warmer temperature inside the host. [4] Yeast cells are phagocytized by immune cells and transported to regional lymph nodes. [5] From there they hematogenous disseminate to multiple organs of the reticuloendothelial system. [6] Risk factors associated with disseminated disease are acquired or congenital T cellular immunity deficiencies.

Even with the development of cell-mediated immunity, patients can have remaining foci of viable *H. capsulatum* in various organs, similar to the situation with tuberculosis. These organisms are held in check by the immune response but are not completely killed, and thus, reactivation of infection years later is possible. [3]

Clinical manifestations of the disease depend on the size of inoculum, age and immune status of the host and the presence of underlying lung disease. [24, 25] Immunocompetent hosts mostly suffer subclinical or mild respiratory infection although acute severe pulmonary disease may occur after inhaling a large inoculum of *H. capsulatum* propagules. Patients with underlying lung conditions, such as chronic obstructive pulmonary disease, may contract chronic pulmonary histoplasmosis, and patients with a compromised immune system may suffer progressive life-threatening disseminated histoplasmosis, which requires prompt diagnosis and treatment. [26, 27] The most common population at risk of progressive disseminated histoplasmosis (PDH) includes those individuals with T-cellular immunity deficiencies, such as patients with HIV/AIDS infection, although patients receiving immunosuppressive therapies, including solid-organ and bone marrow transplantation and tumor-necrosis-factor inhibitors, are also at risk. [28] In these individuals, the infection can disseminate to skin, bone, adrenal glands, the gastrointestinal tract, and the CNS. Recently, with the advent of the COVID-19 pandemic, it became evident that patients with severe COVID-19 at intensive care units are also at risk for histoplasmosis reactivation in endemic areas. [29]

PDH is the most frequent clinical presentation of histoplasmosis in people living with HIV/AIDS (PLHIV) becoming an AIDS-defining illness in 1987. [30.]

Recently, the World Health and Organization broadened their list of neglected tropical diseases to include deep mycoses, of which histoplasmosis is one. [31]

The true global burden of histoplasmosis remains unknown; not only because it is not a notifiable disease [32], but also because clinical symptoms and radiological findings may be similar to those of other diseases, particularly tuberculosis. [33-35] This misdiagnosis may lead to a delayed diagnosis, lack of adequate treatment and subsequent patient death. An annual incidence of over 100,000 cases of PDH in AIDS patients was estimated worldwide, with mortality rates, if treated, ranging between 30-50% and 100% if not. [36] In the Latin American continent where this mycosis is endemic, it is estimated 15,000 new infections and 9,000 deaths among PLHIV. [37] One of the major causes of this high mortality rate is the lack of an early and accurate diagnosis and treatment, as well as to limited access to highly active antiretroviral therapy, which is associated with a reduced risk of developing PDH. In some countries, the prevalence and mortality associated with histoplasmosis are estimated to be equivalent to or higher than that of tuberculosis, indicating that histoplasmosis could be responsible for a significant proportion of the deaths each year in some Latin American countries. [37] Globally, about half a million people get infected with *Histoplasma* every year. [36]

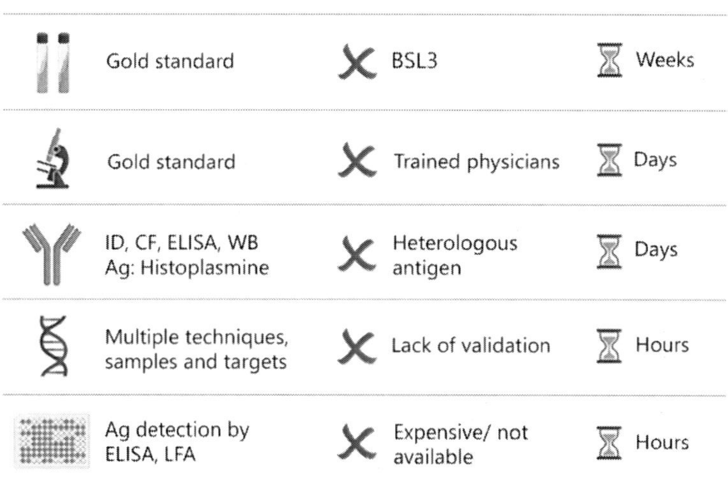

Figure 2. A comparison of the different methods used for diagnosing histoplasmosis.

The definitive diagnosis of histoplasmosis is performed by the isolation of *H. capsulatum* on specific media or by visualization of the yeast cells in direct examination or histopathological samples using specific stains. [38] However, these procedures have several drawbacks: both have limited sensitivity, cultures are time-consuming and need high-level laboratory infrastructure for culture handling (biosecurity level 3), and microscopy identification is sometimes difficult requiring highly trained laboratory staff. [39, 40] Antibody detection assays have played an important role in the diagnosis of histoplasmosis; however, their sensitivity mainly depends on the immune status of the patient and the stage and type of the disease. [41] Antigen detection assays have high sensitivity in PDH cases and great value for patient follow-up, but it is only performed in a few laboratories. [42, 43] Although molecular methods for the identification of fungi play a significant and growing role in clinical mycology due to their high sensitivity and specificity and rapid turnaround time, these methods still lack standardization and a more extensive validation (Figure 2).

There is high variability in the performance and clinical utility of the laboratory tests available for the diagnosis of histoplasmosis. The analytical performance of these assays varies according to disease stage and clinical form of the disease [44] (Table 1).

The present chapter will especially focus on the currently available assays, highlighting their strengths and limitations, as well as addressing the latest approaches to achieve reliable and rapid diagnostic tests.

This chapter is organized into 5 sections. Section 1 is an introductory section. Section 2 addresses virulence factors. Section 3 is concerned with diagnostic tests and the implementation of novel tools to improve the diagnosis of histoplasmosis. Section 4 describes histoplasmosis in animals and their role as reservoirs. Section 5 concludes this chapter with general remarks.

Table 1. Sensitivity of diagnostic tests for the different forms of histoplasmosis

Assay	Acute pulmonary	Subacute pulmonary	Chronic pulmonary	Meni-ngeal	Dissemi-nated	Reference
Microscopy	0 – 47%	9 – 67%	10 – 75%	-	12 – 85%	[43, 45]
Culture	0 – 34%	9 – 82%	65 – 85%	19 – 33%	75 – 92%	[43, 46–48]
Antibody detection	40 – 80%	78 – 92%	65% – 100%	59 – 89% (in CSF)	58 – 73%	[43, 45, 49–51]
Antigen detection	43 – 65%	39%	25 – 80%	42 – 78% (in CSF)	90 – 98%	[43, 45, 46, 52–55]
Nucleotide amplification	50%	-	-	33%	95%	[49, 56–59]

CSF: cerebrospinal fluid

Virulence Factors

It is widely known that pathogenic organisms should meet some basic criteria in order to promote disease, including: (i) thermotolerance (i.e., the ability to grow at or above host temperature); (ii) the capacity to invade or bypass host barriers reaching internal tissues; (iii) the capacity to evade or withstand the immune system, and (d) the expression of a wide diverse enzymatic repertoire to acquire nutrients by hydrolyzing and consuming components of the human tissue. [60]

The dimorphic fungus *H. capsulatum* establishes infection when hyphae and conidia are inhaled into the mammalian respiratory tract. This warm, moist environment triggers conversion of the saprophytic mycelial form to the parasitic yeast form, which is well suited to survival inside alveolar macrophages, thus circumventing a primary defense mechanism of the host: killing and degradation by professional phagocytic cells. This dimorphism reflects a developmental switch in morphology and lifestyle that is necessary for virulence. The dimorphism regulating kinase DRK1 and the *Histoplasma* DNA-binding proteins RYP1, RYP2, RYP3 and RYP4 mediate the thermally induced transition to the pathogenic yeast-phase program. [61-63] Cysteine and other sulfhydryl compounds are also important morphological regulators. [64, 65]

The success of *H. capsulatum* as an intracellular pathogen depends completely on successful conversion of the saprophytic mycelial (mold) form of this fungus to a parasitic yeast form. It is therefore not surprising that yeast phase-specific genes and gene products are proving to be important for survival and proliferation of *H. capsulatum* within macrophages. *Histoplasma* yeasts proliferate within the phagolysosome, a particularly harsh compartment containing many enzymes that are typically effective at destroying microorganisms. However, *H. capsulatum* yeasts maintain the phagolysosomal pH near neutral. [66] Since acidic conditions are required for most lysosomal enzyme activities, modulating the phagolysosomal pH appears to be one of the mechanisms by which *H. capsulatum* survives intracellularly. In this regard, this yeast is thus unique from other intracellular pathogens in its ability to prevent the acidification of the phagolysosome, presumably limiting the antifungal effectiveness of this compartment.

Considerable information has accumulated about specific genes of *H. capsulatum* that are expressed during the process of adaptation when the organism undergoes morphological transition at the onset of infection such as Hcp100, a regulatory protein of 100 kDa of *H. capsulatum* involved in the processes required for fungal adaptation and its survival in the intracellular hostile conditions of the macrophages. [67]

The study of these genes is crucial to identify targets for the development of novel antifungal agents. Virulence in *H. capsulatum*, and its relation to adaptation to elevated temperatures and morphogenesis is of particular interest. *Histoplasma* may also have to contend with surroundings which are low in calcium, iron or copper, meaning that in the infected host, *H. capsulatum* encounters various environmental stresses to which it adapts by regulating the expression of specific genes.

The first *H. capsulatum* virulence factors (CBP-1 [calcium-binding protein-1, important in calcium acquisition during intracellular parasitism] and Yps-3 [yeast-phase specific gene-3, which is related to virulence or morphogenesis, or both]) were identified by searching for high-abundance secreted factors that were produced only by yeast cells. [68, 69]

Regarding CBP-1, yeasts but not mycelial cultures released large quantities of this protein to the culture supernatant, correlating this finding with the dependence of mycelia on calcium for growth. [69] According to this, deprivation of calcium to culture media inhibited the growth of mycelial *H. capsulatum* but had no effect on yeast growth *in vitro*. Therefore, colonization of phagolysosomes of host macrophages by yeasts, potentially implicates that the phagolysosome is a calcium-limiting compartment, suggesting that CBP-1 may function to provide yeasts with calcium when they are in a low-calcium environment, such as the phagolysosomal compartment within macrophages. [69] The fact that the *cbp-1* promoter is only fully active after complete morphological conversion to the yeast form, indicates that CBP-1 is developmentally regulated rather than simply temperature regulated. [70] Continuous activity of the CBP-1 promoter during infection of macrophages supports the hypothesis that CBP-1 secretion plays an important role for *Histoplasma* survival within the phagolysosome. [70] Even more, deletion of CBP-1 allowed for rapid clearance of yeast cells from the lungs of infected mice. [71]

The *yps-3* gene of *H. capsulatum* encodes a 20-kDa protein that is both surface localized in its cell wall and released into the culture medium. This protein is produced only during the pathogenic yeast phase of infection and is also expressed differentially in *H. capsulatum* strains of different virulence levels. The *yps-3* gene is exclusively expressed in the yeast phase of virulent strains, such as G217B (Nam 2), but is not transcribed in either the mycelial or yeast phases of low virulence strains, such as Downs. [68] *Histoplasma* yeast cells produce Yps3 to promote extrapulmonary dissemination. [61]

Expression of the *yps-3* gene thus appears to correlate with virulence, temperature sensitivity, and the speed of the hyphal-to-yeast transition in three non-isogenic *H. capsulatum* strains. [68]

Many virulent strains of *H. capsulatum* also possess α-(1,3)-glucans (glucose homo and hetero-polymers) in the cell wall of the yeast form, although it is absent in the mycelial form. Based on the α-(1,3)-glucan concentration in the yeast cell wall, *H. capsulatum* has been classified as chemotype I and II. [72, 73] A chemotype II cell wall contains a mixture of α- and β-glucans, with glucans predominantly linked in the α-configuration, while chemotype I is entirely β-linked. [74]

Regardless, the presence of α-(1,3)-glucans correlates with strain-specific virulence in a mouse model of infection and influences the dynamics of intracellular survival and proliferation. [14] *H. capsulatum* strains regulate α-(1,3)-glucan production such that it seems to be constitutively synthesized when the yeasts are proliferating inside macrophages. This regulation is in sharp contrast to the modulation of this phenotype during broth culture growth, suggesting that *H. capsulatum* yeast cells release a factor that, when present in sufficient concentration, promotes α-(1,3)-glucan incorporation into the cell wall. [75] This growth-dependent modulation of α-(1,3)-glucan production resembles the "quorum-sensing" phenomenon seen in many bacteria. *Histoplasma* is thus an example of an organism that uses a quorum-sensing mechanism to detect that it is within a host cell compartment. [75]

The binding of *H. capsulatum* to phagocytes might be mediated by its cell wall carbohydrates, glucans, whose glycosydic linkage types (i.e., α- (1,3) and β-(1,3)) differ between the yeast and mycelial phases and have different roles. The α- (1,3)-glucan is considered relevant for *H. capsulatum* virulence, whereas the β-(1,3)-glucan is antigenic and participates in the modulation of the host immune response (i.e., leukocyte recruitment, upregulation of inflammatory mediators, such as nitric oxide synthase, TNF-α and macrophage inflammatory protein-2). [76] Virulent *H. capsulatum* strains contain up to 1,000-fold more of α- (1,3)-glucan than avirulent strains do. Some strains spontaneously produce avirulent variants lacking α- (1,3)-glucan. The α- (1,3)-glucans may contribute to the establishment of intracellular latency, regulate yeast proliferation inside a host macrophage and protect yeast within phagolysosomes. [14, 75, 77-78] The yeast cell wall contains an inner layer of chitin, a polysaccharide composed of β-(1,4)-N-acetyl-glucosamine residues, and an outer fibrous-layer of α-(1,3)-glucan, which topographically overlaps the β-glucan polymer in the yeast cell wall. Thus, yeast α-glucans conceal immunostimulatory cell wall β-glucans from detection by macrophage receptors. The composition of saccharides varies depending on the culture medium composition, environmental conditions and strain types. [72] Genetic loss of the α-(1,3)-glucan covering through mutation or RNA interference of the gene encoding α-(1,3)-glucan synthase (AGS1) severely attenuates *Histoplasma* virulence. [79] Intriguingly, although the majority of *Histoplasma* strains worldwide produce α-glucans, a single phylogenetic group in North America (the NAm 2 group as defined by Kasuga et al. [18] lacks any detectable α-(1,3)-glucan and yet remains virulent. How the NAm 2 group has circumvented the need for the α-glucan mask remains unknown. Possibly other cell surface or secreted molecules such as Yps-3 functionally substitute for α-glucan in the NAm 2 strains. [61] Strikingly, an inverse correlation between strains that express Yps-3 and those that produce α-glucan was described. [61]

Another mechanism by which *Histoplasma* yeasts avoid phagocyte detection is by secreting a β-glucanase, Eng1. [80] In α-glucan-producing *Histoplasma* strains, Eng1 acts in concert with α-glucan to minimize β-glucan exposure: α-glucan provides a masking function by covering the β-glucan-rich cell wall, while Eng1 removes any remaining exposed β-glucans. Thus, *Histoplasma* Eng1 has evolved a specialized pathogenesis function to remove exposed β-glucans, thereby enhancing the ability of yeasts to escape detection by host phagocytes. [80] Recently, Garfoot et al. [80] reported that *Histoplasma* yeasts also secrete the glucanase Exg8, which may serve a similar role as Eng1 in removing exposed β-glucans from the yeast cell surface and showed that Exg8 is an exo-β1,3-glucanase and Eng1 is an endo-β1,3-glucanase. [81] Together, Eng1 and Exg8 account for nearly all of the total secreted glucanase activity of *Histoplasma* yeasts. [81]

H. capsulatum can also directly modulate the immune response exerted by hematopoietic stem and progenitor cells through pattern recognition receptors expressed on their surface, and this interaction could directly affect the process of hematopoiesis, a fact that could explain clinical manifestations such as anemia and pancytopenia in patients with severe histoplasmosis, especially in those with fungal spread to the bone marrow. [82]

Complement receptor-3 (CR3) is considered the main macrophage lectin-like receptor involved in nonopsonic recognition of *H. capsulatum* yeast. [83] CR3 recognizes a single 60-kDa protein present on the surface of *H. capsulatum* yeasts, which was identified as heat shock protein 60 (hsp60) that acts as an adhesin. [83] Signaling via CR3 down-regulates production of interleukin-12 (IL-12), a key mediator of cell-mediated immunity in response of *H. capsulatum*, thus abolishing the protective response of macrophages against this fungus (84). Later, Gómez et al. [85] described that dendritic cells recognize *Histoplasma* yeasts via the VLA-5 receptor and that cyclophilin A, a 20-kDa protein present on the surface of these yeasts, is the corresponding ligand. [85]

The pulmonary collectins, surfactant proteins (SP) A and D are antimicrobial proteins that directly inhibit the growth of *H. capsulatum* by increasing permeability of the organism. However, *H. capsulatum* gains asylum from collectin-mediated killing by rapid entry into pulmonary macrophages. [86]

The interaction between *Histoplasma* yeasts and host phagocytes makes the ability of this fungus to avoid or detoxify reactive oxygen species (ROS), an essential component of its pathogenesis. Activation of macrophages or opsonization of yeasts triggers ROS production. [87, 88] Neutrophils also produce ROS upon encounter with *Histoplasma*. [89] Regardless of the cell type and response, *Histoplasma* yeast are able to survive the ROS challenge. Youseff et al. [90] demonstrated that yeasts produced an extracellular superoxide dismutase (Sod3) that protects *Histoplasma* from macrophage- and neutrophil-generated superoxide and is required for full virulence in a murine model of histoplasmosis. [90] In addition to Sod3, the *Histoplasma* genome encodes three catalase proteins that may potentially assist in combating ROS. [91] CatA is an 80-kDa catalase expressed by mycelia that is highly similar to a large-subunit catalase in *Aspergillus* and *Emericella* species. [91] CatB is an immunodominant 90-kDa extracellular catalase of *Histoplasma* yeasts also known as M antigen, which is similar to catalase B of *Aspergillus* and *Emericella* species. [91] CatP is a 60-kDa intracellular catalase with greatest similarity to known peroxisomal catalases of animals and Saccharomycotina yeasts. [91] Holbrook et al. [92] demonstrated that catB and catP are responsible for the extracellular and intracellular catalase activities of *Histoplasma* yeasts, respectively from hydrogen peroxide *in vitro*. [92]

The 3-hydroxy-methylglutaryl coenzyme A (HMG CoA) lyase (HCL1) is another virulence factor required for macrophage colonization by *H. capsulatum* and replication in the harsh growth environment of the macrophage phagosome. [93]

Furthermore, studies determined the production of iron reductases and siderophores as virulence factors in *Histoplasma* for intracellular iron acquisition in macrophages and host colonization. [94] Disruption of the *SID1* gene, an enzyme important for siderophore production, resulted in a growth defect *in vitro* and attenuation of infections in the murine model of histoplasmosis. [95] Similar, Shen et al. [96] showed that *Histoplasma* yeasts induced the expression of the Ctr3 copper transporter for intramacrophage proliferation and that Ctr3 mediates copper uptake and is required for growth in low copper environment such as the phagolysosome s. [23]

Shen et al. also demonstrated that *Histoplasma* yeasts within macrophages up-regulate the PCK1 gene that encodes a phosphoenolpy-ruvate carboxykinase, related to the first step of gluconeogene-sis, to circumvent the nutritional limitations within macrophages. [96]

In an attempt to identify novel factors that contribute to *Histoplasma* virulence, Holbrook et al. defined the extracellular proteome of pathogenic *Histoplasma* yeast, which include several glycanases, extracellular enzymes related to oxidative stress defense, dehydrogenase enzymes, chaperone-like factors and culture filtrate proteins (Cfps). Among these proteins, Chs1, Exg1, Eng1, Cfp1, Cfp4, Cfp8, CatB, Sod3 and Trl1 were the most abundant. [97] All these exoantigens also represent attractive molecules for diagnostic tests. It should be noted that different phylogenetic groups of *Histoplasma* produce different combinations of extracellular yeast-phase virulence factors. Thus, different strain groups might utilize different strategies for pathogenesis. [97]

Diagnostic Tests and the Implementation of Novel Tools to Improve the Diagnosis of Histoplasmosis

Culture and Microscopy

The definitive diagnosis of histoplasmosis requires the isolation of *H. capsulatum* on specific culture media or the visualization of the yeast form in direct examination of clinical specimens (i.e., bone marrow aspirate or biopsy material, bronchoalveolar lavage (BAL) fluid or biopsy material from lung, sputum, mucocutaneous lesions, peripheral blood), using specific fungal staining techniques, such as Giemsa, Wright, periodic acid–Schiff or Grocott-Gomori's methenamine silver. [38] In clinical samples, the fungus is found as yeast-like cells within macrophages or histiocytes, often in clusters of numerous cells, and, occasionally, in the extracellular compartment, free in tissues.

The sensitivity and specificity of the microscopic examination are limited and depend on the staff with mycology training [98] as well as on the clinical form of the disease (Table 1). Patients with chronic pulmonary or PDH have a higher rate of positive results (<75%) than patients with acute or subacute pulmonary disease (<47%). In addition, the structure of the *Histoplasma* yeasts is similar to other pathogens such as *Candida* spp., *Cryptococcus* spp., *Talaromyces marneffei, Pneumocystis jirovecii, Blastomyces dermatitidis, Leishmania* spp. and *Toxoplasma gondii*, leading to a mistake during the identification for diagnosis purposes. [45, 99] Therefore, it is mandatory to be familiar with the morphology of these pathogens and the staining features of the yeast by different staining techniques. It should be noted that demonstration of *Histoplasma* yeast in tissue may not distinguish active infection from a past infection, as non-viable organisms persist in tissue for long periods following acute infection and often for life.

H. capsulatum isolation from clinical specimens is often performed on a nutrient-poor medium such as Sabouraud agar at 28°C (where it grows macroscopically as smooth colonies that become filamentous, cottony and brownish with age, and microscopically as hyaline hyphae that have tuberculated macroconidia and smooth-walled spherical, pyriform or cigar-shaped microconidia ranging in size from 2-6 μm) or on a nutrient-rich medium such as brain-heart infusion agar supplemented with blood at 37°C (where yeast forms predominate as smooth white to brown colonies that microscopically are observed as ovoid thick-walled cells). The transformation of *H. capsulatum* hyphal cells to yeast cells, or vice versa, can thus be recapitulated in culture simply by only shifting the growth temperature. When *H. capsulatum* cells are grown at 28°C, they grow in the hyphal form. When these cells are shifted to 37°C, they shift to the budding form. However, this laborious task to convert the mold phase to the yeast phase *in vitro* is no longer required for the definitive identification of *H. capsulatum*. [3]

Fungal cultures are time-consuming; *H. capsulatum* commonly grows within two to three weeks but it may take up to eight weeks. This represents a major drawback since most patients with PDH usually die after 10–14 days from the onset of the disease if not treated. [36] Another limitation of this technique is the requirement of biosafety level 3 equipment and facilities due to the infectious risk of *H. capsulatum*.

The sensitivity of a culture-based diagnosis mainly depends on the clinical form of the disease and the specimen tested. The lowest sensitivity values are observed in the acute and subacute forms of pulmonary histoplasmosis, whereas higher values can be found in chronic pulmonary and PDH due to higher fungal burden in the studied specimens. [100] Detection of *H. capsulatum* is possible from blood samples with the chronic and disseminated forms of the disease. However, to improve the recovery of the fungus in histoplasmosis patients with fungemia, several methods were described.

Lysis-centrifugation has been shown to be more effective than conventional biphasic blood systems. However, the BACTEC type machines are highly efficient and provide statistically significant increase compared to lysis-centrifugation for overall recovery of isolates and bloodstream infections. [101-103]

Some molecular assays have been developed to identify *H. capsulatum* from culture. The commercially available AccuProbe test (Gen-Probe Inc, CA, USA) uses a single-stranded DNA probe with a chemiluminescent label targeting the *H. capsulatum* rRNA. [104] Although this test identifies *H. capsulatum*, it requires a sonicator and a luminometer and is not commercially available in developing countries. A fluorescently labeled probe complementary to the rRNA was also developed to detect *H. capsulatum* in blood cultures [105] but further evaluation is still pending. Recently, protein profile databases were constructed for the identification of *H. capsulatum* and other clinically relevant molds by matrix-assisted laser desorption ionization–time of light mass spectrometry (MALDI-TOF MS). [106, 107] MALDI-TOF MS is a rapid and powerful proteome-based technique for the highly accurate identification of many clinical pathogens; however, as well as the hybridization test requires fungal isolation and thus the turnaround time is high.

Antibody Detection Assays

Antibody detection methods are the major tools currently in use for the non-culture diagnosis of histoplasmosis due to their general availability and rapid turnaround time. The two most extensively used antibody detection techniques are complement fixation (CF) and double immunodiffusion (ID) because of convenience, availability, and accuracy of these assays in the diagnosis of subacute and chronic pulmonary histoplasmosis, in which a fourfold rise in antibody titer to *H. capsulatum* can be a diagnostic finding. However, these techniques should not be used in patients with the disseminated form of the disease, since the sensitivity of both assays is limited in immunocompromised patients whose ability to produce antibodies is reduced [43] (Table 1).

Serological tests can also be helpful in *Histoplasma* meningitis, where detection of antibodies in cerebrospinal fluid (CSF) may be the only positive indicator of the diagnosis. However, their utility may be undermined since anti-*Histoplasma* antibodies emerge four to eight weeks after exposure and may persist for years after infection. [108]

Routine serodiagnosis of histoplasmosis is usually performed with the crude supernatant of *H. capsulatum* mycelial cultures known as histoplasmin (HMN). This is composed predominantly of C, H and M antigens. The C-antigen is a heat-stable serologically active polysaccharide, galactomannan (GM) responsible for the cross-reactions observed with other fungal species. [109] According to Azuma et al. [110] the purified water-soluble GM is composed of galactose and mannose in molar ratios of 1.5-3.9:1, with 2,3,4,6-tetra-O-methylgalactofuranose and 2,3,4,6-tetra-O-methyl-mannopyranose as nonreducing terminal sugar residues. [110] The nonreducing terminal of galactofuranosyl residue plays an important role as an immunological determinant of GMs. The H antigen is a β-glucosidase, and the M antigen is a catalase (CatB). [111, 112] These two heat-sensitive glycoproteins are widely used as targets for antibody detection and are typically identified as reference lines in ID tests. Both glycoproteins possess epitopes found in the C-antigen. Most of the carbohydrate chains in the H and M glycoproteins are N-linked to the peptide core and probably belong to the high-mannose-type glycan. It was also reported the presence of terminal α-D-mannose or α-D-glucose residues. [113, 114]

Antibodies directed to the M antigen are the first to arise [115] and may persist for several years after disease resolution, [41] whereas antibodies to the H antigen emerge later and less frequently (<25%) and usually clear within the first six months after the infection [24, 108]. Although the presence of both M and H bands is highly suggestive of active *Histoplasma* infection, the presence solely of M band may represent previous exposure to *H. capsulatum*. [41]

The CF assay detects and titers specific antibodies against yeast and mycelial antigens (a suspension of merthiolate-killed whole *Histoplasma* yeast cells and HMN, respectively). Titers of 1:32 or above with either antigen are suggestive of active histoplasmosis while titers of 1:8 and 1:16 are generally considered presumptive evidence of histoplasmosis and require further testing. [116] Antibody titration can be useful in the follow-up of patients since a four-fold increase in CF antibodies titers suggests progression of the disease. [117] The CF assay is more sensitive but less specific than the ID assay; [24] false-positive results may occur in patients with coccidioidomycosis, paracoccidioidomycosis, aspergillosis, blastomy-cosis, cryptococcosis and tuberculosis as well as in healthy subjects from endemic areas. [118-120] Another drawback is that the CF test has a tedious procedure and requires a complex standardization, being unsuitable for low-volume laboratories. In addition, commercial kits are unavailable for either the ID or the CF test, although individual reagents can be purchased from diagnostic companies.

Enzyme-linked immunosorbent assays (ELISA) and immunoblotting assays may also be used for antibody detection. [54, 121, 122] Most of the ELISA and Western Blot tests were developed in-house also using HMN as reagent. [120-129] Since these techniques have not been commercialized, the standard ID is the only assay available for detection of antibodies.

It should be mentioned that HMN is produced and purified following different protocols. These variabilities make standardization difficult since HMN can differ greatly in its quality and relative content of H, M or C-antigens depending on the protocol of antigenic preparation and the strain of *H. capsulatum* used. [40] In fact, it was suggested that the choice of the fungal strain is the most critical step [130], which is perhaps of some significance, given that various phylogenetic species of *H. capsulatum* circulate in different regions. Due to the presence of cross-reactive carbohydrate components, the sensitivity and specificity of the assays using native HMN is limited. Therefore, different deglycosylation approaches were reported to remove the carbohydrate moieties of the HMN (e.g., chemically by using $NaOI_4$ or enzymatically by using N-glycosidase F, endo-β-N-acetylglucosaminidase H or endo-α-N-acetylgalactosaminidase). [121-122, 129, 131] These treatments increased assay sensitivity (i.e., from 57% to 92%) by exposing the epitopes in the H and M antigens that were hidden by the carbohydrate chains as well as decreased the cross-reactivity produced by the GM and the glycosylation of the H and M proteins (i.e., specificity increased from 93% to 96%). [131] However, false positives still occurred in patients with coccidioidomycosis, paracoccidioidomycosis, blastomycosis, aspergillosis, and tuberculosis. [113, 129, 131]

The only currently available ELISA assay cleared by the Clinical Laboratory Improvement Amendments is the fee-for-service test offered by MiraVista Diagnostics, which is a semi-quantitative ELISA for IgM and IgG antibodies to *Histoplasma* antigen in serum and CSF that reported 88.8% sensitivity in serum samples from patients with acute pulmonary histoplasmosis and 91.0% specificity, with false positive results in patients with blastomycosis, coccidioidomycosis and cryptococcosis. [54] When this ELISA antibody testing is combined with antigen detection testing in serum and urine, the sensitivity increased to 96.3%. Therefore, diagnosis of acute pulmonary histoplasmosis is improved by combining antigen and antibody detection. [54]

Antigen Detection Assays

An alternative approach for immunodiagnosis constitutes the detection of fungal antigens, which is very helpful for the diagnosis of histoplasmosis, particularly, for the acute and disseminated forms of the disease. Recently, a summary of guidelines for diagnosing and managing histoplasmosis among PLHIV was published and the *Histoplasma* antigen testing was included in the WHO list of Essential Diagnostics. [37]

Antigen testing does not rely on the immune responses of the patients, which is especially important in immunocompromised individuals, who are at most risk for the development of disseminated histoplasmosis, and whose humoral response might be attenuated or delayed, leading to falsely negative serology results.

At present, four ELISAs tests are currently used to detect *Histoplasma* GM in urine samples: the Clarus *Histoplasma* GM ELISA from IMMY, USA; the OIDx *Histoplasma* Urinary Antigen EIA from Optimum Imaging Diagnostics, USA; the Niche Diagnostics (ND) *Histoplasma* urine antigen assay from ND, USA; and the MiraVista Diagnostics *Histoplasma* Quantitative EIA test, from MiraVista Diagnostics, USA). All of them are based on the use of monoclonal/polyclonal anti-GM antibodies in urine, although the ELISA developed by MiraVista Diagnostics has also been validated in other clinical samples (i.e., serum, CSF, BAL fluid or bronchial washings). In addition, MiraVista Diagnostics and Optimum Imaging Diagnostics have also developed a rapid test for the detection of urinary antigen (GM) by lateral flow assays (LFA).

Although the detection of circulating *Histoplasma* antigens in urine by ELISA or point-of-care testing (LFA) have proven highly sensitive (67.3-95%) for diagnosing PDH, testing is hampered by the limited availability of commercial *in vitro* diagnostic kits and poor local distribution due to their high cost. [44, 132]

A brief description of the different immunoassays developed for antigen testing is detailed below and summarized in Table 2.

MiraVista Antigen Detection Assays

An enzyme immunoassay (EIA) for the detection of *Histoplasma* antigen in urine, serum, BAL and CSF samples is only performed at the MiraVista

Diagnostics headquarters in Indiana, USA, limiting its use in other parts of the world.

The assay was first described in 1986 as a solid-phase radioimmuno-assay (RIA) and since then, has undergone various modifications. [133]

The Histoplasma antigen has been described as a poorly characterized GM polysaccharide of the fungal cell wall with a molecular weight of less than 10kDa in urine and a higher molecular weight in serum. This antigen is mentioned in the literature as *Histoplasma* polysaccharide antigen (HPA) or GM or C-Ag, and these terms will be used indistinctly in this chapter. The first descriptions about this urinary antigen were reported by Wheat et al. [133], who referred to it as a polysaccharide with low molecular weight, which resists boiling for 15 minutes and treatment with proteinases and nucleases, but it is destroyed by periodate and glycosidase. This antigen also bound to concanavalin A, a lectin (carbohydrate-binding protein), and it was suggested that presumably polysaccharide antigens might be released into blood from infected tissues and subsequently excreted by urine. During an isolated meningeal infection, it might also be released to CSF without reaching high levels in the blood or urine. [133]

Polyclonal antibodies against HPA were obtained by immunizing rabbits with whole formalin-killed yeast cells of *H. capsulatum* followed by boosters with live yeast cells. Then, the IgG fraction from anti-serum positive for both H and M precipitins was purified by ion-exchange chromatography and used as a capture antibody and as a ^{125}I labelled detection antibody. The sensitivity was 91% in PDH, 19% in subacute pulmonary histoplasmosis and 6% in chronic pulmonary histoplasmosis. Specificity was 100%, including healthy subjects and patients with other lung diseases.

In order to avoid the inherent safety problems of working with radioisotopes, the *Histoplasma* antigen RIA was adapted to an ELISA format. After an unsatisfactory attempt using a detection antibody conjugated to alkaline phosphatase or horseradish peroxidase [134], the MiraVista 1st generation EIA was developed in 1997 using a biotin-conjugated detection antibody recognized by a horseradish peroxidase probe. [135] The sensitivity was 89% in PDH and 37% in patients with other clinical forms of histoplasmosis. Specificity was first reported to be 99%; however cross-reactions with paracoccidioidomycosis, blastomycosis and penicilliosis marneffei infection were later documented. In order to reduce the false antigenemia caused by human anti-rabbit antibodies that occurred in approximately 20% of solid organ transplant patients receiving rabbit anti-thymocyte globulin to prevent allograft rejection, a 2nd generation EIA was developed. [136, 137] For this purpose, a biotinylated F(ab)'$_2$ fragment of rabbit anti-*H. capsulatum* IgG diluted in normal rabbit serum was used as the detection antibody. False-positive results caused by human antirabbit antibodies were hence diminished to 95%. However, false positive results caused by other mycoses were still observed in urine and serum samples. [137, 138] In 2006, a quantitative 3rd generation EIA was described using antigen calibrators made of a pool of urine samples with a known concentration of *H. capsulatum* yeast GM. Using this method, antigen levels are reported as ng/ml over a reportable range from 0.4 to 60 ng/ml. [139] Finally, a 4th generation EIA was reported pretreating serum, BAL and CSF samples at 104°C in the presence of EDTA to increase antigen detection sensitivity, probably by the dissociation of antigen-antibody complexes and denaturation of the free antibodies. [46, 53, 140]

The detection of urinary antigen has been a sensitive and convenient alternative method for diagnosing histoplasmosis, particularly PDH among immunocompromised individuals since other methods such as culture, histopathology or nucleotide amplification techniques often require invasive procedures to collect specimens (e.g., BAL or biopsy). In addition, antigen detection in CSF and BAL samples has been an aid for the diagnosis of *Histoplasma* meningitis and acute pulmonary histoplasmosis, respectively. [48, 141] It should be noted that antigen may not appear in the urine of some patients with focal sites of dissemination, such as chronic meningitis, or patients with mild forms of nonprogressive disseminated disease. [133]

In addition to being useful for rapid diagnosis of histoplasmosis, *Histoplasma* antigen has also been proven to be useful for monitoring the effect of therapy and for relapse detection. [142] Antigenemia provides a more sensitive and earlier y marker for therapy response than antigenuria, since antigen clearance is more rapid in serum than in urine after successful therapy. [42] It was reported that antigen levels in urine may not decline significantly during the first 2 weeks of effective treatment in some patients and may remain positive in low levels even in asymptomatic patients with completed antifungal treatment. [42, 47]

Most studies evaluated the effectiveness of the MiraVista *Histoplasma* Antigen Quantitative EIA in patients with AIDS and PDH, in which antigen quantification is based on the identification of the terminal (1-6)-α-D-galactofuranose, a major component of *Histoplasma* GM, found in the fungal cell wall. [43, 139-140, 143] Sensitivity of this quantitative EIA among patients with AIDS and PDH was 94.6-100% in urine and 92.3-100% in serum with antigen levels correlating with severity. Sensitivity was lower in patients with disseminated histoplasmosis and no underlying immunosuppression (63.3%) and with chronic (25-80%), subacute (38.9%) or acute (0-68.6%) pulmonary histoplasmosis. [43, 53, 55] In acute pulmonary histoplasmosis, higher sensitivity was achieved by testing both urinary and serum antigen and by testing BAL samples. [53-55] However, quantification of antigen in BAL fluids is inaccurate due to the variations in the amount of liquid used in the lavage process. [53]

Detection of GM in CSF has been an aid for the diagnosis of *Histoplasma* meningitis. [47] In a recent retrospective multicenter study of patients with CNS histoplasmosis cases occurring, mostly between 1997 and 2010, GM antigen was detected in CSF samples of 30/37 (81%) and 5/16 (31%) patients with and without immunosuppression, respectively. Among all studied patients with CNS histoplasmosis, antigen was detected in the urine of 44/60 (73%) patients and in the serum in 14 of 28 (50%) that were tested (51). Wheat et al. [144] recommends that both urine and serum might be tested to provide the highest sensitivity for diagnosis and CSF should be tested when chronic meningitis is suspected. [144]

Despite the MiraVista *Histoplasma* quantitative EIA exhibits 80% cross-reactivity with *Paracoccidioides brasiliensis* and *T. marneffei*, 70% with *B. dermatitidis,* 60% with *Coccidioides immitis* and, less frequently, with other unrelated fungi, such as in aspergillosis and sporotrichosis, they do not limit the usefulness of the test to detect histoplasmosis. [53, 139, 145] In addition, the antifungal treatment for all the aforementioned mycoses is generally similar. [109] Special care should be prompted in the evaluation of patients with positive results in serum but negative results in urine, due to false-positive results related with rheumatoid factors in serum. [146]

Since patients with histoplasmosis might test falsely negative for *H. capsulatum* antigenuria, because antigen is present at levels below the limit of detection of the assay, Egan et al. [147] reported that ultrafiltration of samples could improve sensitivity. [147] In this regard, antigen could be detected in 73.8% of falsely negative specimens after ultrafiltration using 5,000-molecular-weight-cutoff Amicon Ultra centrifugal filter tubes.

In recent years, MiraVista developed the first point-of-care test for the diagnosis of histoplasmosis (*Histoplasma* Urine Antigen LFA, MiraVista Diagnostics, USA). The assay is an immunochromatographic LFA for the visual and rapid detection of *Histoplasma* GM antigen in urine. Minimal laboratory equipment is needed, and results can be available in less than one hour. Although the LFA kit package insert indicated its use in urine, it has been evaluated in 24 serum samples from Colombian patients with AIDS and disseminated histoplasmosis. [148] High analytical performance was observed either by the naked eye or with an automated reader; however, higher sensitivity values (96% *vs* 92%) were achieved using the former. Cross-reactions were observed among patients with paracoccidioidomycosis and salmonellosis and in one patient with toxoplasmosis and tuberculosis. Further studies should be carried out to assess the performance of this test in both urine and serum samples of a larger population including patients with other clinical forms of histoplasmosis and other fungal infections. Other studies showed a sensitivity of 78.8-96% and a specificity of 96-99.3%. [149, 150] Cross reactions were noted with paracoccidioidomycosis and blastomycosis.

CDC Antigen Detection Assay

In 2007 the Centers for Disease Control and Prevention (CDC) developed an in-house *H. capsulatum* antigen-capture quantitative ELISA. [151] The capture and detection antibodies were produced by immunizing rabbits intravenously with whole, killed *H. capsulatum* yeast cells. The concentration of relative *H. capsulatum* antigen was quantified using a calibration curve of a common cell wall antigen, the C-antigen, obtained after purification mycelial culture filtrates by cation-exchange chromatography. The assay was evaluated in urine samples from patients with HIV/AIDS and PDH from Guatemala, Colombia and Brazil, with sensitivity and specificity values of 81-100% and 91.4-95%, respectively [152-154] (Table 2). However, the reagents for this test are no longer available, and no further distribution was planned in the regions where histoplasmosis is endemic. [52]

IMMY Antigen Detection Assays

In 2006, a diagnostic kit for HPA detection in urine samples was approved for clinical use by the Food and Drug Administration (FDA), becoming commercially available a year later (IMMY ALPHA *Histoplasma* Antigen EIA, IMMY, USA). The assay was a "sandwich" ELISA that used rabbit polyclonal IgG antibodies for both capture and detection. [155] Antibodies were developed in New Zealand rabbits immunized with a mixture of three clinical isolates of *H. capsulatum* in the yeast form. Several laboratories of different countries have evaluated the assay and reported low performance 9% sensitivity and 79.3-84% specificity), thus limiting its clinical utility in the diagnosis of histoplasmosis (Table 2). [156-159] False-positive results were observed in patients with *B. dermatitidis, C. immitis, P. brasiliensis,* disseminated *Cryptococcus neoformans* infection and with tuberculosis. [155, 159]

In 2013, another ELISA for the detection of HPA in urine samples became commercially available (IMMY/Clarus *Histoplasma* GM EIA, IMMY, USA). This ELISA kit, originally developed as an analyte-specific reagent, is a single-monoclonal-antibody sandwich ELISA that detects *Histoplasma* GM with a sensitivity of 88-100% and a specificity of 95-98.7%. [52, 160] There are two procedures on the Clarus *Histoplasma* GM EIA. The quantitative standard procedure, also known as "standard curve procedure," uses a seven-concentration standard curve, and provides quantitative results in ng/ml. This quantitative standard procedure uses a cut-off ≥ 0.20 ng/mL for positive results. The second procedure uses a calibrator for the calculation of an index. This procedure is considered a semi-quantitative assay and is also known as "calibrator cut-off procedure". The semi-quantitative assay reports results in EIA units, and based on manufacturer, this procedure uses a cut-off of ≥ 1 EIA units for positive results. The semi-quantitative assay allows to test a greater number of specimens per kit, resulting in cost-benefit due to the reduction of reagents used during testing. However, the semi-quantitative assay can be less sensitive in comparison with the results obtained with the quantitative assay. [160] Cross-reactions with paracoccidioidomycosis have been reported in the Clarus *Histoplasma* GM EIA. [52] False-negative results were described for a patient treated with trimethoprim/sulfamethoxazole as PCP prophylaxis, in whom this medication could have lowered the fungal burden, subsequently reducing the level of circulating urinary antigen. [52]

The *Histoplasma* GM EIA assay can even be performed in middle-equipped laboratories in less than 3 h, significantly reducing the time for PDH diagnosis. However, results must be thoroughly analyzed since a negative result does not rule out histoplasmosis and false-positive results may occur in patients with other mycoses. Further studies are needed in order to fully evaluate its clinical performance in other clinical samples (e.g., CSF, BAL and serum), in patients with other clinical forms of histoplasmosis as well as in other non-HIV immunocompromised patients at risk for PDH. The applicability of the *Histoplasma* GM EIA in the monitoring of antifungal therapy also deserves further investigation.

A recent multicenter, prospective, double-blinded study done in ten Mexican hospitals compared the diagnostic accuracy of detecting *H. capsulatum* antigen in urine of 391 specimens using the IMMY ALPHA

Histoplasma EIA kit, *Clarus Histoplasma* GM EIA and MiraVista *Histoplasma* Urine Antigen LFA and the sensitivity/specificity values obtained were 67.3%/96.2% for IMMY ALPHA *Histoplasma* EIA kit, 91.3%/90.9% for *Clarus Histoplasma* GM EIA and 90.4%/92.3% for MiraVista *Histoplasma* Urine Antigen LFA. [132]

A similar study carried out by Andreani et al. (2022) showed that both *Clarus Histoplasma* GM EIA and MiraVista *Histoplasma* Urine Antigen LFA have a similar analytical performance, with a sensitivity of 94%, specificity of 100%, positive predictive value of 100%, negative predictive value of 97%, and an accuracy of 98%. [161] Therefore, both assays had high analytical performance; they provided rapid diagnosis of histoplasmosis with minimal requirements for laboratory training, equipment, and laboratory infrastructure.

Niche Diagnostics Antigen Detection Assays

A recent study evaluated the performance of a monoclonal antibody-based *Histoplasma* urine antigen ELISA manufactured by Niche Diagnostics (Niche Diagnostics, LLC, Scarborough, USA) in a collection of 250 specimens previously tested by the MiraVista assay, 21 of which belonged to patients with histoplasmosis. The assay showed 90.5% positive agreement and 99.6% negative agreement with the MiraVista assay. However further evaluation is needed in order to fully establish its clinical utility. [162]

OIDx Histoplasma Urinary Antigen Detection Assays

Recently, in 2021, a sandwich enzyme immunoassay (EIA) for the detection of *Histoplasma* antigens (Ag) in urine was evaluated. [163] This assay was developed by Optimum Imaging Diagnosis (OIDx, Scarborough, Maine, USA) in agreement with the CDC's Mycotic Diseases Branch, using a rabbit monoclonal antibody for the detection of *Histoplasma* GM in the urine from 78 PLHIV from Colombia. The assay displayed a sensitivity of 92%, specificity of 32% and accuracy of 51%. In this study, the OIDx *Histoplasma* urinary Ag EIA displayed high sensitivity, however, in non-histoplasmosis cases this EIA displayed false-positive results in 68% of specimens tested.

In 2022, a LFA has become available with a reported in-house performance of 96% sensitivity and 89% specificity (Optimum Imaging Diagnostics, 2022). A study carried out in Ghana showed that the OIDx

Histoplasma LFA displayed a high concordance (98.4%) with the IMMY *Histoplasma* EIA. [164] This LFA was also used for detecting three probable cases of PDH in HIV/AIDS patients in Cameroon. [165]

Table 2. Summary of antigen detection assays for the diagnosis of histoplasmosis

Assay	Specimen	Sensitivity	Specificity	Cross-reactions	References
MiraVista 4th generation EIA	Urine, serum*, BAL*	U: 42.7-95.0% S: 63.3-100% B: 95.2%	U: 99.0% S: 99.0% B: NR	*B. dermatitidis*	[43, 53–55, 140]
MiraVista LFA	Urine, serum*	U: 94% S: 92-96%	U: 100% S: 90%-94%	*P. brasiliensis*, *Salmonella* infection and in a patient with toxoplasmosis and tuberculosis	[148, 161]
Clarus IMMY GM EIA	Urine	71.5-98%	97-98%	*P. brasiliensis*	[52, 166]
Niche Diagnostics EIA	Urine	90.5% positive agreement with MVista	99.6% negative agreement with MVista	*B. dermatitidis*	[162]
OIDx EIA	Urine	92%	32%	NR	[163]

B/BAL: Bronchoalveolar lavage; EIA: Enzyme immunoassay; NR: Not reported; S: Serum; U: Urine.
*Pretreated with EDTA and heat.

Potential Novel Antigens

As mentioned above, current diagnosis of PDH utilizes an ELISA/LFA-based assay for an extracellular polysaccharide antigen (GM). For serological assays, the M and H antigens which are the culture filtrate molecules CatB and β-glucosidase, respectively, are used in the serological tests for diagnosing histoplasmosis.

Despite the continuous development of those immunodiagnostic tests, improving the serological and urinary biomarkers is necessary to make these methods efficient tools for definitive diagnosis of histoplasmosis. In addition, several other protein antigens or exoantigens have been reported in *H. capsulatum*, as attractive molecules for diagnostic tests in order to improve sensitivity and specificity of assays.

For instance, Chandrashekar et al. reported that a 60-kDa antigen of *H. capsulatum* which is a β-galactosidase (GH17) might be useful for the diagnosis of histoplasmosis in humans, since this antigen was recognized by antibodies in 18 of 18 sera from histoplasmosis patients but not by antibodies in sera from patients or animals infected with other fungi by Western blot. [167]

Toyotome et al. explored the potential diagnostic utility of several proteins from 50 to 100 kDa obtained from *H. capsulatum* yeast cells. Of them, eight were seroreactive proteins that reacted with sera from patients with histoplasmosis: Hsp60, aconitase, CatP, dihydrolipoamide dehydrogenase, protein disulfide isomerase, the ATP synthase β-subunit, Hsp70 and N-acetylated α-linked acidic dipeptidase (NAALADase). [168] These proteins were identified by mass spectrometry and expressed in *E. coli* as His-tagged proteins and used for ELISA for detecting antibodies. Results showed, that only in the ELISA using recombinant NAALADase, the titer of the groups of patients with histoplasmosis was significantly higher than that of healthy volunteers, suggesting that NAALADase is recognized as a major antigen during histoplasmosis, like the H and M antigens.

The extracellular proteome of the yeast phase of *H. capsulatum* was investigated by Holbrook et al. who identified 33 proteins. [97] The proteins include glycanases (i.e., Eng1, Chs1, Exg1), extracellular enzymes related to oxidative stress defense (i.e., CatB, Sod3, Trl1), dehydrogenase enzymes (i.e., Mpd1, Gdh1, Hom1), chaperone-like factors (i.e., Hsp60, Ssa1, Hsp82), and five-novel culture filtrate proteins (Cfp1, Cfp4, Cfp7, Cfp8, Cfp11). Five of the Cfps secreted by yeasts lacked significant homology to other identified proteins from other organisms [169]. At the protein level, Cfp4 was one of the most abundant extracellular proteins, second to the Cbp1 secreted factor. The Cfp4 protein is a heavily glycosylated protein expressed exclusively by the pathogenic phase. Human immune sera recognize the *Histoplasma* Cfp4 protein, confirming Cfp4 production during infection of human hosts. These results suggest the potential utility of Cfp4 as a diagnostic exoantigen for histoplasmosis. [169] As an abundantly secreted protein, Cfp4 could potentially be a target for antigen detection-based diagnostics, but further studies to establish its utility as a biomarker will be required.

By an immunoproteomic approach Almeida et al. (2020) detected 132 reactive proteins to antibodies present in the sera of patients with histoplasmosis. [170] Among them, 127 were recognized also by antibodies present in sera from normal healthy donors or from patients with other pulmonary infections living in endemic areas of histoplasmosis. Only three antigens were specifically recognized by antibodies of histoplasmosis patients as potential antigenic candidates: CatB, CatP and Yps-3 proteins.

Recently, Toscanini et al. have demonstrated the role of the recombinant antigen Hcp100, as a useful tool in the serological diagnosis of chronic histoplasmosis tested by immunodiffusion. In addition, polyclonal antibodies against this recombinant antigen allowed detecting this antigen in urine samples from AIDS patients with PDH. [171] It should be pointed out that recombinant proteins may improve the performance of diagnostic tests by offering a defined antigen that can be produced in large quantities with little variability in quality, in contraposition to the use of native antigens such as HMN. In this regard, current methods for the production of *H. capsulatum* antigens are problematic in terms of standardization, specificity, stability, repeatability and reproducibility. [40]

An inhibition ELISA has been developed for the detection of a 69-70 kDa cytoplasmatic *H. capsulatum* yeast antigen in urine and serum using a species-specific murine monoclonal antibody. [172] The test overall sensitivity was moderate (71.4%) in serum and low in urine (44%) and exhibited cross-reactions in patients with paracoccidioidomycosis, aspergillosis, cryptococcosis and tuberculosis. Another report showed that the inhibition ELISA can be used for monitoring antigenemia of non-AIDS patients during the treatment of acute pulmonary and disseminated histoplasmosis, complementing existing means of follow-up. [173] However, no further studies validating this assay in a larger number of patients were published.

An exploratory study carried out by Kushnir et al. evaluated differences among excretory proteins in urine from patients with histoplasma antigenuria, healthy individuals and patients with proteinuria of other causes. [174] The number of unique proteins identified in the samples from patients with histoplasmosis was 23. Among them, the most abundant were six enzymes (glutaredoxin, carbonic anhydrase, kallikrein, acid alpha-glucosidase, ribonuclease T2 precursor, quiescin Q6), four plasma membrane proteins (peptidoglycan recognition protein, brain abundant signal protein, carcinoembryonic antigen-related cell adhesion molecule, vascular cell adhesion molecule) and five immunoglobulins (Ig kappa chain).

By a comparative nanospray tandem mass spectrometry (LC-MS/MS) analysis of urine specimens from infected and noninfected patients with *H. capsulatum*, Crocket et al. identified several potential protein and peptide markers specific to *H. capsulatum* infection in human urine. [175] In total 52 peptides were identified, which belongs to 37 known and predicted *Histoplasma* proteins, such as YPS-3.

Nucleic Acid Amplification Assays

Nucleic acid amplification diagnostic techniques including polymerase chain reaction (PCR) are commercially available and are increasingly used in clinical practice. However, for histoplasmosis, all PCRs assays have been developed as "in-house" methods and have not yet been established as regular diagnostic tools. So far, no nucleic acid assay is commercially available for use in clinical samples, and the existing assays have not yet been fully standardized and validated by multi-centric studies. [176]

The reported molecular assays for histoplasmosis varied in the target gene, the sample tested, the DNA extraction method and the amplification technique. These assays target multi-copy genes, such as the ribosomal DNA (rDNA) genes (18S, 28S and 5.8S) and the intervening internal transcribed spacer (ITS) regions; and single-copy genes, such as those coding for the Hcp100 protein, the H and M antigens, the NAALADase, the GAPDH, and the 1281-1283$_{220}$ sequence-characterized amplified region (SCAR) marker.

The most common gene coding for a specific protein used for molecular diagnosis of histoplasmosis has been the gene coding for Hcp100 that had been described by Porta et al. [67]

In 2002 Bialek et al. reported two nested PCR assays for detecting H. capsulatum DNA in formalin-fixed and paraffin-embedded tissues. [177] One of the nested PCR assays used specific primers for the Hcp100 gene, which detected *H. capsulatum* in 69% of tissues from *Histoplasma*-positive patients and in none of the *Histoplasma*-negative specimens. The other nested PCR assay used primers for the 18S rDNA gene and detected *H. capsulatum* in 89.6% of samples from *Histoplasma*-positive individuals but also in 54.5% of samples from *Histoplasma*-negative individuals. Furthermore, products amplified with primers for the 18S rDNA gene have to be confirmed by sequencing, because ribosomal genes are conserved regions in the kingdom fungi, bearing the risk of nonspecific amplifications. In a clinical context, this needs for sequencing for confirming the amplification product would increase costs and delay the reporting of results.

The nested PCR assay that targets the gene coding for Hcp100 was further validated using a variety of human samples, including respiratory samples, fresh biopsies, bone marrow, serum and blood samples reporting sensitivity and specificity values ranging from 18-100% and 93.6-100%, respectively. [56, 178-182] In all cases, the low sensitivity values observed in serum samples (18%) may be explained by the fact that *H. capsulatum* is an intracellular pathogen and thus, the amount of free DNA is low.

A recent study carried out by Martínez-Gamboa et al. showed that the sensitivity and specificity values for the Hcp100 nested PCR among PLHIV were 62.9%/89.5% in blood samples, 65.9%/89.0% in bone marrow samples, 62.1%/82.6% in tissue samples and 34.9%/67.3% of urine samples. [132] For the 1281-1283$_{220}$SCAR nested PCR developed by Frias De León et al., the sensitivity/specificity values obtained for the same samples were 65.3%/ 58.8%, 70.8%/52.9%, 71.4%/40.4% and 18.1%/90.4%, respectively. [183]

A semi-nested PCR that partially amplifies the *H. capsulatum* H antigen gene was developed by Bracca et al. and showed concordance with culture methods in 1/2 tissue samples, 3/3 mucocutaneous lesions and 2/2 blood samples. [184] However, in 22 culture-negative blood samples for *H. capsulatum*, 2 rendered positive results with this semi-nested PCR. The M antigen has been used to detect *H. capsulatum* DNA from culture with sensitivity and specificity values of 100%. [185] The use of these gene targets remains very limited at this time in spite of their promise as targets for diagnosis and more evaluation is necessary.

Tang et al. developed a colorimetric microtiter plate PCR-EIA for the detection of *H. capsulatum* in urine. However, the sensitivity of this assay in urine samples positive for *Histoplasma* antigen testing was low (7.8%). [186] This PCR assay detects DNA from *Histoplasma* yeasts with high sensitivity (2 yeasts/reaction or 10^2yeasts/ml) but does not detect antigen because antigens contain no DNA. DNA was only detected in specimens from which the *Histoplasma* organism could be isolated by culture.

Lopez et al. standardized three real time PCR protocols for the detection of *H. capsulatum* in fresh and formalin-fixed, paraffin-embedded lung tissues from infected mice targeting the genes that code for Hcp100 and the H and M antigens. [187] This assay exhibited 100% analytical sensitivity and specificity using isolates from *H. capsulatum* and other medically relevant pathogens. The results of the Hcp100 and H antigen rt-PCR highly agreed with colony-forming unit counts and histopathological analysis but their clinical utility for the diagnosis of histoplasmosis still has to be evaluated.

Some research groups developed real time PCR assays targeting the ITS region using different probe systems (i.e., TaqMan® and Light Cycler® platforms), with sensitivity values that varied depending on the type of clinical specimen tested (37.5-100%) and specificity values of 96-100%. [188-190]

The ITS region has also been used as target in a multiplex real time PCR assay to simultaneously detect in a single-tube three fungal species that frequently cause pneumonia in AIDS patients: *H. capsulatum, P. jirovecii* and *C. neoformans/C. gattii*. [191] The assay was evaluated in 40 HIV patients with proven fungal infections, 14 of whom suffered from histoplasmosis, achieving 90.7% sensitivity and 100% specificity.

Other attempts to identify multiple microorganisms from a single sample involve next generation sequencing (NGS) techniques. [192-194] However, further studies need to be carried out in order to evaluate its utility in fungal diagnosis. In addition, the high cost of NGS methods makes it difficult to implement in the near future.

Isothermal nucleic acid amplification techniques appear to be an appealing tool for a rapid and low-cost diagnosis. Since amplification occurs at a single temperature, this step can be performed in a heat block or a water bath. In addition, results can be observed in the reaction tube by using several simple strategies. [195] Despite its advantages, limited attempts have been made to develop these assays for the diagnosis of histoplasmosis. Two loop-mediated isothermal amplification (LAMP) assays targeting the ITS region [179] and thc Hcp100 gene [196] were designed to detect *H. capsulatum* DNA in a few clinical samples of AIDS patients with PDH, including urine. The ITS LAMP assay results agreed in 6 of 7 positive results obtained with ITS nested-PCR, whereas the Hcp100 LAMP was positive in only 4 of 6 of the antigen positive urine samples tested. The low sensitivity yield in urine may be explained for its low content of complete fungal DNA, making urine an unsuitable sample for DNA detection, as mentioned above. [186, 196]

Another isothermal nucleic acid amplification technique developed for histoplasmosis diagnosis was the rolling circle amplification (RCA) of the ITS region. [197] Despite the excellent analytical sensitivity and specificity values reported, this assay involves an amplification step by PCR, which increases the cost and contamination risk and decreases its utility in resource-challenged regions.

Overall, nucleotide amplification techniques have demonstrated rapid turnaround times, which is greatly important in the diagnosis of PDH. In addition, based on the results of a recent meta-analysis study involving the Hcp100 nested-PCR and the ITS rt-PCR, the overall sensitivity of PDH diagnosis in HIV+ patients of molecular methods was higher than that calculated for culture methods (95.4% vs 77%). [49] These techniques could be effective in non-endemic regions with inadequate culture facilities and limited experience in isolating *H. capsulatum*. In these regions, the antigen detection tests are commonly unavailable, therefore, molecular tests could contribute to rapid diagnosis and therapy. Additionally, it has been suggested that nucleotide amplification methods could be useful in the follow-up of patients, since it seems to be a correlation between clinical improvement and

DNA negativization. [180] Nucleotide amplification techniques may also represent a suitable alternative for the detection of *H. capsulatum* in environmental samples, instead of using experimental animals, also decreasing costs and turnaround times. Furthermore, molecular assays might allow the identification of *H. capsulatum* organisms that cannot be easily identified by direct microscopic examination and isolates with atypical phenotypic characteristics. [198]

A pending challenge for nucleotide amplification assays is to obtain fungal DNA in high quality and quantity from clinical samples. The extraction step is usually performed using commercial kits— which increases costs [179] — and, in some cases, boiling and freezing cycles to facilitate the fungal wall rupture. [56, 180] This step is also important to remove polymerase inhibitors (e.g., hemoglobin and EDTA), which would cause false-negative results. False-positive results in molecular tests may be due to mutations in the targeted *H. capsulatum* gene; thus, primers and probes must be thoroughly designed regarding the sequences of the different clades reported.

Histoplasmosis in Animals

H. capsulatum infects numerous mammalian hosts, including humans. The infection is also very common in wild (e.g., marsupials, rodents, armadillos, lamas, sea mammals, sloths, bats) and domestic animals (e.g., dogs and cats) in endemic areas. [199, 200] However, mammals appear to be dead-end hosts of *Histoplasma* since there is no person-to-person or animal-to-person spread. Bats have been proposed as a vector of spread, both because the fungus grows well in soil contaminated with bat guano and because bats themselves can be colonized with this fungus. [201] *H. capsulatum* has been found in the soil of dog kennels, under porches of old houses, under trees and bushes frequented by birds in the daytime and prefers the undisturbed litter in and around old chicken houses or in undisturbed droppings under bird roosts. It has also been found in isolated caves and hollow trees. It apparently is capable of competing very well with other organisms found in the ground if the ground is enriched by fecal material of chickens, other birds or bats. It is quite significant that histoplasmosis is not found in chickens or in fresh chicken droppings. Work done by Menges showed that chickens and probably all birds are not susceptible to natural infection. [202] This may be due to their high body temperatures, that ranges from 40 to 42°C. Reptiles none were proved to have histoplasmosis. [202]

Recently, *H. capsulatum* was molecularly detected in penguin excreta and ornithogenic soil samples in the Antarctic Peninsula, showing that this pathogen occurs more broadly than suspected. Its presence might be related either to human intervention in the region or to the migratory behavior of birds. During migration, birds have the potential to disperse microorganisms that can be dangerous to humans and a threat to animals. [203]

As mentioned in the introductory section, *H. capsulatum* var. *capsulatum* causes pulmonary and systemic infections in a diversity of mammals. *H. capsulatum* var. *duboisii* causes lymphadenopathy, and dissemination to the skin and bones, mainly in humans and other primates. *H. capsulatum* var. *farciminosum* affects the skin and the subcutaneous lymphatic system in equids (horses, donkeys, and mules) but has also been recovered from humans, dogs, cats and badgers.

Despite all mammals are susceptible to histoplasmosis, cases have been reported most often in dogs, cats, and horses. As in humans, disease outcome is variable and depends on the immune status of the host, inoculum size, and the virulence of the isolate. [200] Histoplasmosis affects dogs and cats of all ages but is reported predominantly in younger animals: mean age of 3.9 years in cats and 4.3 years in dogs. [204-207] Several dog breeds have been shown to have an increased risk of histoplasmosis, including the Pointer, Weimeraner and Brittany spaniel. [208] Among cats, Persian cats are slightly overrepresented, while Siamese cats are marginally under-represented. [207] Interestingly, indoor-only cats remain at risk for histoplasmosis. [209] In a review of 571 cats with deep mycotic infections, histoplasmosis (16.7%) was the second most commonly reported fungal disease after cryptococcosis (46.1%). [207]

As in humans, the severity of clinical manifestations correlates with the intensity of exposure and the underlying health of the exposed individual. While histoplasmosis is self-limited in over 95% of healthy humans, chronic granulomatous disease and/or progressive disease may occur more often in animals. In this regard, 31 to 44% of euthanized dogs and cats in endemic areas had evidence for histoplasmosis. [210-212]

Cole described rapidly progressive fatal course over two to four weeks in 10% of dogs with histoplasmosis, and chronic progressive course over two to 20 months in 90%. [209] Histoplasmosis in dogs is commonly multisystemic. Like humans and cats, most canine gastrointestinal histoplasmosis is thought to be a part of disseminated disease.

Syndromes most commonly identified include pneumonia, mediastinal lymphadenitis, and PDH. Bone lesions are common in cats. [205] CNS and ocular lesions may be found in all animal species. Although intestinal lesions are prominent in dogs with PDH, experimental infection by gastric inoculation failed to induce disease in dogs, ruling out the oral route as an additional possible via for acquiring infection. [213]

Among horses, infections in the fetus or neonatal foal may occur, causing the mare to abort or the foal to die soon after birth. [214-216] Pulmonary and disseminated involvement usually are present in the fetus or newborn. [216] In most cases the mare appears healthy, but the placenta is involved.

Cytology is the most valuable tool for the diagnosis of histoplasmosis in veterinary medicine. However, organisms can be missed cytologically with low organism burdens and nonrepresentative aspirates. Fungal culture of affected tissues is not routinely relied upon clinically because of the slow growing of the organism and the requirement of specialized laboratories. Serologic tests, including complement fixation and immunodiffusion are available, but are associated with poor sensitivity

Histoplasma antigen detection using the EIA-based third-generation *Histoplasma* antigen Assay (MiraVista Diagnostics) was described to be clinically useful test to support the diagnosis of histoplasmosis in dogs and cats, specifically in regions where there is a high prevalence of disease. [217-221] Noteworthy, a retrospective study in cats suggested that a compromised renal function may lower urinary antigen levels. [222] Using the monoclonal antibody based IMMY urine *Histoplasma* antigen for the diagnosis of histoplasmosis in cats, Rothenburg et al. reported a sensitivity of 89%, specificity of 80% and accuracy of 83%. However, using the MiraVista EIA to compare the performance of the IMMY EIA, the sensitivity was 94%, the specificity was 97% and the accuracy was 96%. [221]

Veterinarians should be aware that histoplasmosis is the most frequent endemic mycosis among dogs, cats, raccons, thoroughbred horses and other animals, in at least the United States and Canada. [223]

Conclusion

Understanding the uses and limitations of all the diagnostic methods and techniques used in the laboratory setting is essential for diagnosing histoplasmosis.

In Latin America, *H. capsulatum* has been a silent killer, causing more deaths in PLHIV than tuberculosis and this problem is evolving under the radars of healthcare systems in the vast majority of countries. [224] The HIV/AIDS pandemic, along with the growing number of patients under immunosuppressive treatments, increased the population at risk of contracting the life-threatening disseminated form of histoplasmosis. The problem is even more serious in Latin America, where patients continue to die from a treatable disease due to the lack of accurate diagnostic methods.

Histoplasma antigen detection immunoassays have represented a step forward in the rapid diagnosis of PDH. However, despite the fact that this assay has been included in the Model List of Essential In Vitro Diagnostics for PLHIV [225], commercial kits are only used in some highly specialized reference laboratories and are not yet registered in most countries. [44] Although detecting *Histoplasma* antigen from urine samples has highly improved sensitivity and represents an aid in the diagnosis of PDH, the European Organization for Research and Treatment of Cancer and the Mycoses consensus declared that it is not sufficient evidence of proven histoplasmosis, because *Histoplasma* antigen is also found in specimens of patients with coccidioidomycosis and blastomycosis. [38]

The search for novel antigens, particularly for protein antigens, is an alternative that deserves further investigation because their production by recombinant-DNA technology would guarantee an unlimited supply of high-quality reagents. In addition, the standardization and validation of nucleotide amplification assays would also suppose an advance in obtaining rapid and reliable methods for the diagnosis of PDH, especially in high-income laboratories.

Regardless of the technique used, efforts from commercial companies and research laboratories should be focused on developing high-quality reproducibly produced diagnostic kits or reagents for the rapid diagnosis of histoplasmosis -as well as other fungal diseases-, and on making those kits commercially available worldwide at reasonable cost. This cooperation road is necessary to achieve the goal established in the Manaus Declaration, which aims that all laboratories in the Americas could have access to rapid antigen or molecular tests for the diagnosis of histoplasmosis by the year 2025. [44]

References

[1] Darling ST. A Protozoon General Infection Producing Pseudotubercles in the Lungs and Focal Necroses in the Liver, Spleen and Lymphnodes. *J Am Clin Assoc.* 1906 Apr 28;1283–5. Available from: http://jama.jamanetwork.com/

[2] De Monbreun WA. The cultivation and cultural characteristics of Darling's *Histoplasma capsulatum*. *J Trop Med.* 1934;14(2).

[3] Kauffman CA. Histoplasmosis: A clinical and laboratory update. Vol. 20, *Clinical Microbiology Reviews.* 2007. p. 115–32.

[4] Emmons CW. Isolation of *Histoplasma capsulatum* from soil. *Public Heal Reports.* 1949;892–6.

[5] Maresca, B, Carratù L, Kobayashi GS. Morphological transition in the human fungal pathogen *Histoplasma capulatum*. *Trends Microbiol.* 1994;2(4):110–4.

[6] Klugman HB, Lurie HI. Systemic histoplasmosis in South Africa. A review of the previous cases and a report of an additional case--the first successfully treated. *S Afr Med J.* 1963;37:29–31.

[7] Oladele RO, Ayanlowo OO, Richardson MD, Denning DW. Histoplasmosis in Africa: An emerging or a neglected disease? *PLoS Negl Trop Dis.* 2018 Jan 18;12(1).

[8] Randhawa HS, Gugnani HC. Occurrence of Histoplasmosis in the Indian Sub-Continent: An Overview and Update. *J Med Res Pract.* 2018;7(3):71–83.

[9] McLeod DSA, Mortimer RH, Perry-Keene DA, Allworth A, Woods ML, Perry-Keene J, McBride WJH, Coulter C, Robson JMB. Histoplasmosis in Australia: Report of 16 cases and literature review. *Medicine* (Baltimore). 2011 Jan;90(1):61–8.

[10] Pan B, Chen M, Pan W, Liao W. Histoplasmosis: A new endemic fungal infection in China? Review and analysis of cases. *Mycoses.* 2013 May;56(3):212–21.

[11] Baker J, Setianingrum F, Wahyuningsih R, Denning DW. Mapping histoplasmosis in South East Asia–implications for diagnosis in AIDS. *Emerg Microbes Infect.* 2019 Jan 1;8(1):1139–45.

[12] Confalonieri M, Gandola L, Aiolfi S, Mazzoni A. Histoplasmin sensitivity among a student population in Crema, Po Valley, Italy. *New Microbiol.* 1994 Apr;17(2):151–3.

[13] Sotgiu G, Mantovani A, Mazzoni A. Histoplasmosis in Europe. *Mycopathol Mycol Appl.* 1970 Sep;41(1–2):53–74.

[14] Eissenberg LG, Goldman WE. *Histoplasma* variation and adaptive strategies for parasitism: new perspectives on histoplasmosis. *Clin Microbiol Rev.* 1991;4(4):411–21. Available from: https://pubmed.ncbi.nlm.nih.gov/1747859/

[15] Loulergue P, Bastides F, Baudouin V, Chandenier J, Mariani-Kurkdjian P, Dupont B, Viard JP, Dromer F, Lortholary O. Literature Review and Case Histories of *Histoplasma capsulatum* var. *duboisii* Infections in HIV-infected Patients. *Emerg Infect Dis.* 2007;13(11):1647. Available from:/pmc/articles/PMC3375808/

[16] Pakasa N, Biber A, Nsiangana S, Imposo D, Sumaili E, Muhindo H, Buitrago MJ, Barshack I, Schwartz E. African histoplasmosis in HIV-negative patients, Kimpese, Democratic Republic of the Congo. *Emerg Infect Dis.* 24(11):2068.

[17] Selim SA, Soliman R, Osman K, Padhye AA, Ajello L. Studies on Histoplasmosis Farciminosi (Epizootic Lymphangitis) in Egypt: Isolation of *Histoplasma farciminosum* from Cases of Histoplasmosis Farciminosi in Horses and Its Morphological Characteristics. *Eur J Epidemiol.* 1985 Jun;1(2):84–9. Available from: https://www.jstor.org/stable/3520809

[18] Kasuga T, White TJ, Koenig G, McEwen J, Restrepo A, Castañeda E, Da Silva Lacaz C, Heins-Vaccari EM, De Freitas RS, Zancopé-Oliveira RM, Qin Z, Negroni R, Carter DA, Mikami Y, Tamura M, Taylor ML, Miller GF, Poonwan N, Taylor JW. Phylogeography of the fungal pathogen *Histoplasma capsulatum. Mol Ecol.* 2003;12(12):3383–401.

[19] Kasuga T, Taylor JW, White TJ. Phylogenetic relationships of varieties and geographical groups of the human pathogenic fungus *Histoplasma capsulatum* Darling. *J Clin Microbiol.* 1999;37(3):653–63.

[20] Teixeira Mde M, Patané JS, Taylor ML, Gómez BL, Theodoro RC, de Hoog S, Engelthaler DM, Zancopé-Oliveira RM, Felipe MS, Barker BM. Worldwide Phylogenetic Distributions and Population Dynamics of the Genus *Histoplasma*. *PLoS Negl Trop Dis.* 2016 Jun 1;10(6).

[21] Sepúlveda VE, Márquez R, Turissini DA, Goldman WE, Matute DR. Genome sequences reveal cryptic speciation in the human pathogen *Histoplasma capsulatum. MBio.* 2017 Nov 1;8(6).

[22] Kroetz DN, Deepe GS. The role of cytokines and chemokines in *Histoplasma capsulatum* infection. *Cytokine.* 2012;58(1):112–7.

[23] Shen Q, Beucler MJ, Ray SC, Rappleye CA. Macrophage activation by IFN-γ triggers restriction of phagosomal copper from intracellular pathogens. *PLoS Pathog.* 2018;14(11):e1007444.

[24] Wheat J, French ML, Kohler RB, Zimmerman SE, Smith WR, Norton JA, Eitzen HE, Smith CD, Slama TG. The diagnostic laboratory tests for histoplasmosis. Analysis of experience in a large urban outbreak. *Ann Intern Med.* 1982;97(5):680–5.

[25] Wheat LJ, Azar MM, Bahr NC, Spec A, Relich RF, Hage C. Histoplasmosis. *Infect Dis Clin North Am.* 2016;30(1):207–27.

[26] Wheat LJ, Slama TG, Norton JA, Kohler RB, Eitzen HE, French ML, Sathapatayavongs B. Risk factors for disseminated or fatal histoplasmosis. Analysis of a large urban outbreak. *Ann Intern Med.* 1982;96(2):159–63.

[27] Sil A, Andrianopoulos A. Thermally dimorphic human fungal pathogens—polyphyletic pathogens with a convergent pathogenicity trait. *Cold Spring Harb Perspect Med.* 2015;5(8):a019794.

[28] Homei A, Worboys M. *Fungal Disease in Britain and the United States 1850–2000: Mycoses and Modernity.* Springer Nature. Basingstoke, UK: Palgrave Macmillan; 2013.

[29] Toscanini MA, Barberis F, Benedetti MF, Garrido AV, Posse GB, Capece P, Daneri GL, Nusblat AD, Cuestas ML. Detection of anti-*Histoplasma capsulatum* antibodies and seroconversion patterns in critically ill patients with COVID-19 : An underdiagnosed fungal entity complicating COVID-19? *Med Mycol.* 2022;60(February):1–8.

[30] Centers for Disease Control. Revision of the CDC surveillance case definition for acquired immunodeficiency syndrome. Council of State and Territorial Epidemiologists; AIDS Program, Center for Infectious Diseases. *MMWR Suppl.* 1987 Aug;36(1):1S-15S.

[31] WHO. *Mycetoma, chromoblastomycosis amd other deep mycoses.* 2017 [cited 2020 Jul 2]. Available from: https://www.who.int/medical_devices/publications/Standalone_document_v8.pdf?ua=1

[32] Nacher M, Blanchet D, Bongomin F, Chakrabarti A, Couppié P, Demar M, Denning DW, Djossou F, Epelboin L, Govender N, Leitão T, Mac Donald S, Mandengue C, Marques da Silva SH, Oladele R, Panizo MM, Pasqualotto A, Ramos R, Swaminathan S, Rodriguez-Tudela JL, Vreden S, Zancopé-Oliveira R, Adenis A. *Histoplasma capsulatum* antigen detection tests as an essential diagnostic tool for patients with advanced HIV disease in low and middle income countries: A systematic review of diagnostic accuracy studies. *PLoS Negl Trop Dis.* 2018;12(10):1–12.

[33] Wheat LJ. Endemic mycoses in AIDS: A clinical review. *Clin Microbiol Rev.* 1995;8(1):146–59.

[34] Nacher M, Adenis A, Mc Donald S, Do Socorro Mendonca Gomes M, Singh S, Lopes Lima I, Malcher Leite R, Hermelijn S, Wongsokarijo M, Van Eer M, Marques Da Silva S, Mesquita Da Costa M, Silva M, Calvacante M, do Menino Jesus Silva Leitao T, Gómez BL, Restrepo A, Tobon A, Canteros CE, Aznar C, Blanchet D, Vantilcke V, Vautrin C, Boukhari R, Chiller T, Scheel C, Ahlquist A, Roy M, Lortholary O, Carme B, Couppié P, Vreden S. Disseminated Histoplasmosis in HIV-Infected Patients in South America: A Neglected Killer Continues on Its Rampage. *PLoS Negl Trop Dis.* 2013;7(11):7–9.

[35] Adenis A, Nacher M, Hanf M, Basurko C, Dufour J, Huber F, Aznar C, Carme B, Couppie P. Tuberculosis and Histoplasmosis among Human Immunodeficiency Virus-Infected Patients: A Comparative Study. *Am J Trop Med Hyg.* 2014;90(2):216–23.

[36] Denning DW. Minimizing fungal disease deaths will allow the UNAIDS target of reducing annual AIDS deaths below 500 000 by 2020 to be realized. *Philos Trans R Soc B Biol Sci.* 2016 Dec 5;371(1709). Available from: https://pubmed.ncbi.nlm.nih.gov/28080991/

[37] Perez F, Caceres DH, Ford N, Ravasi G, Gomez BL, Pasqualotto AC, Hine P, Adenis AA, Nacher M, Chiller T, Baddley J, For The Guideline Development Group For Diagnosing And Managing Disseminated Histoplasmosis Among People Living With Hiv. Summary of Guidelines for Managing Histoplasmosis among People Living with HIV. *J Fungi.* 2021;7(134).

[38] Donnelly JP, Chen SC, Kauffman CA, Steinbach WJ, Baddley JW, Verweij PE, Clancy CJ, Wingard JR, Lockhart SR, Groll AH, Sorrell TC, Bassetti M, Akan H, Alexander BD, Andes D, Azoulay E, Bialek R, Bradsher RW, Bretagne S, Calandra T, Caliendo AM, Castagnola E, Cruciani M, Cuenca-Estrella M, Decker CF, Desai SR, Fisher B, Harrison T, Heussel CP, Jensen HE, Kibbler CC, Kontoyiannis DP, Kullberg BJ, Lagrou K, Lamoth F, Lehrnbecher T, Loeffler J, Lortholary O,

Maertens J, Marchetti O, Marr KA, Masur H, Meis JF, Morrisey CO, Nucci M, Ostrosky-Zeichner L, Pagano L, Patterson TF, Perfect JR, Racil Z, Roilides E, Ruhnke M, Prokop CS, Shoham S, Slavin MA, Stevens DA, Thompson GR, Vazquez JA, Viscoli C, Walsh TJ, Warris A, Wheat LJ, White PL, Zaoutis TE, Pappas PG. Revision and Update of the Consensus Definitions of Invasive Fungal Disease From the European Organization for Research and Treatment of Cancer and the Mycoses Study Group Education and Research Consortium. *Clin Infect Dis an Off Publ Infect Dis Soc Am.* 2020 Sep 12;71(6):1367–76. Available from: www.fpcri.eu

[39] Falci DR, Hoffmann ER, Paskulin DD, Pasqualotto AC. Progressive disseminated histoplasmosis: a systematic review on the performance of non-culture-based diagnostic tests. *Brazilian J Infect Dis.* 2017;21(1):7–11. Available from: http://dx.doi.org/10.1016/j.bjid.2016.09.012

[40] de Freitas RS, Kamikawa CM, Vicentini AP. Fast protocol for the production of *Histoplasma capsulatum* antigens for antibody detection in the immunodiagnosis of histoplasmosis. *Rev Iberoam Micol.* 2018;35(1):27–31. Available from: http://dx.doi.org/10.1016/j.riam.2017.04.004

[41] Kauffman CA. Diagnosis of histoplasmosis in immunosuppressed patients. *Curr Opin Infect Dis.* 2008;21(4):421–5.

[42] Hage CA, Kirsch EJ, Stump TE, Kauffman CA, Goldman M, Connolly P, Johnson PC, Wheat LJ, Baddley JW. *Histoplasma* antigen clearance during treatment of histoplasmosis in patients with AIDS determined by a quantitative antigen enzyme immunoassay. *Clin Vaccine Immunol.* 2011;18(4):661–6.

[43] Hage CA, Ribes JA, Wengenack NL, Baddour LM, Assi M, McKinsey DS, Hammoud K, Alapat D, Babady NE, Parker M, Fuller D, Noor A, Davis TE, Rodgers M, Connolly PA, El Haddad B, Wheat LJ. A multicenter evaluation of tests for diagnosis of histoplasmosis. *Clin Infect Dis.* 2011;53(5):448–54.

[44] Cáceres DH, Adenis A, de Souza JVB, Gomez BL, Cruz KS, Pasqualotto A, Ravasi G, Perez F, Chiller T, de Lacerda M.V.G. The Manaus Declaration: Current Situation of Histoplasmosis in the Americas, Report of the II Regional Meeting of the International Histoplasmosis Advocacy Group. *Curr Fungal Infect Rep.* 2019;13(4):244–9.

[45] Wheat LJ. Improvements in diagnosis of histoplasmosis. *Expert Opin Biol Ther.* 2006;6(11):1207–21.

[46] Bloch KC, Myint T, Raymond-Guillen L, Hage CA, Davis TE, Wright PW, Chow FC, Woc-Colburn L, Khairy RN, Street AC, Yamamoto T, Albers A, Wheat LJ. Improvement in diagnosis of *Histoplasma* meningitis by combined testing for *Histoplasma* antigen and immunoglobulin G and immunoglobulin M anti-*Histoplasma* antibody in cerebrospinal fluid. *Clin Infect Dis.* 2018;66(1):89–94.

[47] Wheat LJ, Freifeld AG, Kleiman MB, Baddley JW, McKinsey DS, Loyd JE, Kauffman CA; Infectious Diseases Society of America. Clinical Practice Guidelines for the Management of Patients with Histoplasmosis: 2007 Update by the Infectious Diseases Society of America. *Clin Infect Dis.* 2007 Oct 1;45(7): 807–25.

[48] Wheat LJ, Kohler RB, Tewari RP, Garten M, French MLV. Significance of *Histoplasma* Antigen in the Cerebrospinal Fluid of Patients With Meningitis. *Arch Intern Med.* 1989;149(2):302–4.

[49] Cáceres DH, Knuth M, Derado G, Lindsley MD. Diagnosis of progressive disseminated histoplasmosis in advanced HIV: A meta-analysis of assay analytical performance. *J Fungi.* 2019;5(3):1–13.

[50] Schestatsky P, Chedid MF, Amaral OB, Unis G, Oliveira FM, Severo LC. Isolated central nervous system histoplasmosis in immunocompetent hosts: A series of 11 cases. *Scand J Infect Dis.* 2006;38(1):43–8.

[51] Wheat J, Myint T, Guo Y, Kemmer P, Hage C, Terry C, Azar MM, Riddell J, Ender P, Chen S, Shehab K, Cleveland K, Esguerra E, Johnson J, Wright P, Douglas V, Vergidis P, Ooi W, Baddley J, Bamberger D, Khairy R, Vikram HR, Jenny-Avital E, Sivasubramanian G, Bowlware K, Pahud B, Sarria J, Tsai T, Assi M, Mocherla S, Prakash V, Allen D, Passaretti C, Huprikar S, Anderson A. Central nervous system histoplasmosis. *Med* (United States). 2018;97(13):1–8.

[52] Cáceres DH, Samayoa BE, Medina NG, Tobón AM, Guzmán BJ, Mercado D, Restrepo A, Chiller T, Arathoon EE, Gómez BL. Multicenter validation of commercial antigenuria reagents to diagnose progressive disseminated histoplasmosis in people living with HIV/AIDS in two Latin American countries. *J Clin Microbiol.* 2018;56(6):1–10.

[53] Hage CA, Davis TE, Fuller D, Egan L, Witt JR 3rd, Wheat LJ, Knox KS. Diagnosis of histoplasmosis by antigen detection in BAL fluid. *Chest.* 2010;137(3):623–8.

[54] Richer SM, Smedema ML, Durkin MM, Herman KM, Hage CA, Fuller D, Wheat LJ. Improved diagnosis of acute pulmonary histoplasmosis by combining antigen and antibody detection. *Clin Infect Dis.* 2016;62(7):896–902.

[55] Swartzentruber S, Rhodes L, Kurkjian K, Zahn M, Brandt ME, Connolly P, Wheat LJ. Diagnosis of acute pulmonary histoplasmosis by antigen detection. *Clin Infect Dis.* 2009;49(12):1878–82.

[56] Maubon D, Simon S, Aznar C. Histoplasmosis diagnosis using a polymerase chain reaction method. Application on human samples in French Guiana, South America. *Diagn Microbiol Infect Dis.* 2007;58(4):441–4.

[57] Muñoz C, Gómez BL, Tobón A, Arango K, Restrepo A, Correa MM, Muskus C, Cano LE, González A. Validation and clinical application of a molecular method for identification of *Histoplasma capsulatum* in human specimens in Colombia, South America. *Clin Vaccine Immunol.* 2010;17(1):62–7.

[58] Muraosa Y, Toyotome T, Yahiro M, Watanabe A, Shikanai-Yasuda MA, Kamei K. Detection of *Histoplasma capsulatum* from clinical specimens by cycling probe-based real-time PCR and nested real-time PCR. *Med Mycol.* 2016; 54(4):433–8.

[59] Ohno H, Tanabe K, Umeyama T, Kaneko Y, Yamagoe S, Miyazaki Y. Application of nested PCR for diagnosis of histoplasmosis. *J Infect Chemother.* 2013;19(5):999–1003.

[60] Köhler JR, Hube B, Puccia R, Casadevall A, Perfect J. Fungi that infect humans. *Microbiol Spectr.* 2017;5(3):5–3.

[61] Holbrook ED, Rappleye CA. *Histoplasma capsulatum* pathogenesis: making a lifestyle switch. *Curr Opin Microbiol.* 2008;11(4):318–24.

[62] Webster RH, Sil A. Conserved factors Ryp2 and Ryp3 control cell morphology and infectious spore formation in the fungal pathogen *Histoplasma capsulatum. Proc Natl Acad Sci.* 2008;105(38):14573–8.

[63] Beyhan S, Gutierrez M, Voorhies M, Sil A. A temperature-responsive network links cell shape and virulence traits in a primary fungal pathogen. *PLoS Biol.* 2013;11(7):e1001614.

[64] Maresca B, Medoff G, Schlessinger D, Kobayashi GS, Medoff J. Regulation of dimorphism in the pathogenic fungus *Histoplasma capsulatum. Nature.* 1977;266(5601):447–8.

[65] Sacco M, Medoff G, Lambowitz AM, Kumar BV, Kobayashi GS, Painter A. Sulfhydryl induced respiratory" shunt" pathways and their role in morphogenesis in the fungus, *Histoplasma capsulatum.* J Biol Chem. 1983;258(13):8223–30.

[66] Eissenberg LG, Goldman WE, Schlesinger PH. *Histoplasma capsulatum* modulates the acidification of phagolysosomes. *J Exp Med.* 1993 Jun 1;177(6):1605–11. Available from: https://pubmed.ncbi.nlm.nih.gov/8496679/

[67] Porta A, Colonna-Romano S, Callebaut I, Franco A, Marzullo L, Kobayashi GS, Maresca B.An homologue of the human 100-kDa protein (p100) is differentially expressed by *Histoplasma capsulatum* during infection of murine macrophages. *Biochem Biophys Res Commun.* 1999;254(3):605–13.

[68] Keath EJ, Abidi FE. Molecular cloning and sequence analysis of yps-3, a yeast-phase-specific gene in the dimorphic fungal pathogen *Histoplasma capsulatum. Microbiology.* 1994;140(4):759–67.

[69] Batanghari JW, Goldman WE. Calcium dependence and binding in cultures of *Histoplasma capsulatum*. *Infect immunity,* 1997;65(12):5257–61.

[70] Kügler S, Young B, Miller VL, Goldman WE. Monitoring phase-specific gene expression in *Histoplasma capsulatum* with telomeric GFP fusion plasmids. *Cell Microbiol.* 2000;2(6):537-547.

[71] Sebghati TS, Engle JT, Goldman WE. Intracellular parasitism by *Histoplasma capsulatum*: fungal virulence and calcium dependence. *Science* (80-). 2000;290(5495):1368–72.

[72] Domer JE, Hamilton JG, Harkin JC. Comparative study of the cell walls of the yeastlike and mycelial phases of *Histoplasma capsulatum. J Bacteriol.* 1967;94(2):466–74.

[73] Domer JE. Monosaccharide and chitin content of cell walls of *Histoplasma capsulatum* and *Blastomyces dermatitidis. J Bacteriol.* 1971;107(3):870–7.

[74] Davis Jr TE, Domer JE, Li YT. Cell wall studies of *Histoplasma capsulatum* and *Blastomyces dermatitidis* using autologous and heterologous enzymes. *Infect Immun.* 1977;15(3):978–87.

[75] Kügler S, Sebghati TS, Eissenberg LG, Goldman WE. Phenotypic variation and intracellular parasitism by *Histoplasma capsulatum. Proc Natl Acad Sci.* 2000;97(16):8794–8.

[76] Gorocica P, Taylor ML, Alvarado-Vásquez N, Pérez-Torres A, Lascurain R, Zenteno E. The interaction between *Histoplasma capsulatum* cell wall

carbohydrates and host components: relevance in the immunomodulatory role of histoplasmosis. *Mem Inst Oswaldo Cruz.* 2009;104:492–6.

[77] Eissenberg LG, Poirier S, Goldman WE. Phenotypic variation and persistence of *Histoplasma capsulatum* yeasts in host cells. *Infect Immun.* 1996;64(12):5310–4.

[78] Eissenberg LG, Moser SA, Goldman WE. Alterations to the cell wall of *Histoplasma capsulatum* yeasts during infection of macrophages or epithelial cells. *J Infect Dis.* 1997;175(6):1538–44.

[79] Rappleye CA, Engle JT, Goldman WE. RNA interference in *Histoplasma capsulatum* demonstrates a role for α-(1, 3)-glucan in virulence. *Mol Microbiol.* 2004;53(1):153–65.

[80] Garfoot AL, Shen Q, Wüthrich M, Klein BS, Rappleye CA. The Eng1 β-glucanase enhances *Histoplasma* virulence by reducing β-glucan exposure. *MBio.* 2016;7(2):e01388-15.

[81] Garfoot AL, Dearing KL, VanSchoiack AD, Wysocki VH, Rappleye CA. Eng1 and Exg8 are the major β-glucanases secreted by the fungal pathogen *Histoplasma capsulatum*. *J Biol Chem.* 2017;292(12):4801.

[82] Rodríguez-Echeverri C, Gómez BL, González Á. *Histoplasma capsulatum* Activates Hematopoietic Stem Cells and Their Progenitors through a Mechanism Dependent on TLR2, TLR4, and Dectin-1. *J Fungi.* 2022;8(10):1108.

[83] Long KH, Gomez FJ, Morris RE, Newman SL. Identification of heat shock protein 60 as the ligand on *Histoplasma capsulatum* that mediates binding to CD18 receptors on human macrophages. *J Immunol.* 2003;170(1):487–94.

[84] Marth T, Kelsall BL. Regulation of interleukin-12 by complement receptor 3 signaling. *J Exp Med.* 1997;185(11):1987–95.

[85] Gomez FJ, Pilcher-Roberts R, Alborzi A, Newman SL. *Histoplasma capsulatum* cyclophilin A mediates attachment to dendritic cell VLA-5. *J Immunol.* 2008;181(10):7106–14.

[86] McCormack FX, Gibbons R, Ward SR, Kuzmenko A, Wu H, Deepe GS. Macrophage-independent fungicidal action of the pulmonary collectins. *J Biol Chem.* 2003;278(38):36250–6.

[87] Eissenberg LG, Goldman WE. *Histoplasma capsulatum* fails to trigger release of superoxide from macrophages. *Infect Immun.* 1987;55(1):29–34.

[88] Wolf JE, Kerchberger V, Kobayashi GS, Little JR. *Modulation of the macrophage oxidative burst by Histoplasma capsulatum.* (Baltimore, Md 1950), 138(2). 1987;138(2):582–6.

[89] Schnur RA, Newman SL. The respiratory burst response to *Histoplasma capsulatum* by human neutrophils. Evidence for intracellular trapping of superoxide anion. *J Immunol.* 1990;144(12):4765–72.

[90] Youseff BH, Holbrook ED, Smolnycki KA, Rappleye CA. Extracellular superoxide dismutase protects *Histoplasma* yeast cells from host-derived oxidative stress. *PLoS Pathog.* 2012 May;8(5). Available from: https://pubmed.ncbi.nlm.nih.gov/22615571/

[91] Johnson CH, Klotz MG, York JL, Kruft V, McEwen JE. Redundancy, phylogeny and differential expression of *Histoplasma capsulatum* catalases. *Microbiology.* 2002;148(4):1129–42.

[92] Holbrook ED, Smolnycki KA, Youseff BH, Rappleye CA. Redundant catalases detoxify phagocyte reactive oxygen and facilitate *Histoplasma capsulatum* pathogenesis. *Infect Immun.* 2013;81(7):2334–46.

[93] Isaac DT, Coady A, Van Prooyen N, Sil A. The 3-hydroxy-methylglutaryl coenzyme A lyase HCL1 is required for macrophage colonization by human fungal pathogen *Histoplasma capsulatum. Infect Immun.* 2013;81(2):411–20.

[94] Hilty J, George Smulian A, Newman SL. *Histoplasma capsulatum* utilizes siderophores for intracellular iron acquisition in macrophages. *Med Mycol.* 2011;49(6):633–42.

[95] Hwang LH, Mayfield JA, Rine J, Sil A. *Histoplasma* requires SID1, a member of an iron-regulated siderophore gene cluster, for host colonization. *PLoS Pathog.* 2008;4(4):e1000044.

[96] Shen Q, Ray SC, Evans HM, Deepe Jr GS, Rappleye CA. Metabolism of gluconeogenic substrates by an intracellular fungal pathogen circumvents nutritional limitations within macrophages. *MBio.* 2020;11(2):e02712-19.

[97] Holbrook ED, Edwards JA, Youseff BH, Rappleye CA. Definition of the extracellular proteome of pathogenic-phase *Histoplasma capsulatum. J Proteome Res.* 2011;10(4):1929–43.

[98] Caceres DH, Zuluaga A, Arango-Bustamante K, de Bedout C, Tobón ÁM, Restrepo Á, Gómez BL, Cano LE, González Á. Implementation of a training course increased the diagnosis of histoplasmosis in Colombia. *Am J Trop Med Hyg.* 2015;93(3):662–7.

[99] Guimarães AJ, Nosanchuk JD, Zancopé-Oliveira RM. Diagnosis of histoplasmosis. Vol. 37, *Brazilian Journal of Microbiology.* 2006. p. 1–13.

[100] Wheat LJ, Kauffman CA. Histoplasmosis. *Infect Dis Clin North Am.* 2003; 17(1):1–19.

[101] Murray PR. Comparison of the lysis-centrifugation and agitated biphasic blood culture systems for detection of fungemia. *J Clin Microbiol.* 1991;29(1):96–8.

[102] Santiago AR, Hernández B, Rodríguez M, Romero H. A comparative study of blood voncentional method vs. a modified lysis/centrifugation technique for the diagnosis of fungemias. *Rev Iberoam Micol.* 2004;21(4):198–201.

[103] Gaur A, Giannini MA, Flynn PM, Boudreaux JW, Mestemacher MA, Shenep JL, Hayden RT. Optimizing blood culture practices in pediatric immunocompromised patients: evaluation of media types and blood culture volume. *Pediatr Infect Dis J.* 2003;22(6):545–52.

[104] Gen-Probe Incorporated. *AccuProbe Histoplasma capsulatum Culture Identification Test.* Growth (Lakeland). San Diego, CA: Gen-Probe Incorporated; 2011.

[105] da Silva RM Jr, da Silva Neto JR, Santos CS, Cruz KS, Frickmann H, Poppert S, Koshikene D, de Souza JV. Fluorescent in situ hybridization of pre-incubated blood culture material for the rapid diagnosis of histoplasmosis. *Med Mycol.* 2015;53(2):160–4.

[106] Lau AF, Drake SK, Calhoun LB, Henderson CM, Zelazny AM. Development of a clinically comprehensive database and a simple procedure for identification of

molds from solid media by matrix-assisted laser desorption ionization-Time of flight mass spectrometry. *J Clin Microbiol.* 2013;51(3):828–34.
[107] Valero C, Buitrago MJ, Gago S, Quiles-Melero I, Garćia-Rodríguez J. A matrix-assisted laser desorption/ionization time of flight mass spectrometry reference database for the identification of *Histoplasma capsulatum. Med Mycol.* 2018;56(3):307–14.
[108] Wheat LJ. Histoplasmosis in Indianapolis. *Clin Infect Dis.* 1992;14(Suppl 1):S91–9.
[109] Wheat J, Wheat H, Connolly P, Kleiman M, Supparatpinyo K, Nelson K, Bradsher R, Restrepo A. Cross-Reactivity in *Histoplasma capsulatum* variety *capsulatum* Antigen Assays of Urine Samples from Patients with Endemic Mycoses. *Clin Infect Dis.* 1997;24(6):1169–71.
[110] Azuma I, Kanetsuna F, Tanaka Y, Yamamura Y, Carbonell LM. Chemical and immunological properties of galactomannans obtained from *Histoplasma duboisii, Histoplasma capsulatum, Paracoccidioides brasiliensis* and *Blastomyces dermatitidis*. *Mycopathol Mycol Appl.* 1974;54(1):111–25.
[111] Deepe GS, Durose GG. Immunobiological activity of recombinant H antigen from *Histoplasma capsulatum*. *Infect Immun.* 1995;63(8):3151–7.
[112] Zancopé-Oliveira RM, Reiss E, Lott TJ, Mayer LW, Deepe GS. Molecular cloning, characterization, and expression of the M antigen of *Histoplasma capsulatum. Infect Immun.* 1999;67(4):1947–53.
[113] Zancopé-Oliveira RM, Bragg SL, Reiss E, Wanke B, Peralta JM. Effects of histoplasmin M antigen chemical and enzymatic deglycosylation on cross-reactivity in the enzyme-linked immunoelectrotransfer blot method. *Clin Diagn Lab Immunol.* 1994;1(4):390–3.
[114] Zancopé-Oliveira RM, Bragg SL, Reiss E, Peralta JM. Immunochemical analysis of the H and M glycoproteins from *Histoplasma capsulatum. Clin Diagn Lab Immunol.* 1994;1(5):563.
[115] Kaufman L, Kovacs JA, Reiss E. Clinical immunomycology. In: de Macario EC, Folds JD, Lane HC, Nakamura RM, editors. *Manual of clinical laboratory immunology.* 5th ed. Washington, DC: American Society for Microbiology; 1997. p. 575–84.
[116] Lindsley MD. The future of fungal serology. *Curr Fungal Infect Rep.* 2013;7(3):161–70.
[117] Kaufman L. Serological tests for histoplasmosis: their use and interpretation. In: *Histoplasmosis: Proceedings of the Second National Conference held at the Center for Disease Control, Atlanta, Georgia.* Springfield, Illinois: Charles C Thomas; 1971. p. 321.326.
[118] Picardi JL, Kauffman CA, Schwarz J, Phair JP. Detection of precipitating antibodies to *Histoplasma capsulatum* by counterimmunoelectrophoresis. *Am Rev Respir Dis.* 1976;114(1):171–6.
[119] George RB, Lambert RS. Significance of serum antibodies to *Histoplasma capsulatum* in endemic areas. *South Med J.* 1984;77(2):161–3.

[120] Raman C, Khardori N, Tewari RP, Von Behren LA, Wheat LJ. Evaluation of an ELISA for the detection of anti-*Histoplasma* ribosomal and antihistoplasmin antibodies in histoplasmosis. *J Clin Lab Anal.* 1990;4(3):199–207.

[121] Guimarães AJ, Pizzini CV, de Matos Guedes HL, Albuquerque PC, Peralta JM, Hamilton AJ, Zancopé-Oliveira RM. ELISA for early diagnosis of histoplasmosis. *J Med Microbiol.* 2004;53(6):509–14.

[122] Almeida MA, Damasceno LS, Pizzini CV, Muniz M de M, Almeida-Paes R, Zancope-Oliveira RM. Role of western blot assay for the diagnosis of histoplasmosis in AIDS patients from a National Institute of Infectious Diseases in Rio de Janeiro, Brazil. *Mycoses.* 2019;62(3):261–7.

[123] Sharma A, Johri BN, Shriniwas. An Enzyme Immunoassay for yeast and mycelial phase-specific antibodies in histoplasmosis. *J Immunol Methods.* 1982; 50(1982):115–21.

[124] Brock EG, Reiss E, Pine L, Kaufman L. Effect of periodate oxidation on the detection of antibodies against the M-antigen of histoplasmin by enzyme immunoassay (EIA) inhibition. *Curr Microbiol.* 1984;10(3):177–80.

[125] Zimmerman SE, French MLV, Kleiman MB, Wheat LJ. Evaluation of an enzyme-linked immunosorbent assay that uses ferrous metal beads for determination of antihistoplasmal immunoglobulins G and M. *J Clin Microbiol.* 1990;28(1):59–64.

[126] Torres M, Díaz H, Herrera T, Sada E. Evaluation of enzyme linked immunosorbent-assay and western blot for diagnosis of histoplasmosis. *Rev Invest Clin.* 1993;45(2):155–60.

[127] Pizzini CV, Zancopé-Oliveira RM, Reiss E, Hajjeh R, Kaufman L, Peralta JM. Evaluation of a western blot test in an outbreak of acute pulmonary histoplasmosis. *Clin Diagn Lab Immunol.* 1999;6(1):20–3.

[128] Almeida Mde A, Pizzini CV, Damasceno LS, Muniz Mde M, Almeida-Paes R, Peralta RH, Peralta JM, Oliveira Rde V, Vizzoni AG, de Andrade CL, Zancopé-Oliveira RM. Validation of western blot for *Histoplasma capsulatum* antibody detection assay. *BMC Infect Dis.* 2016;16(1):1–8. http://dx.doi.org/10.1186/s12879-016-1427-0

[129] Alvarado P, Pérez-Rojas Y, Zambrano EA, Gonzatti MI, Roschman-González A. Improved serodiagnosis of histoplasmosis by use of deglycosylated extracellular released antigens of *Histoplasma capsulatum. J Microbiol Methods.* 2020;175(June):105981. https://doi.org/10.1016/j.mimet.2020.105981

[130] Pine L, Boone CJ, McLaughlin D. Antigenic Properties of the Cell Wall and Other Fractions of the Yeast Form of *Histoplasma capsulatum. J Bacteriol.* 1966;91(6):2158–68.

[131] Guimarães AJ, Pizzini CV, Almeida MDA, Peralta JM, Nosanchuk JD, Zancope-Oliveira RM. Evaluation of an enzyme-linked immunosorbent assay using purified, deglycosylated histoplasmin for different clinical manifestations of histoplasmosis. *Microbiol Res (Pavia).* 2010;1(1):7–14.

[132] Martínez-Gamboa A, Niembro-Ortega MD, Torres-González P, Santiago-Cruz J, Velázquez-Zavala NG, Rangel-Cordero A, Crabtree-Ramírez B, Gamboa-Domínguez A, Reyes-Gutiérrez E, Reyes-Terán G, Lozano-Fernandez VH, Ahumada-Topete VH, Martínez-Ayala P, Manríquez-Reyes M, Ramírez-Hinojosa

JP, Rodríguez-Zulueta P, Hernández-León C, Ruíz-Quiñones J, Rivera-Martínez NE, Chaparro-Sánchez A, Andrade-Villanueva J, González-Hernández LA, Cruz-Martínez S, Flores-Barrientos O, Gaytán-Martínez JE, Magaña-Aquino M, Cervantes-Sánchez A, Olivas-Martínez A, Araujo-Meléndez J, Del Rocío Reyes-Montes M, Duarte-Escalante E, Frías-De León MG, Ramírez JA, Taylor ML, de León-Garduño AP, Sifuentes-Osornio J. Diagnostic accuracy of antigen detection in urine and molecular assays testing in different clinical samples for the diagnosis of progressive disseminated histoplasmosis in patients living with hiv/aids: A prospective multicenter study in Mexico. *PLoS Negl Trop Dis.* 2021;15(3):1–26.

[133] Wheat LJ, Kohler RB, Tewari RP. Diagnosis of disseminated histoplasmosis by detection of *Histoplasma capsulatum* antigen in serum and urine specimens. *New Engl J Med.* 1986;314(2):83–8.

[134] Zimmerman SE, Connolly Stringfield P, Wheat LJ, French MLV, Kohler RB. Comparison of Sandwich Solid-Phase Radioimmunoassay and Two Enzyme-Linked Immunosorbent Assays for Detection of *Histoplasma capsulatum* Polysaccharide Antigen. *J Infect Dis.* 1989;160(4):678–85.

[135] Durkin MM, Connolly PA, Wheat LJ. Comparison of radioimmunoassay and enzyme-linked immunoassay methods for detection of *Histoplasma capsulatum* var. *capsulatum* Antigen. *J Clin Microbiol.* 1997;35(9):2252–5.

[136] Wheat LJ, Connolly P, Durkin M, Book BK, Tector AJ, Fridell J, Pescovitz MD. False-positive *Histoplasma* antigenemia caused by antithymocyte globulin antibodies. *Transpl Infect Dis.* 2004;6(1):23–7.

[137] Wheat LJ, Connolly PA, Durkin M, Book BK, Pescovitz MD. Elimination of false-positive *Histoplasma* antigenemia caused by human anti-rabbit antibodies in the second-generation *Histoplasma* antigen assay. *Transpl Infect Dis.* 2006;8(1):219–21.

[138] Wheat LJ, Witt J, Durkin M, Connolly P. Reduction in false antigenemia in the second generation *Histoplasma* antigen assay. *Med Mycol.* 2007;45(2):169–71.

[139] Connolly PA, Durkin MM, LeMonte AM, Hackett EJ, Wheat LJ. Detection of *Histoplasma* antigen by a quantitative enzyme immunoassay. *Clin Vaccine Immunol.* 2007;14(12):1587–91.

[140] Swartzentruber S, LeMonte A, Witt J, Fuller D, Davis T, Hage C, Connolly P, Durkin M, Wheat LJ. Improved detection of *Histoplasma* antigenemia following dissociation of immune complexes. *Clin Vaccine Immunol.* 2009;16(3):320–2.

[141] Wheat LJ, Connolly-Stringfield P, Williams B, Connolly K, Blair R, Bartlett M, Durkin M. Diagnosis of histoplasmosis in patients with the acquired immunodeficiency syndrome by detection of *Histoplasma capsulatum* polysaccharide antigen in bronchoalveolar lavage fluid. *Am Rev Respir Dis.* 1992; 145(6):1421–4.

[142] Wheat LJ, Connolly P, Blair R, Connolly K, Garringer T, Katz BP. Histoplasmosis relapse in patients with AIDS: Detection using *Histoplasma capsulatum* variety *capsulatum* antigen levels. *Ann Intern Med.* 1991;115(12):936–41.

[143] Gutierrez ME, Canton A, Connolly P, Zarnowski R, Wheat LJ. Detection of *Histoplasma capsulatum* antigen in Panamanian patients with disseminated histoplasmosis and AIDS. *Clin Vaccine Immunol.* 2008;15(4):681–3.

[144] Wheat LJ, Garringer T, Brizendine E, Connolly P. Diagnosis of histoplasmosis by antigen detection based upon experience at the histoplasmosis reference laboratory. *Diagn Microbiol Infect Dis.* 2002;43(1):29–37.

[145] Assi M, Lakkis IE, Wheat LJ. Cross-reactivity in the *Histoplasma* antigen enzyme immunoassay caused by sporotrichosis. *Clin Vaccine Immunol.* 2011 Oct;18(10):1781–2.

[146] Wheat LJ, Connolly P, Haddad N, Le Monte A, Brizendine E, Hafner R. Antigen clearance during treatment of disseminated histoplasmosis with itraconazole versus fluconazole in patients with AIDS. *Antimicrob Agents Chemother.* 2002;46(1):248–50.

[147] Egan L, Connolly PA, Fuller D, Davis TE, Witt J 3rd, Knox KS, Hage CA, Wheat LJ.Detection of *Histoplasma capsulatum* antigenuria by ultrafiltration of samples with false-negative results. *Clin Vaccine Immunol.* 2008;15(4):726–8.

[148] Cáceres DH, Gómez BL, Tobón AM, Chiller TM, Lindsley MD. Evaluation of a *Histoplasma* antigen lateral flow assay for the rapid diagnosis of progressive disseminated histoplasmosis in Colombian patients with AIDS. *Mycoses. 2020;63(2):139–44.*

[149] Abdallah W, Myint T, LaRue R, Minderman M, Gunn S, Wheat LJ, Hage CA. Diagnosis of Histoplasmosis Using the MVista *Histoplasma* Galactomannan Antigen Qualitative Lateral Flow–Based Immunoassay: A Multicenter Study. *Open Forum Infect Dis.* 2021 Sep 1;8(9):1–32. Available from: https:///doi/10.1093/ofid/ofab454/6360396

[150] Cáceres DH, Gómez BL, Tobón ÁM, Minderman M, Bridges N, Chiller T, Lindsley MD. Validation and Concordance Analysis of a New Lateral Flow Assay for Detection of *Histoplasma* Antigen in Urine. *J Fungi.* 2021 Sep 24;7(10):799.

[151] Lindsley MD, Holland HL, Bragg SL, Hurst SF, Wannemuehler KA, Morrison CJ. Production and evaluation of reagents for detection of *Histoplasma capsulatum* antigenuria by enzyme immunoassay. *Clin Vaccine Immunol.* 2007;14(6):700–9.

[152] Scheel CM, Samayoa B, Herrera A, Lindsley MD, Benjamin L, Reed Y, Hart J, Lima S, Rivera BE, Raxcaco G, Chiller T, Arathoon E, Gómez BL. Development and evaluation of an enzyme-linked immunosorbent assay to detect *Histoplasma capsulatum* antigenuria in immunocompromised patients. *Clin Vaccine Immunol.* 2009;16(6):852–8.

[153] Caceres DH, Scheel CM, Tobón AM, Ahlquist Cleveland A, Restrepo A, Brandt ME, Chiller T, Gómez BL. Validation of an enzyme-linked immunosorbent assay that detects *Histoplasma capsulatum* antigenuria in colombian patients with AIDS for diagnosis and follow-up during therapy. *Clin Vaccine Immunol.* 2014;21(9):1364–8.

[154] Hoffmann ER, Daboit TC, Paskulin DD, Monteiro AA, Falci DR, Linhares T, Flores JM, Goldani LZ, de Melo MG, Behar PR, Pasqualotto AC. Disseminated histoplasmosis and AIDS: a prospective and multicentre study to evaluate the performance of different diagnostic tests. *Mycoses.* 2017;60(1):20–4.

[155] Cloud JL, Bauman SK, Neary BP, Ludwig KG, Ashwood ER. Performance characteristics of a polyclonal enzyme immunoassay for the quantitation of

Histoplasma antigen in human urine samples. *Am J Clin Pathol.* 2007;128(1):18–22.

[156] LeMonte A, Egan L, Connolly P, Durkin M, Wheat LJ. Evaluation of the IMMY ALPHA *Histoplasma* antigen enzyme immunoassay for diagnosis of histoplasmosis marked by antigenuria. *Clin Vaccine Immunol.* 2007;14(6):802–3.

[157] Zhang X, Gibson B, Daly TM. Evaluation of commercially available reagents for diagnosis of Histoplasmosis infection in Immunocompromised patients. *J Clin Microbiol.* 2013;51(12):4095–101.

[158] Zhang C, Lei GS, Lee CH, Hage CA. Evaluation of two new enzyme immunoassay reagents for diagnosis of histoplasmosis in a cohort of clinically characterized patients. *Med Mycol.* 2015;53(8):868–73.

[159] Torres-González P, Niembro-Ortega MD, Martínez-Gamboa A, Ahumada-Topete VH, Andrade-Villanueva J, Araujo-Meléndez J, Chaparro-Sánchez A, Crabtree-Ramírez B, Cruz-Martínez S, Gamboa-Domínguez A, Flores-Barrientos OI, Gaytán-Martínez JE, González-Hernández LA, Hernández-León C, Lozano-Fernandez VH, Manríquez-Reyes M, Magaña-Aquino M, Martínez-Ayala P, Ramírez-Hinojosa JP, Rangel-Cordero A, Rivera-Martínez NE, Reyes-Gutiérrez E, Reyes-Terán G, Rodríguez-Zulueta P, Ruíz-Quiñones J, Santiago-Cruz J, Velázquez-Zavala NG, Sifuentes-Osornio J, Ponce de León A. Diagnostic accuracy cohort study and clinical value of the *Histoplasma* urine antigen (ALPHA *Histoplasma* EIA) for disseminated histoplasmosis among HIV infected patients: A multicenter study. *PLoS Negl Trop Dis.* 2018;12(11):1–16.

[160] Blan BDS, Poester VR, Basso RP, Benelli JL, Sanchotene KO, Caceres DH, Doherty B, Pasqualotto AC, Xavier MO. Optimization of a commercial *Histoplasma* galactomannan EIA test in a population from an endemic area of histoplasmosis in southern Brazil. *Mycoses.* 2022;

[161] Andreani M, Frola CE, Caceres DH, Canteros CE, Rolón MJ, Chiller T, Guelfand L. Validation of a Lateral Flow Assay for Rapid Diagnosis of Histoplasmosis in Advanced HIV Disease, Buenos Aires, Argentina. *Appl Microbiol.* 2022 Nov 15;2(4):950–5.

[162] Persaud SP, Lawton T, Burnham C-AD, Anderson NW. Comparison of Urine Antigen Assays for the Diagnosis of *Histoplasma capsulatum* Infection. *J Appl Lab Med.* 2019 Nov;4(3):370–82.

[163] Cáceres DH, Gómez BL, Tobón ÁM, Chiller TM, Lindsley MD. Evaluation of OIDx *Histoplasma* Urinary Antigen EIA. *Mycopathologia.* 2022 Feb 1;187 (1):129–31.

[164] Ocansey BK, Otoo B, Asamoah I, Ganu V, Berko KP, Oladele O, Amankwa EA, Opoku-Asare B, Agyei M, George L, Kotey FCN, Kosmidis C, Puplampu P, Opintan JA, Denning DW. Cryptococcal and *Histoplasma* Antigen Screening among People with Human Immunodeficiency Virus in Ghana and Comparative Analysis of OIDx *Histoplasma* Lateral Flow Assay and IMMY *Histoplasma* Enzyme Immunoassay. *Open Forum Infect Dis.* 2022 Jul 1;9(7).

[165] Kuate MPN, Abessolo Abessolo H, Denning DW, Stone NR, Ndip RN, Cáceres DH. Evaluation of OIDx *Histoplasma* Urinary Antigen EIA. *Ther Adv Infect Dis.* 2022 Feb 1;9(1):129–31.

[166] Falci DR, Monteiro AA, Braz Caurio CF, Magalhães TCO, Xavier MO, Basso RP, Melo M, Schwarzbold AV, Ferreira PRA, Vidal JE, Marochi JP, Godoy CSM, Soares RBA, Paste A, Bay MB, Pereira-Chiccola VL, Damasceno LS, Leitão TDMJS, Pasqualotto AC. Histoplasmosis, An Underdiagnosed Disease Affecting People Living with HIV/AIDS in Brazil: Results of a Multicenter Prospective Cohort Study Using Both Classical Mycology Tests and *Histoplasma* Urine Antigen Detection. *Open Forum Infect Dis.* 2019;6(4).

[167] Chandrashekar R, Curtis KC, Rawot BW, Kobayashi GS, Weil GJ. Molecular cloning and characterization of a recombinant *Histoplasma capsulatum* antigen for antibody-based diagnosis of human histoplasmosis. *J Clin Microbiol.* 1997;35(5):1071–6.

[168] Toyotome T, Watanabe A, Ochiai E, Kamei K. N-acetylated α-linked acidic dipeptidase is identified as an antigen of *Histoplasma capsulatum*. *Biochem Biophys Res Commun.* 2015;458(3):483–7.

[169] Holbrook ED, Kemski MM, Richer SM, Wheat LJ, Rappleye CA. Glycosylation and immunoreactivity of the *Histoplasma capsulatum* Cfp4 yeast-phase exoantigen. *Infect Immun.* 2014;82(10):4414–25.

[170] Abreu Almeida M, Almeida-Paes R, Guimarães AJ, Valente RH, de Almeida Soares CM, Zancopé-Oliveira RM. Immunoproteomics Reveals Pathogen's Antigens Involved in *Homo sapiens–Histoplasma capsulatum* Interaction and Specific Linear B-Cell Epitopes in Histoplasmosis. *Front Cell Infect Microbiol.* 2020 Oct 29;10.

[171] Toscanini MA, Maglio DG, Capece P, Posse G, Iovannitti CA, Nusblat AD, Cuestas ML. *Histoplasma capsulatum* 100-kilodalton antigen: recombinant production, characterization, and evaluation of its possible application in the diagnosis of histoplasmosis. *Appl Microbiol Biotechnol.* 2020;104(13):5861–5872.

[172] Gomez BL, Figueroa JI, Hamilton AJ, Ortiz BL, Robledo MA, Restrepo A, Hay RJ. Development of a novel antigen detection test for histoplasmosis. *J Clin Microbiol.* 1997;35(10):2618–22.

[173] Gómez BL, Figueroa JI, Hamilton AJ, Diez S, Rojas M, Tobón A, Restrepo A, Hay RJ. Detection of the 70-kilodalton *Histoplasma capsulatum* antigen in serum of histoplasmosis patients: Correlation between antigenemia and therapy during follow-up. *J Clin Microbiol.* 1999;37(3):675–80.

[174] Kushnir MM, Crockett DK, Cloud JL, Ashwood ER, Rockwood AL. Exploratory study of proteins in urine of patients with *histoplasma* antigenuria. *J Chromatogr B Anal Technol Biomed Life Sci.* 2012;883–884:147–54.

[175] Crockett DK, Kushnir MM, Cloud JL, Ashwood ER, Rockwood AL. Identification of *Histoplasma* -specific peptides in human urine. *Int J Pept.* 2012;2012(621329).

[176] Gómez BL. Molecular diagnosis of endemic and invasive mycoses: Advances and challenges. *Rev Iberoam Micol.* 2014;31(1):35–41.

[177] Bialek R, Feucht A, Aepinus C, Robertson VJ, Hohle R. Evaluation of two nested PCR assays for detection of *Histoplasma capsulatum* DNA in human tissue. *J Clin Microbiol.* 2002;40(5):1644–7.

[178] Collela MT, Mata S, Hartung C, Pérez C, Roselló A, Olaizola C, Fernandez C, Magaldi S, Toro F. Detection of *Histoplasma capsulatum* by Nested-PCR in Clinical Specimens. *Kasmera.* 2007;35(2):156–63.

[179] Zatti MDS, Arantes TD, Fernandes JAL, Bay MB, Milan EP, Naliato GFS, Theodoro RC. Loop-mediated Isothermal Amplification and nested PCR of the Internal Transcribed Spacer (ITS) for *Histoplasma capsulatum* detection. *PLoS Negl Trop Dis.* 2019;13(8):1–20.

[180] Toranzo AI, Tiraboschi IN, Fernández N, Ibarra-Camou B, Rivas MC, Lee W, Davel G, Canteros CE. Diagnóstico molecular de histoplasmosis humana en muestras de sangre entera. *Rev Argent Microbiol.* 2009;41(1):20–6.

[181] Muñoz C, Cano L, Gonzalez A. Detection and identification of the fungal pathogen *Histoplasma capsulatum* : from conventional to molecular methods. *Infection.* 2010;14(S2):145–58.

[182] Dantas KC, De Freitas RS, da Silva MV, Criado PR, Luiz O do C, Vicentini AP. Comparison of diagnostic methods to detect *Histoplasma capsulatum* in serum and blood samples from AIDS patients. *PLoS One.* 2018;13(1):1–12.

[183] Frías De León MG, López GA, Taylor ML, Altamirano GA, Del Rocío Reyes-Montes M. Development of specific sequence-characterized amplified region markers for detecting *Histoplasma capsulatum* in clinical and environmental samples. *J Clin Microbiol.* 2012;50(3):673–9.

[184] Bracca A, Tosello ME, Girardini JE, Amigot SL, Gomez C, Serra E. Molecular detection of *Histoplasma capsulatum* var. *capsulatum* in human clinical samples. *J Clin Microbiol.* 2003;41(4):1753–5.

[185] Guedes HL, Guimarães AJ, Muniz Mde M, Pizzini CV, Hamilton AJ, Peralta JM, Deepe GS Jr, Zancopé-Oliveira RM. PCR assay for identification of *Histoplasma capsulatum* based on the nucleotide sequence of the M antigen. *J Clin Microbiol.* 2003;41(2):535–9.

[186] Tang YW, Li H, Durkin MM, Sefers SE, Meng S, Connolly PA, Stratton CW, Wheat LJ. Urine polymerase chain reaction is not as sensitive as urine antigen for the diagnosis of disseminated histoplasmosis. *Diagn Microbiol Infect Dis.* 2006;54(4):283–7.

[187] López LF, Muñoz CO, Cáceres DH, Tobón ÁM, Loparev V, Clay O, Chiller T, Litvintseva A, Gade L, González Á, Gómez BL. Standardization and validation of real time PCR assays for the diagnosis of histoplasmosis using three molecular targets in an animal model. *PLoS One.* 2017;12(12):1–15.

[188] Martagon-Villamil J, Shrestha N, Sholtis M, Isada CM, Hall GS, Bryne T, Lodge BA, Reller LB, Procop GW. Identification of *Histoplasma capsulatum* from culture extracts by Real-Time PCR. *J Clin Microbiol.* 2003;41(3):1295–8.

[189] Buitrago MJ, Berenguer J, Mellado E, Rodríguez-Tudela JL, Cuenca-Estrella M. Detection of imported histoplasmosis in serum of HIV-infected patients using a real-time PCR-based assay. *Eur J Clin Microbiol Infect Dis.* 2006;25(10):665–8.

[190] Simon S, Veron V, Boukhari R, Blanchet D, Aznar C. Detection of *Histoplasma capsulatum* DNA in human samples by real-time polymerase chain reaction. *Diagn Microbiol Infect Dis.* 2010;66(3):268–73.

[191] Gago S, Esteban C, Valero C, Zaragoza Ó, De La Bellacasa JP, Buitrago MJ. A multiplex real-time PCR assay for identification of *Pneumocystis jirovecii*, *Histoplasma capsulatum*, and *Cryptococcus neoformans/Cryptococcus gattii* in samples from AIDS patients with opportunistic pneumonia. *J Clin Microbiol.* 2014;52(4):1168–76.

[192] Frickmann H, Künne C, Hagen RM, Podbielski A, Normann J, Poppert S, Looso M, Kreikemeyer B. Next-generation sequencing for hypothesis-free genomic detection of invasive tropical infections in poly-microbially contaminated, formalin-fixed, paraffin-embedded tissue samples - A proof-of-principle assessment. *BMC Microbiol.* 2019;19(1):1–19.

[193] McTaggart LR, Copeland JK, Surendra A, Wang PW, Husain S, Coburn B, Guttman DS, Kus JV. Mycobiome sequencing and analysis applied to fungal community profiling of the lower respiratory tract during fungal pathogenesis. *Front Microbiol.* 2019;10(MAR):1–12.

[194] Zhang HC, Zhang QR, Ai JW, Cui P, Wu HL, Zhang WH, Wang T. The role of bone marrow metagenomics next-generation sequencing to differential diagnosis among visceral leishmaniasis, histoplasmosis, and talaromycosis marneffei. *Int J Lab Hematol.* 2020;42(2):e52–4.

[195] Becherer L, Borst N, Bakheit M, Frischmann S, Zengerle R, Von Stetten F. Loop-mediated isothermal amplification (LAMP)-review and classification of methods for sequence-specific detection. *Anal Methods.* 2020 Feb 14;12(6):717–46.

[196] Scheel CM, Zhou Y, Theodoro RC, Abrams B, Balajee SA, Litvintseva AP. Development of a loop-mediated isothermal amplification method for detection of *Histoplasma capsulatum* DNA in clinical samples. *J Clin Microbiol.* 2014;52(2):483–8.

[197] Furuie JL, Sun J, do Nascimento MM, Gomes RR, Waculicz-Andrade CE, Sessegolo GC, Rodrigues AM, Galvão-Dias MA, de Camargo ZP, Queiroz-Telles F, Najafzadeh MJ, de Hoog SG, Vicente VA. Molecular identification of *Histoplasma capsulatum* using rolling circle amplification. *Mycoses.* 2016;59(1):12–9.

[198] Elías NA, Cuestas ML, Sandoval M, Poblete G, Lopez-Daneri G, Jewtuchowicz V, Iovannitti C, Mujica MT. Rapid identification of *Histoplasma capsulatum* directly from cultures by multiplex PCR. *Mycopathologia.* 2012;174(5–6):451–6.

[199] Emmons CW. Histoplasmosis: animal reservoirs and other sources in nature of pathogenic fungus, *Histoplasma. Am J Public Heal Nations Heal.* 1950;40 (4):436–40.

[200] Seyedmousavi S, Bosco SMG, de Hoog S, Ebel F, Elad D, Gomes RR, Jacobsen ID, Jensen HE, Martel A, Mignon B, Pasmans F, Piecková E, Rodrigues AM, Singh K, Vicente VA, Wibbelt G, Wiederhold NP, Guillot J. Fungal infections in animals: a patchwork of different situations. *Med Mycol.* 2018;56(supl 1):S165-S187.

[201] Hoff GL, Bigler WJ. The role of bats in the propagation and spread of histoplasmosis: a review. *J Wildl Dis.* 1981;17(2):191–6.

[202] Rw M, Rt H. Experimental avian histoplasmosis. *Am J Vet Res.* 1955.

[203] Moreira LM, Meyer W, Chame M, Brandão ML, Vivoni AM, Portugal J, Wanke B, Trilles L. Molecular Detection of *Histoplasma capsulatum* in Antarctica. *Emerg Infect Dis.* 2022 Oct;28(10):2100–4.

[204] Mitchell M, Stark DR. Disseminated canine histoplasmosis: a clinical survey of 24 cases in Texas. *Can Vet J = La Rev Vet Can.* 1980 Mar;21(3):95–100.

[205] Clinkenbeard KD, Cowell RL, Tyler RD. Disseminated histoplasmosis in dogs: 12 cases (1981-1986). *J Am Vet Med Assoc.* 1987 Dec 1;193(11):1443–7.

[206] Hodges RD, Legendre AM, Adams LG, Willard MD, Pitts RP, Monce K, Needels CC, Ward H. Itraconazole for the Treatment of Histoplasmosis in Cats. *J Vet Intern Med.* 1994 Nov;8(6):409–13.

[207] Davies C, Troy G. Deep mycotic infections in cats. *J Am Anim Hosp Assoc.* 1996 Sep 1;32(5):380–91.

[208] Selby LA, Becker SV, Hayes HW. Epidemiologic risk factors associated with canine systemic mucoses. *Am J Epidemiol.* 1981 Feb;113(2):133–9.

[209] Cole CR, Farrell RL, Chamberlain DM, Prior JA, Saslaw S. Histoplasmosis in animals. *J Am Vet Med Assoc.* 1953;122(915):471–3.

[210] Rowley DA, Haberman RT, Emmons CW. Histoplasmosis: pathologic studies of fifty cars and fifty dogs from Loudoun County, Virginia. *J Infect Dis.* 1954;95(1):98–108.

[211] Fattal RL, Shwartz J, Straub S. Isolation of *Histoplasma capsulatum* from lymph nodes of spontaneously infected dofs. *Am J Clin Pathol.* 1961;36:119–24.

[212] Turner C, Smith C, Furcolow ML. The efficiency of serologic and cultural methods in the detection of infection with *Histoplasma* and *Blastomyces* in mongrel dogs. *Sabouraudia J Med Vet Mycol.* 1972;10(1):1–5.

[213] Farrell RL, Cole CR, Prior JA, Saslaw S. Experimental histoplasmosis, I. Methods for production of histoplasmosis in dogs. *Proc Soc Exp Biol Med.* 1953;84(1):51–4.

[214] Hall AD. An equine abortion due to histoplasmosis. *Vet Med Small Anim Clin* 1979 Feb;74(2):200–1.

[215] Saunders JR, Matthiesen RJ, Kaplan W. Abortion due to histoplasmosis in a mare. *J Am Vet Med Assoc.* 1983;183(10):1097–9.

[216] Rezabek GB, Donahue JM, Giles RC, Petrites-Murphy MB, Poonacha KB, Rooney JR, Smith BJ, Swerczek TW, Tramontin RR. Histoplasmosis in horses. *J Comp Pathol.* 1993 Jul;109(1):47–55.

[217] Cook AK, Cunningham LY, Cowell AK, Wheat LJ. Clinical evaluation of urine *Histoplasma capsulatum* antigen measurement in cats with suspected disseminated histoplasmosis. *J Feline Med Surg.* 2012;14(8):512–5.

[218] Cunningham L, Cook A, Hanzlicek A, Harkin K, Wheat J, Goad C, Kirsch E. Sensitivity and specificity of *Histoplasma* antigen detection by enzyme immunoassay. *J Am Anim Hosp Assoc.* 2015;51(5):306–10.

[219] Hanzlicek AS, Meinkoth JH, Renschler JS, Goad C, Wheat LJ. Antigen Concentrations as an Indicator of Clinical Remission and Disease Relapse in Cats with Histoplasmosis. *J Vet Intern Med.* 2016;30(4):1065–73.

[220] Fielder SE, Meinkoth JH, Rizzi TE, Hanzlicek AS, Hallman RM. Feline histoplasmosis presenting with bone and joint involvement: clinical and diagnostic findings in 25 cats. *J Feline Med Surg.* 2019;21(10):887–92.

[221] Rothenburg L, Hanzlicek AS, Payton ME. A monoclonal antibody-based urine *Histoplasma* antigen enzyme immunoassay (IMMY®) for the diagnosis of histoplasmosis in cats. *J Vet Intern Med.* 2019;33(2):603–10.

[222] McGill JE, Hanzlicek AS, Kukanich KS, Norsworthy GD, Cook AK. Pretreatment *Histoplasma capsulatum* urine enzymatic immunoassay concentrations do not correlate with outcome but may be influenced by renal function in cats with histoplasmosis. *J Feline Med Surg.* 2018;20(12):1177–9.

[223] MiraVista Veterinary Diagnostics. *Histoplasmosis in Veterinary Medicine 2020.* 2020 [cited 2022 Dec 14]. Available from: https://miravistavets.com/fungal-diseases/histoplasma/review-histoplasmosis/

[224] Adenis AA, Valdes A, Cropet C, McCotter OZ, Derado G, Couppie P, Chiller T, Nacher M. Burden of HIV-associated histoplasmosis compared with tuberculosis in Latin America: a modelling study. *Lancet Infect Dis.* 2018;18(10):1150–9.

[225] WHO. *Second WHO Model List of Essential In Vitro Diagnostics.* 2019 [cited 2020 Jul 2]. Available from: https://www.who.int/medical_devices/publications/Standalone_document_v8.pdf?ua=1

Chapter 5

Radiological Findings in Histoplasmosis

Mikael Mir[1,*], BA
Taylor Benedict[1], BS
Sydney Boike[1], BS
Noura Attallah[2], MD
Jessica Sheehy[3], PA
Eric Gomez Urena[3], MD
and Syed Anjum Khan[2], MD

[1]Department of Medicine; University of Minnesota Medical School, Minneapolis, Minnesota, USA
[2]Critical Care Medicine, Mayo Clinic Health System, Mankato, Minnesota, USA
[3]Department of Infectious Disease, Mayo Clinic Health System, Mankato, Minnesota, USA

Abstract

Histoplasmosis is a fungal infection that can manifest itself in various forms, including acute and chronic pulmonary histoplasmosis, and disseminated or extrapulmonary histoplasmosis. Accurate diagnosis of histoplasmosis infections is aided by imaging studies such as chest radiography and computed tomography (CT). Consideration of the diverse ways in which histoplasmosis manifests on imaging is important to the management, especially considering the extra-pulmonary and disseminated forms of the disease. The goal of this chapter is to provide knowledge regarding the imaging findings and provide insight into how these findings can aid in diagnosis and management. Further research and continued education on the imaging findings associated with

* Corresponding Author's Email: mir00013@umn.edu.

In: Histoplasmosis
Editors: Salim Surani, Syed Anjum Khan and Reena Shah
ISBN: 979-8-89113-129-3

histoplasmosis will be important in ensuring accurate and prompt diagnosis and effective treatment.

Keywords: computed tomography, histoplasmosis, histoplasmoma, interstitial infiltrates, hilar lymphadenopathy, cavitation, hepatomegaly, splenomegaly, Addison's disease, acute peritoneal histoplasmosis

Introduction

Histoplasmosis is a type of fungal infection due to the inhalation of spores from the soil contaminated with the *Histoplasma capsulatum* fungus. This infection can manifest in various forms, including acute pulmonary histoplasmosis, chronic pulmonary histoplasmosis, and extrapulmonary (disseminated) histoplasmosis, each with its own characteristic symptoms and imaging findings. Imaging studies, such as chest radiography, computed tomography (CT) scans, and other modalities, are crucial in diagnosing and managing histoplasmosis. This chapter will provide a comprehensive overview of the imaging findings seen in all forms of histoplasmosis, including acute pulmonary histoplasmosis, chronic pulmonary histoplasmosis, and disseminated or extrapulmonary histoplasmosis. This section aims to increase understanding of the imaging findings associated with histoplasmosis and provide insight into how these findings can aid in diagnosing and managing this complex and sometimes difficult-to-diagnose infection.

Acute Pulmonary Histoplasmosis

The most common subtype of histoplasmosis presentation is acute pulmonary histoplasmosis, with around 10% of people exposed developing this pathologic subtype [1]. This presentation is known to be the most benign, typically manifesting as a lack of significant symptomology in most patients [2], involving fever, dry cough, and shortness of breath [1, 2]. However, this can progress into more serious disease pathways, including mediastinal fibrosis, histoplasmoma, and broncholithiasis, though this is considered rare [2]. Most commonly, acute pulmonary histoplasmosis clinically presents in an *immunocompetent* host who has been exposed to *H. capsulatum*. The incubation period is typically 7-21 days, and individuals may then develop mild flu-like symptoms, though it is important to note that some individuals will not have any symptoms [2]. Patients at the extremes of age, immunocompromised patients, and those exposed to a large amount of inoculum are more likely to have a symptomatic or severe disease course [3].

Imaging in those with acute pulmonary histoplasmosis is well-established and can be utilized in making a confident diagnosis. On radiography, one can observe pneumonitis patches with interstitial infiltrate areas (Figure 1) [2, 3]. These images will often also have hilar or mediastinal lymphadenopathy [2]. On computed tomography scanning (CT), commonly observed phenomena include enlarged mediastinal and hilar lymph nodes as well as solitary or multiple pulmonary nodules (Figure 2) [4]. Additionally, in those who have inhaled a large amount of inoculum, one may observe significant reticulonodular infiltrates with nodules [5]. As the disease process begins to clear, calcifications may be seen on imaging, leading to what is known as a "buckshot" appearance [5]. Some have also noted a "snowstorm" appearance on CT [6], depicted by the lymphadenopathy previously discussed and included in Figure 3.

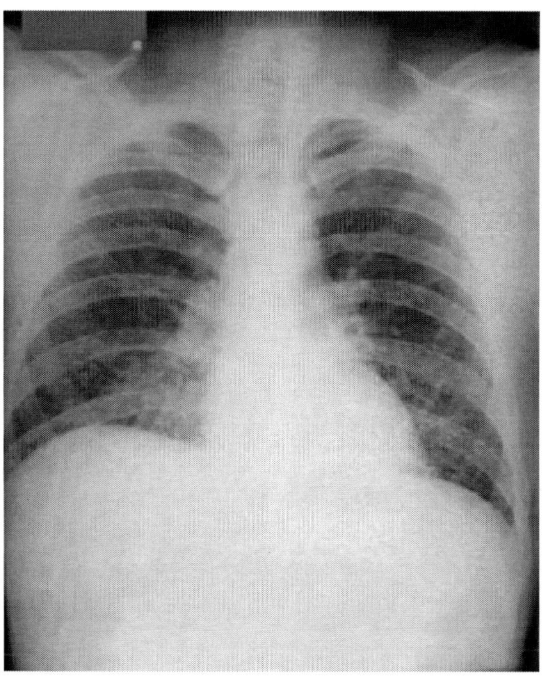

Figure 1. An anteroposterior (AP) chest x-ray of an individual with acute pulmonary histoplasmosis with diffuse bilateral pulmonary infiltrates caused by Histoplasma capsulatum [3]. 3 Image from the CDC and M. Renz. https://phil.cdc.gov/details.aspx?pid=3954.

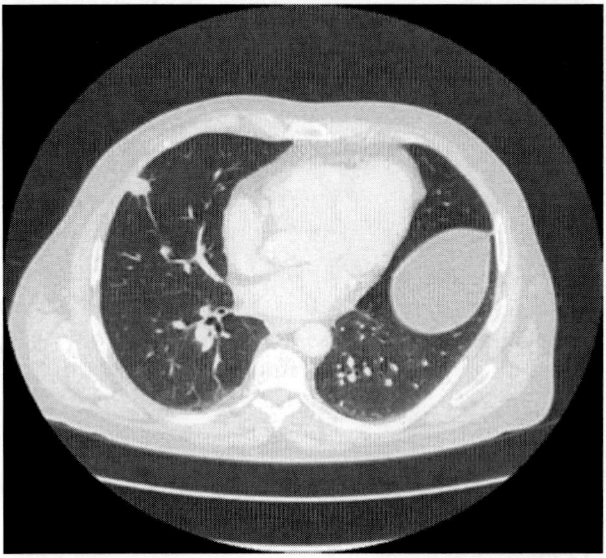

Figure 2. Histoplasmoma. Transaxial CT showing a lung nodule that was concerning for a neoplastic process. On lung biopsy noted to have yeast-like organisms consistent with Histoplasma.

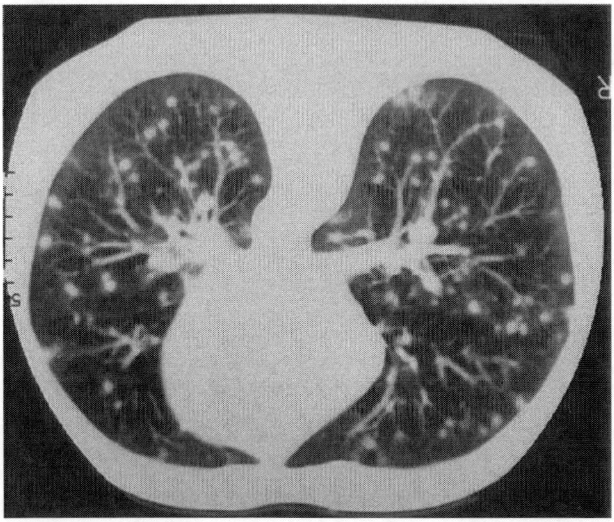

Figure 3. A transaxial computed tomography (CT) scan of the thoracic cavity from the CDC. Showing the classic snowstorm appearance of both the left and right lung fields caused by the H. capsulatum fungus [6]. Image from CDC. https://phil.cdc.gov/Details.aspx?pid=472.

Chronic Pulmonary Histoplasmosis

Chronic pulmonary histoplasmosis (CPH) is a rare occurrence among those infected with histoplasmosis. In 1976, Goodwin et al., defined chronic pulmonary histoplasmosis infection as a complication of an acute infection characterized by persistent cavitation, low-grade chronic disease, and a predisposition to developing pulmonary fibrosis and often progressive pulmonary insufficiency [7]. A more recent retrospective case series defined CPH based on the duration of clinical symptoms and explicit confirmation of the diagnosis irrespective of the radiological results [8]. One review noted two outbreaks of histoplasmosis in the United States and found that amongst those with a diagnosed acute histoplasmosis infection, only 8% developed CPH. Within that group, CPH can be further divided into either cavitary chronic pulmonary histoplasmosis (CCPH) or non-cavitary chronic pulmonary histoplasmosis (NCPH) [2]. Due to a tendency of the cavitations to appear in the upper lobes of the lungs, CCPH is often said to be similar to a reactivated tuberculosis infection which can lead to CCPH being misidentified on imaging as TB [2, 9, 10].

As more teams have studied CPH, it has been realized that the rate of cavitation vs. non-cavitation varies, with more recent studies finding lower cavitation rates than previously documented. Initial studies claimed that cavitary disease rates in CPH have been as high as 87% [8, 9]. This is partly due to the criteria used to discriminate between CCPH and NCPH. In the past, studies defined CPH patients as those with cavitary lesions on chest x-ray or those suspected to have tuberculosis, leading to a higher occurrence of CCPH in their study groups. Still, with modern studies basing the inclusion criteria on the length of chronicity of symptoms for the patient, the rate of cavitation has shown to be much less at 39-40% [8, 11]. Some studies have found cavitation rates to be as low as 28% and 30% [8, 9].

The Goodwin et al., article was also able to find several characteristics that were common to CPH. These included an interstitial infiltrate, necrotic component, progressive enlargement of the cavity, spillover phenomenon, early nodular infiltrate, peribronchial streaking, emphysema, cavity formation, persistent cavitation, "marching" cavities, and secondary infection with aspergillus - though this is typically in the Tennessee area [7]. The necrotic component, which, when present, appears early in the disease course and can be seen as dense pneumonic shadows situated within the area of interstitial pneumonitis, sometimes as single central areas but often as scattered focal lesions [7]. Upper lobe cavitation, especially on the right, is another prevalent finding in CPH (Figure 4) [2, 9, 11]. Hilar lymphadenopathy, a common finding in acute pulmonary disease, tends to be rare in CPH (2.2%) [9, 12].

These characteristics are supported in other studies, which found that the most common findings on chest X-rays were: nodules (74%), infiltrates (61%), lymphadenopathy (41%), fibrosis (37%), thickened pleura (35%), volume loss (24%), hyperinflation/emphysema (15%), atelectasis (11%), and bronchiectasis (7%) [8]. Additionally, on CT images, common findings include nodules (93%), lymphadenopathy (67%), infiltrate (60%), cavitary disease (30%), emphysema (23%), bronchiectasis (10%), and bronchopleural fistula (3%) [8]. These results demonstrate that nodules were the most common finding on both chest x-ray and CT within this patient set.

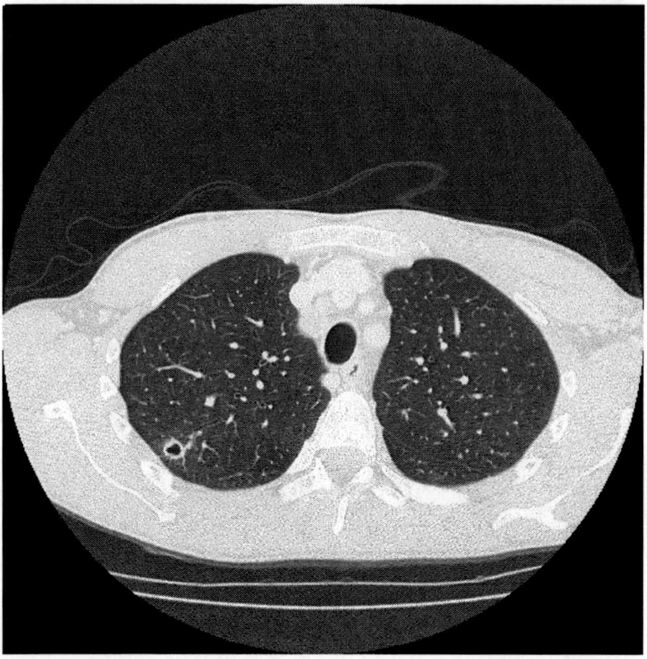

Figure 4. Right upper lobe cavitation in a patient with chronic pulmonary histoplasmosis three months into treatment.

Previous literature defined CPH as having cavitation on imaging in the presence of preexisting lung diseases such as emphysema and low-grade chronic illness. Newer studies are finding that basing the diagnosis of CPH upon the presence of cavitation on imaging is an insufficient metric. New data suggest that CCPH is less common than NCPH and that the first signs of chronic pulmonary histoplasmosis are nodules and pulmonary infiltrates. According to previous case studies by Wheat et al., upper lobe cavitation is a highly associated finding in CPH, with nearly 100% of patients showing upper lobe cavities, with the majority involving the right side (84%) [9]. However, this should not be a defining radiographic characteristic of CPH due to the increasing evidence that cavitation is not evident in even half of CPH cases, and upper lobe cavitations can be associated with other conditions such as tuberculosis and aspergillosis [9]. Rather, the Kennedy and Limper classification style of prioritizing the presence of nodules on both CT and chest x-ray in the light of positive cultures or *H. capsulatum* antibody titers and the presence of symptoms suggestive of pulmonary histoplasmosis for six or more weeks allows a more accurate count of CPH while still including those with and without cavitation.

Disseminated and Extrapulmonary Histoplasmosis

Most patients with *H. capsulatum infection* develop asymptomatic hematogenous dissemination within the reticuloendothelial system due to the organism remaining inside infected macrophages. Nonspecific symptoms such as fever, anorexia, malaise, and weight loss are all symptoms of disseminated histoplasmosis [13]. Radiographs of the chest may show diffuse reticulonodular infiltrates, or they could be varied, nonspecific, or normal [14]. Normal chest radiograph findings do not exclude disseminated histoplasmosis or involvement of the lungs. Some manifestations of disseminated histoplasmosis that can be seen on contrast-enhanced chest computed tomography (CT) include mediastinal lymphadenopathy and bilateral fibrotic lung lesions [15].

Abdominal findings of disseminated histoplasmosis are common in both endemic and non-endemic areas. Similar to chest radiographs, these findings are often nonspecific but warrant consideration of histoplasmosis when found on imaging. Abdominal CT findings include hepatomegaly, splenomegaly, diffuse hypoattenuation of the spleen, enlarging lymph nodes, and bilateral adrenal gland enlargement [16]. In patients with AIDS, a demographic at risk for disseminated or extrapulmonary histoplasmosis, colonic manifestations can be similar to carcinoma. CT in these patients can reveal circumferential thickening of the colonic wall with proximal lymphadenopathy of variable attenuation, and barium enema can show an apple-core pathological pattern in the transverse, descending, and ascending colon [17].

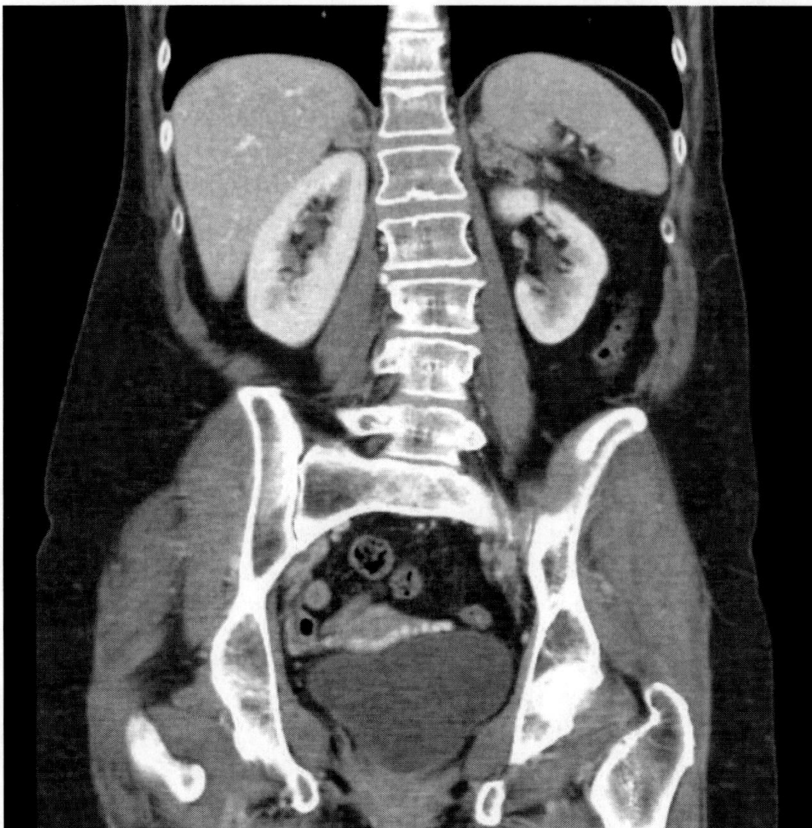

Figure 5a. Bilateral thickening of adrenal glands, hypodense centrally with peripherally enhancing margins. Case courtesy of Francis Fortin, Radiopaedia.org, rID: 68894.24.

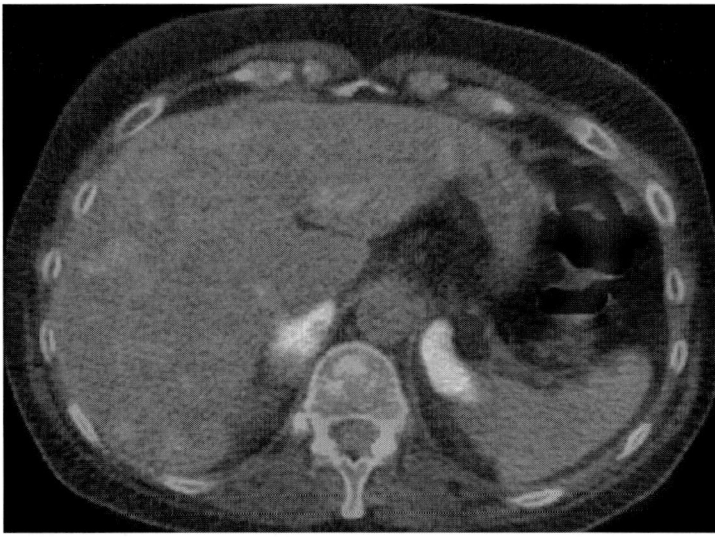

Figure 5b. The adrenal thickening shows high FDG uptake on PET-CT. Case courtesy of Francis Fortin, Radiopaedia.org, rID: 68894.24.

Central nervous system (CNS) involvement can manifest as a disseminated infection or as an isolated local infection [18]. This manifestation occurs due to hematogenous dissemination to the CNS brain and meninges and commonly manifests as chronic meningitis defined by basilar meningeal involvement, which can cause communicating hydrocephalus [13]. In these cases, small ring-enhancing lesions are found on MRI throughout the spinal cord and brain [13]. These lesions can occur with meningitis or as isolated brain lesions with no meningeal involvement. In addition, there are reports of disseminated histoplasmosis brain masses mimicking brain tumors at initial presentation due to altered mental status and focal neurological findings in the patient [19, 20]. MRI often shows an enhancing mass, and patients may or may not present with classic signs and symptoms of meningitis. Only after biopsy or resection can the mass be confirmed to be of histoplasmosis origin. Focal neurological findings often correlate with the lesions seen on MRI, but at other times patients may be entirely asymptomatic [13].

Several unique manifestations of disseminated histoplasmosis are essential to consider. These findings often only occur with disseminated *H. capsulatum* infection and not with other disseminated infections by other fungal organisms [13]. For example, severe destruction of the bilateral adrenal glands due to the condition has been shown to lead to Addison's disease [21]. In these cases, a CT scan can show significantly enlarged adrenal glands, often with central necrosis and dense calcification [21-24]. This manifests as thickened, hypodense adrenal glands with peripherally enhancing margins and high FDG uptake on PET-CT (Figure 5). Other CT findings can be present as minimal enlargement with faint areas of calcium or moderate enlargement with focal low-attenuation lesions. These findings are often bilateral and symmetrical, and the shape of the adrenal glands is usually preserved. Hyponatremia, hyperkalemia, and eosinophilia are typically present, and patients are at risk for adrenal insufficiency, a frequent cause of death in those cases [13].

Some other uncommon manifestations recently described in the literature include acute peritoneal histoplasmosis. Acute peritoneal histoplasmosis has typically affected individuals receiving continuous ambulatory peritoneal dialysis. Acute peritoneal histoplasmosis can also occur in patients undergoing therapy with immunomodulators such as infliximab, and this can mimic ovarian cancer complications. CT findings, in this case, included ascites, diffuse omental caking, and soft tissue stranding across the omentum with no definite peritoneal or ovarian masses [25].

Conclusion

Histoplasmosis is a fungal infection that can manifest in various forms, including acute pulmonary histoplasmosis, chronic pulmonary histoplasmosis, and disseminated or extrapulmonary histoplasmosis. Imaging studies, such as chest radiography, computed tomography (CT) scans, and other modalities, are crucial in diagnosing and managing histoplasmosis. A thorough understanding of the imaging findings associated with each form of histoplasmosis is essential for accurate diagnosis and effective management of this infection. Further research and continued education on the imaging findings associated with histoplasmosis will be important in ensuring accurate and prompt diagnosis and effective treatment.

References

[1] Araúz A. B., Papineni P. Histoplasmosis. *Infect Dis Clin North Am*. 2021;35(2):471-491. doi: https://doi.org/10.1016/j.idc.2021.03.011.

[2] Tobón A. M., Gómez B. L. Pulmonary Histoplasmosis. *Mycopathologia.* 2021;186(5):697-705. doi: https://doi.org/10.1007/s11046-021-00588-4.

[3] Details - *Public Health Image Library* (PHIL). (n.d.). Retrieved January 29, 2023, from https://phil.cdc.gov/details.aspx?pid=3954.

[4] Azar M. M., Hage C. A. Clinical Perspectives in the Diagnosis and Management of Histoplasmosis. *Clin Chest Med.* 2017;38(3):403-415. doi: https://doi.org/10.1016/j.ccm.2017.04.004.

[5] Dylewski J. Acute pulmonary histoplasmosis. *CMAJ.* 2011;183(14):E1090. doi: https://doi.org/10.1503/cmaj.110203.

[6] Details - *Public Health Image Library* (PHIL). (n.d.). Retrieved January 29, 2023, from https://phil.cdc.gov/Details.aspx?pid=472.

[7] Goodwin R. A. Jr, Owens F. T., Snell J. D., Hubbard W. W., Buchanan R. D., Terry R. T., Des Prez R. M. Chronic pulmonary histoplasmosis. *Medicine* (Baltimore). 1976;55(6):413-452. doi: https://doi.org/10.1097/00005792-197611000-00001.

[8] Kennedy C. C., Limper A. H. Redefining the clinical spectrum of chronic pulmonary histoplasmosis: a retrospective case series of 46 patients. *Medicine* (Baltimore). 2007;86(4):252-258. doi: https://doi.org/10.1097/MD.0b013e318144b1d9.

[9] Baker J., Kosmidis C., Rozaliyani A., Wahyuningsih R., Denning D. W. Chronic Pulmonary Histoplasmosis-A Scoping Literature Review. *Open Forum Infect Dis.* 2020;7(5):ofaa119. Published 2020 Apr 6. doi: https://doi.org/10.1093/ofid/ofaa119.

[10] Aidé M. A. Capítulo 4: histoplasmose. *Jornal Brasileiro de Pneumologia* (Chapter 4: Histoplasmosis. *Brazilian Journal of Pulmonology*). 2009;35(11):1145-51.

[11] Akram S. M., Koirala J. Histoplasmosis [Internet]. *StatPearls Publishing.* 2022. Available from: https://www.ncbi.nlm.nih.gov/books/NBK448185/?report=classic.

[12] Kunin J. R., Flors L., Hamid A., Fuss C., Sauer D., Walker C. M. Thoracic Endemic Fungi in the United States: Importance of Patient Location [published correction appears in Radiographics. 2021 Nov-Dec;41(7):E211]. *Radiographics.* 2021;41(2):380-398. doi: https://doi.org/10.1148/rg.2021200071.

[13] Kauffman C. A. Histoplasmosis: a clinical and laboratory update. *Clin Microbiol Rev.* 2007 Jan;20(1):115-32. doi: https://doi.org/10.1128/CMR.00027-06. PMID: 17223625; PMCID: PMC1797635.

[14] Conces D. J. J., Stockberger S. M., Tarver R. D., Wheat L. J. Disseminated histoplasmosis in AIDS: findings on chest radiographs. *American Journal of Roentgenology.* 1993;160: 15-19. doi: https://doi.org/10.2214/ajr.160.1.8416614.

[15] Grover S. B., Midha N., Gupta M., Sharma U., Talib V. H. Imaging spectrum in disseminated histoplasmosis: case report and brief review. *Australas Radiol.* 2005;49(2):175-178. doi: https://doi.org/10.1111/j.1440-1673.2005.01369.x.

[16] Radin D. R. Disseminated histoplasmosis: abdominal CT findings in 16 patients. *American Journal of Roentgenology.* 1991;157: 955-958. doi: https://doi.org/10.2214/ajr.157.5.1927816.

[17] Balthazar E. J., Megibow A. J., Barry M., Opulencia J. F. Histoplasmosis of the colon in patients with AIDS: imaging findings in four cases. *American Journal of Roentgenology.* 1993;161: 585-587. doi: https://doi.org/10.2214/ajr.161.3.8352111.

[18] Wheat L. J., Musial C. E., Jenny-Avital E. Diagnosis and management of central nervous system histoplasmosis. *Clin Infect Dis.* 2005;40(6):844-852. doi: https://doi.org/10.1086/427880.

[19] Klein C. J., Dinapoli R. P., Temesgen Z., Meyer F. B. Central nervous system histoplasmosis mimicking a brain tumor: difficulties in diagnosis and treatment. *Mayo Clin Proc.* 1999;74(8):803-807. doi: https://doi.org/10.4065/74.8.803.

[20] Andrade A. I., Donato M., Previgliano C., Hardjasudarma M. Histoplasmosis Brain Abscesses in an Immunocompetent Adult:A Case Report and Literature Review. *The Neuroradiology Journal.* 2014;27(3):334-8.

[21] Wilson D. A., Muchmore H. G., Tisdal R. G., Fahmy A., Pitha J. V. Histoplasmosis of the adrenal glands studied by CT. *Radiology.* 1984;150(3):779-783. https://doi.org/10.1148/radiology.150.3.6695079.

[22] Levine E. CT evaluation of active adrenal histoplasmosis. *Urol Radiol.* 1991;13(2):103-106. https://doi.org/10.1007/BF02924600.

[23] Wilson D. A., Nguyen D. L., Tytle T. L., Swaney C. M., Muchmore H. G. Sonography of the adrenal glands in chronic disseminated histoplasmosis. *J Ultrasound Med.* 1986;5(2):69-73. https://doi.org/10.7863/jum.1986.5.2.69.

[24] Fortin F., Adrenal histoplasmosis. Case study, Radiopaedia.org (Accessed on 07 Feb 2023) https://doi.org/10.53347/rID-68894.

[25] Szvalb A. D., Yepez Guevara E., Euscher E., Nahmod K. A., Kontoyiannis D. P. Acute Peritoneal Histoplasmosis Mimicking Ovarian Cancer and Review of the Literature on Histoplasma Peritonitis. *Open Forum Infectious Diseases*. 2023;10(1).

Chapter 6

The Histopathology of Histoplasma

Gude Geethanjali[1]
Lisa Centeno[2]
Lia Nandi[3]
Namratha Seetharam Meda[4]
Karuna Bista[5]
Esraa Hassan[6]
Mool Chand[6]
Aishwarya Reddy Korsapati[7]
Shika M Jain[8]
Sydney Boike[9]
Hasnain Saifee Bawaadam[10]
Syed Anjum Khan[6]
Sri J. Obulareddy[11]
and Nitesh Kumar Jain[6,*]

[1]Department of Histopathology, Postgraduate Institute of Medical Education and Research, Chandigarh, India
[2]Department of Medicine; University of Santo Tomas Faculty of Medicine and Surgery, Manila, Philippines
[3]Department of Medicine; Kasturba Medical College, Manipal, India
[4]Department of Medicine; MedStar Washington Hospital Center, NW, Washington, D.C., USA
[5]Department of Medicine; Nepal Medical College, Kathmandu, Nepal

[*] Corresponding author's Email: jain.nitesh@mayo.edu.

In: Histoplasmosis
Editors: Salim Surani, Syed Anjum Khan and Reena Shah
ISBN: 979-8-89113-129-3

[6]Department of Hospital Medicine, Mayo Clinic Health System, Mankato, Minnesota, USA
[7]Department of Medicine, University of Buckingham Medical School, Buckingham, UK
[8]Department of Medicine, MVJ Medical College and Research Hospital, Karnataka, India
[9]Department of Medicine, University of Minnesota, Minneapolis, Minnesota, USA
[10]Department of Pulmonary & Critical Care Medicine, Aurora Medical Center, Kenosha, Wisconsin, USA
[11]Department of Oncology and Hematology, University of Arkansas for Medical Sciences, Little Rock, Arkansas, USA

Abstract

Histoplasmosis is a systemic fungal infection, caused by inhalation of conidia of thermally dimorphic fungus *Histoplasma capsulatum*. It is an intracellular pathogen affecting cells of the reticuloendothelial system and produces a broad spectrum of clinical manifestations, ranging from self-limited pulmonary infection in immunocompetent patients which can rarely lead to life-threatening complications and disseminated disease in immunocompromised hosts. Heavy inoculum can produce severe disease even in healthy persons and chronic manifestations of healed infection can also be problematic. The clinical manifestations of disseminated Histoplasmosis are non-specific, often lead to diagnostic difficulty with differential diagnosis of tuberculosis or malignancy. Culture remains the gold standard for diagnosis but requires a lengthy incubation period and BSL3 laboratory. Histopathology provides a rapid presumptive diagnosis of the fungus while waiting for the fungal culture results. Quicker results can be obtained by identification of yeast phase by direct microscopic examination of clinical specimens such as sputum, bronchoalveolar lavage fluid, and smears of fine needle aspiration or biopsy specimens from lesions in the lungs, skin, gastrointestinal tract, liver, and adrenal glands. The histopathologic examination allows study of the fungal morphology with special staining procedures and the host tissue response thereby permits to distinguish Histoplasma from similar illnesses such as tuberculosis, and other opportunistic fungal and protozoal infections

Keywords: histoplasmosis, dimorphic fungus, histopathology, granuloma, intracellular yeast, diagnosis

Introduction

Histoplasmosis is caused by two similar fungi, the classic small-celled *Histoplasma capsulatum var. capsulatum* and large-celled *Histoplasma capsulatum var. duboisii (*African Histoplasmosis*)*. The two species have different geographic distribution and clinical presentation but share morphological similarities [1]. The clinical spectrum of histoplasmosis depends on the extent of exposure and the immune status of the host. The majority of new infections in an immunocompetent host are asymptomatic pulmonary infections which heal without treatment. Symptomatic disease may present as acute pulmonary disease, chronic progressive pulmonary disease or disseminated disease [2]. A wide variety of systems may be involved in disseminated disease. In disseminated disease, the lesions are seen in the gastrointestinal tract, liver, spleen, lymph nodes and bone marrow. The clinical presentation of Histoplasmosis can overlap with infections like tuberculosis, endemic fungal infections, sarcoidosis, and malignancy. Therefore, diagnosis of histoplasmosis requires an integrated diagnostic approach utilizing clinical, radiologic and laboratory evidence. In acutely ill and symptomatic patients' tissue biopsy or fine needle aspiration from the organ involved should be done as soon as possible to look for H. *capsulatum.*

Histopathology

H. capsulatum is a dimorphic fungus growing as yeast at body temperature and mycelium at room temperature. *H. capsulatum* exists as a septate hypha in the environment and forms a tan, white, brown wooly mold on Sabouraud dextrose agar at 25 to 30 °C. Two types of conidia are formed – microconidia and macroconidia (Figure 1). The macroconidia or tuberculate conidia (also known as ship's wheel) are 8 to 15 µm in diameter and have a thick wall with projections on the surface; the microconidia are smaller smooth structures that are 2 to 4 µm in diameter and are the infectious form. At 37 °C in vitro and in tissues, the organism converts into the yeast phase [3]. Infection is through inhalation of conidia or mycelial fragments. The fungi germinate in the alveoli and yeast like cells are formed, which then proliferate and disseminates to various organs via lymphatics. The organism is phagocytized by the macrophages of the lymphoreticular tissue thereby removing the organism from the circulation [4].

In hematoxylin and eosin (H&E) sections, after it is phagocytized, Histoplasma is visualized as an intracellular basophilic yeast form present within a histocyte (Figure 2A). The yeast is small and oval, ranges in size from 2 to 5 μm. Multiplication by narrow based budding from the end of the parent cell can be seen. Histoplasma is unencapsulated, but an artefactual pseudocapsule appears on H & E stain, which is an artifact of formalin fixation [5]. The pseudocapsule appears due to the clear space created by the retraction of the basophilic cytoplasm from the poorly stained cell. The organism is readily demonstrated by any of the fungal special stains, which are Grocott' s Gomori methenamine silver stain (GMS, figure 2B), Gridley's fungus and periodic acid-Schiff stain. GMS stain is preferred for screening as it gives better contrast and also stains degenerated and non-viable fungus. The artefactual halo of histoplasma is not seen in the GMS stain.

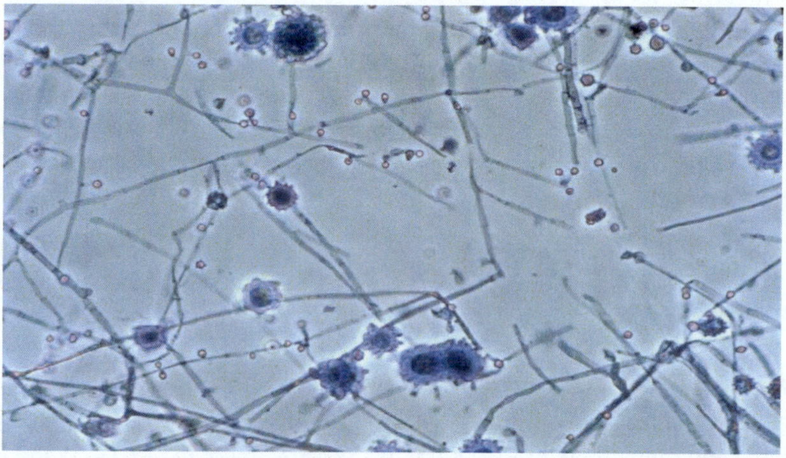

Figure 1. Photomicrograph showing mycelium of H. capsulatum with septate hyphae, large tuberculate macroconidia, and small smooth round microconidia (Source: Center for disease control. ID #10963; https://phil.cdc.gov/Details.aspx?pid=10963).

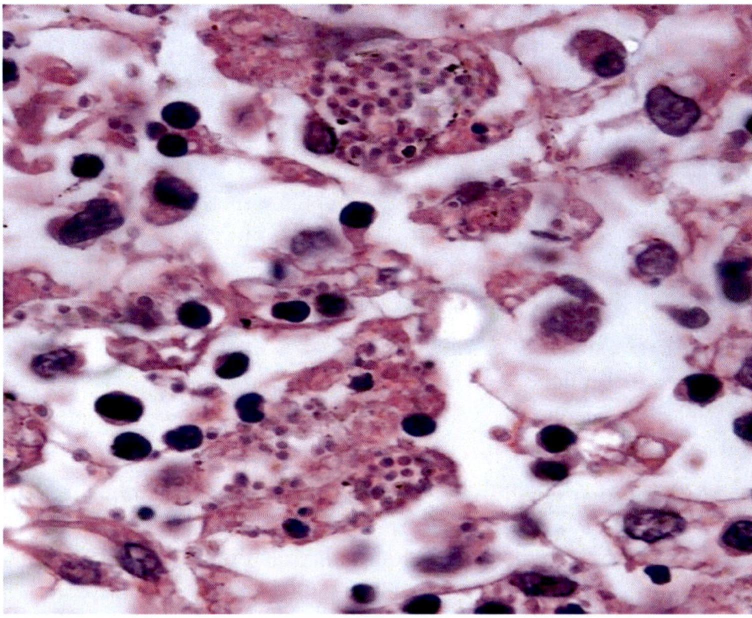

A

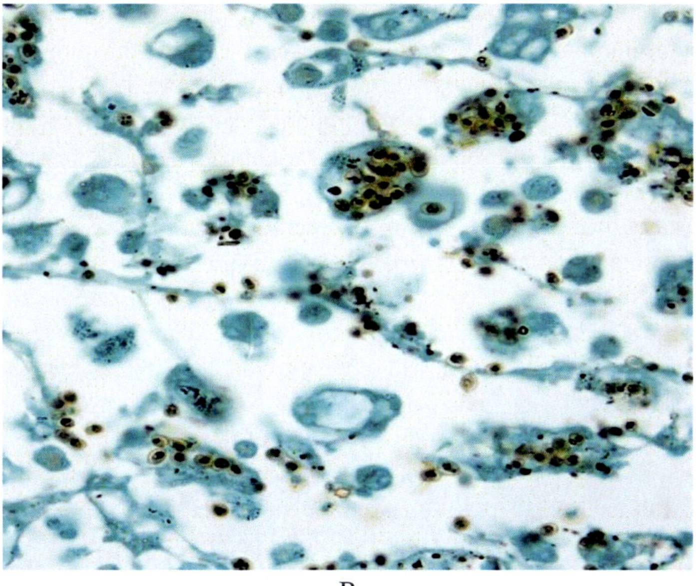

B

Figure 2. (A) Oil immersion magnification showing histiocytes with intracellular basophilic yeast forms of Histoplasma in (H & E, 1000x). (B) Grocott' s Gomori methenamine silver stain highlights the intracellular and few extracellular fungal profiles (GMS, 1000x).

The host reaction to Histoplasma infection depends on the inoculum dose, age, and immunological status of the host. Seventy five percent of patients with new infections are asymptomatic. The other twenty five percent develop symptomatic disease that present as acute pulmonary disease, chronic pulmonary disease, disseminated disease and fibrosing mediastinitis [4-6]. In acute histoplasmosis, lungs show bronchopneumonia with dense neutrophilic inflammation along with macrophages and plasma cells. Hilar lymph node involvement is seen. Unusual histologic findings such as diffuse alveolar damage, pulmonary alveolar proteinosis and bronchocentric granulomatosis are described in acute stage infection [7]. Acute histoplasmosis is self-limited and presents as bronchopneumonia unless the inoculum dose is large. Biopsy is not usually needed for diagnosis in this form of disease, but serologic testing is still useful.

Chronic pulmonary infection has predilection to involve the apices of lungs. Radiologically four patterns are described – Infiltrative, cavitary, fibrosis with emphysema and solitary nodular presentation [8]. The fibro-cavitary lesion appears similar to tuberculosis. Bronchiectasis and pleural fibrosis are also seen in the lung grossly. The solitary nodular presentation of histoplasmoma often resembles carcinoma. Granuloma formation with or without central caseous necrosis is the characteristic histologic lesion of chronic progressive pulmonary histoplasmoma (Figure 3). The granuloma is surrounded by fibrosis with lymphoid aggregates and sometimes multinucleated giant cells. The central caseous necrotic region can become calcified, progressively fibrotic, and rarely osseous metaplasia can develop. The yeast forms are found in the central necrotic area [4, 5, 9-11]. Granulomatous inflammation is also seen in hilar and peribronchial lymph nodes. Given the pathologic presentation of this form of .infection, other pathologies such as tuberculosis may be considered. However, fungal infections are more common than tuberculosis in the USA, while tuberculosis is frequent in other parts of world [12, 13]. Non-necrotizing granulomas are associated with sarcoidosis. Demonstration of the organism on the biopsy is often essential for diagnosis. GMS stain is often required for screening and identifying the organism as it may not be visualized in H & E sections. Ziehl Neelsen should be performed to screen for tuberculosis.

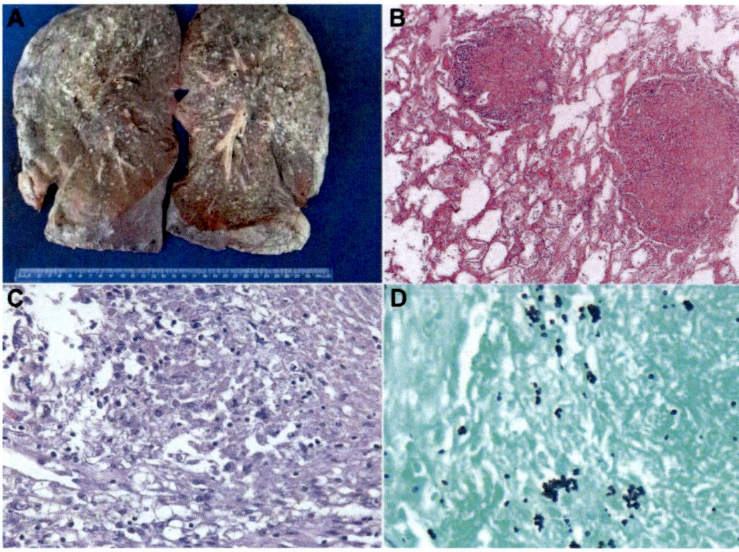

Figure 3. (A) Formalin-fixed autopsy specimen of lung specimen showing numerous yellowish nodular lesions. (B) Lung alveoli with two ill-defined granulomatous nodules with peripheric inflammatory infiltrate simulating tuberculous lesions (H & E 200x). (C) Higher magnification of lung lesions reveals granulomatous infiltrate with caseous-like necrosis (H & E 400x). (D) *H. Capsulatum* yeast forms highlighted in GMS stain (GMS stain 600x). Courtesy of open-source article [9].

Based on presence / absence of active granulomas, fibrous rim and lymphoid aggregates, a grading system was proposed to stratify the lesions of Histoplasma granulomas (see Table 1). The Grade 2 (resolving) and Grade 3 (resolved) granulomas do not benefit from additional laboratory studies and/or antifungal therapy. The grading system was developed to provide clinicians with information regarding disease resolution and hence useful for making therapeutic decisions [14].

The epithelioid, giant cell and granulomatous inflammation occurs in immunocompetent hosts with chronic progressive disease. In immunosuppressed host and very young patients, there is a predominantly histiocytic response with many intracellular yeast forms, and there may be minimal to no granulomas with wide dissemination. Extracellular lakes of yeast forms in the background of necrosis can also be seen in cases of profound lack of cell mediated immunity, for example, as in AIDS, hematologic malignancies, and post-transplant patients [15]. Serologic tests are of limited diagnostic value in immunosuppressed individuals. The most useful diagnostic method is bone marrow biopsy and microscopic examination for H.

capsulatum. Biopsy of other involved organs including lymph node, lung and liver are also beneficial as organismal growth in culture occurs too slowly for diagnosis in ill patients [16].

Table 1. Recommended grading of histoplasma granulomas

Grade	Granulomas	Fibrous rim	Fibrous rim associated lymphoid clusters
Grade 1 (Active)	Present With or without caseous necrosis	Minimal or absent	Absent
Grade 2 (Resolving)	Present But diminished	Present and associated with remaining granulomas	None to minimal
Grade 3 (Resolved)	Absent	Present	Present, well formed

Fibrosing mediastinitis is a fatal rare complication of histoplasmosis. Collagen deposition is seen entrapping the mediastinal structures including heart, great vessels, and esophagus. No granulomas or organisms are identified in these fibrotic deposits [17].

Gastrointestinal histoplasmosis is seen in 80% of patients with disseminated histoplasmosis. GI illness without concomitant pulmonary involvement and normal chest radiographs is also noted [18, 19]. Dissemination to the GI and liver occurs through reticuloendothelial cells. The ileum which has rich lymphatic network and numerous Peyer's patches is the most common site of involvement in the gastrointestinal tract (GIT). Any portion of the GIT including jejunum, colon, esophagus, and stomach can be involved in Histoplasma infection. Grossly, an ulcerative, plaque like, nodular or tumor like lesion can be seen on the mucosa. Unlike the pulmonary involvement, well-formed granulomas are rare in the GIT. Histologically there is diffuse lymphohistiocytic infiltration in the mucosa and submucosa. The yeast forms are found intracellularly in the macrophages (Figure 4). There is rare extension of inflammation into muscularis propria, serosa or mesentery. The lesion is characteristically present over the Peyer's patches with ulceration or nodularity of the overlying mucosa. In addition to lymphocytes and macrophages, eosinophils, plasma cells and neutrophils are also found. Giant cells are seen rarely [20]. In immunocompromised patients and infants, Histoplasma can also be seen extracellularly with minimal tissue reaction.

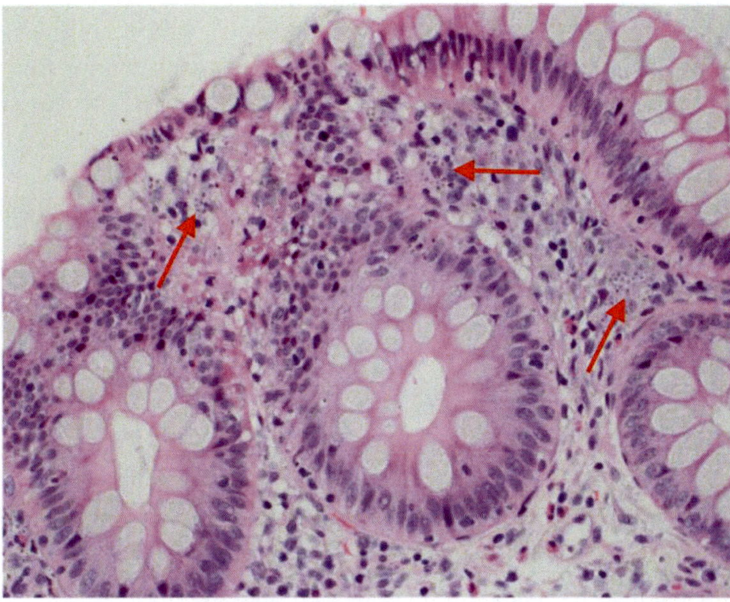

A

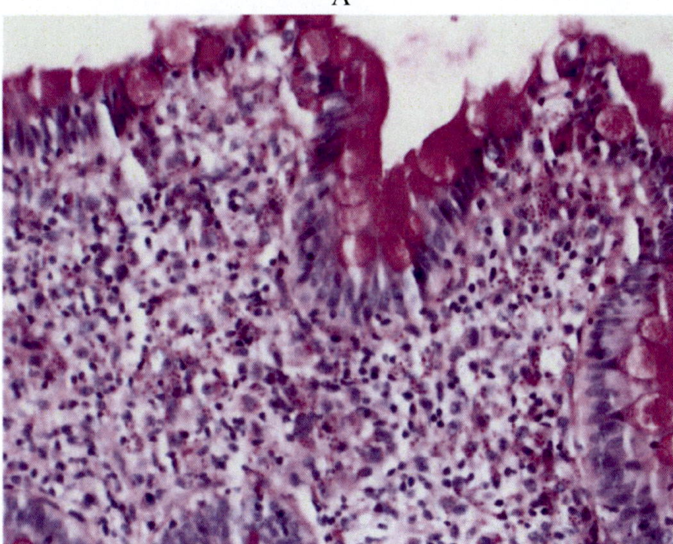

B

Figure 4. (A) Photomicrograph showing histiocytes with *H. Capsulatum* yeast forms in the lamina propria (H & E 200x). (B) Periodic acid-Schiff stain highlights the fungal organisms (PAS 200x). Courtesy of open-source article [19].

The liver in histoplasmosis is enlarged and congested. There are distended sinusoids with Kupffer cell hyperplasia and yeast containing macrophages. Portal tracts also show lympho-histiocytic inflammation with Histoplasma yeast forms present in the histiocytes. In some cases, portal-based epithelioid cell granulomas can be seen with or without necrosis (Figure 5) [20, 21].

Cutaneous involvement with H. *capsulatum* in immunocompetent patients is uncommon, it occurs more often in immunocompromised patients. Mucosal involvement with oral, vaginal, and penile ulcers has been reported [22-24]. Rare primary cutaneous infection due to direct inoculation presenting as nodules, ulcers, cellulitis, or lymphangitis have also been reported. Histologically, granulomatous reaction is usually seen in the reticular dermis. Necrosis is less common in cutaneous lesions. In addition, inflammation by polymorphs, plasma cells and a few eosinophils are seen. Patients with HIV/AIDS lack granuloma formation and show minimal inflammation with mild perivascular lymphocytic inflammation and few histiocytes. Areas of necrosis and karyorrhectic debris can also be seen. Diagnosis is based on the identification of the characteristic yeast forms of Histoplasma.

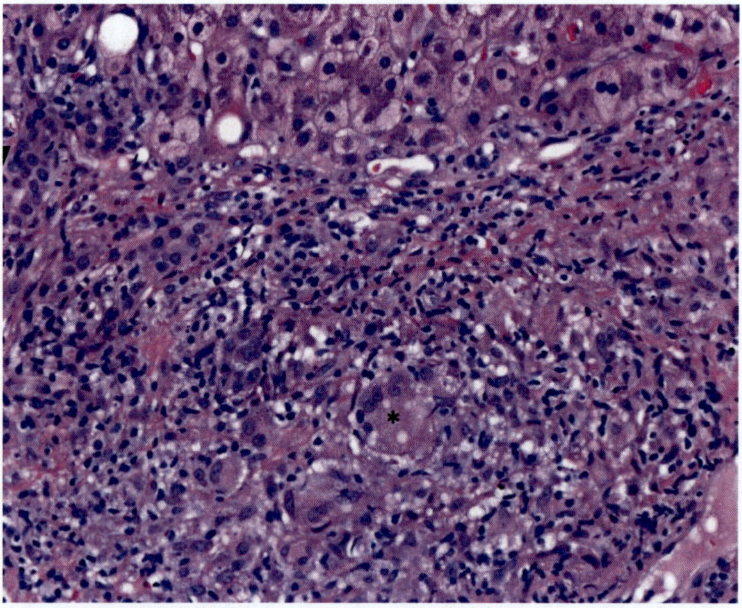

A

Figure 5. (Continued)

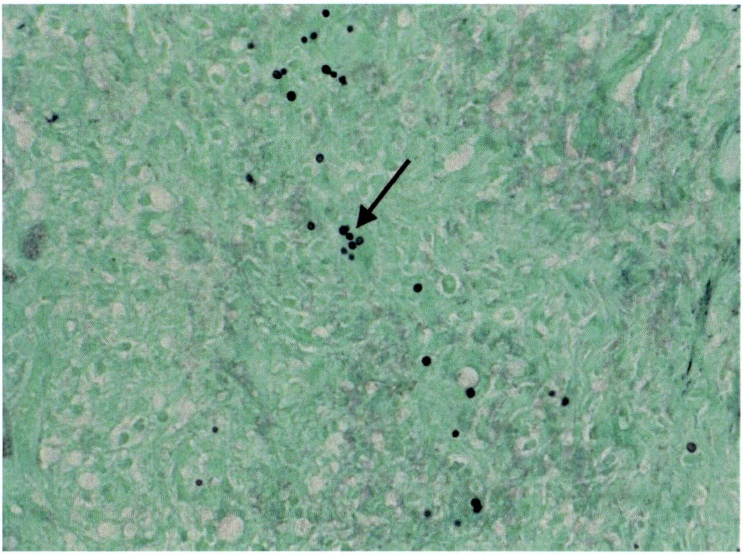

B

Figure 5. (A) Photomicrograph showing portal tract lympho-histiocytic inflammation with non- necrotising granulomas and giant cells () (H & E 200x). (B) GMS stain highlights scattered fungal yeast forms in portal area (GMS 400x). Courtesy of open-source article [21].

Histoplasma involves every organ during its asymptomatic course of dissemination. Addison's disease with electrolyte abnormalities due to bilateral destruction of adrenal glands is more common in Histoplasma than any other disseminated fungal infection [25]. Genitourinary involvement is seen in autopsy cases of disseminated histoplasmosis, however its rarely symptomatic. Osteoarticular involvement is another uncommon manifestation of histoplasmosis [26]. Histoplasma endocarditis is another rare manifestation. Infection can occur on native or prosthetic valve and also atrial myxoma [27]. A few patients develop CNS disease and one third of these cases occur in immunocompetent patients [28]. The most common CNS manifestation is chronic basal meningitis with grey, yellow exudate and mass cerebral lesions. Histopathology is characterized by granulomatous inflammation with large areas of caseous necrosis seen in intracerebral lesions. Endarteritis obliterans is also identified similar to tuberculosis which leads to areas of necrosis in the brain [29, 30]. With severely impaired cell mediated immunity diffuse histiocytic infiltration along with bland caseous necrosis is seen. Small intracellular ovoid yeast forms can be seen in histiocytes [31].

Fine needle aspiration (FNA) from the clinically accessible sites is an increasingly important test in the diagnosis of Histoplasma as cytopathologic examination has a quick turnaround time. Endobronchial ultrasound (EBUS) and endoscopic ultrasound (EUS) FNA techniques can allow clinicians to sample difficult areas in the lung and GIT to facilitate rapid diagnosis [32]. The smears are stained with Romanowsky or Papanicolaou stains. GMS can also be performed directly on the smear. The cytological findings range from bland acellular necrosis, epithelioid cell granulomas, histocytes, giant cells and neutrophilic response. Intracellular yeast forms can be seen in the histiocytes, and even extracellular organisms can be identified in the necrotic material (Figure 6) [33, 34]. Bronchoalveolar lavage (BAL) is also a relatively cost-effective technique for the examination of lung disease in immunocompromised patients. BAL also allows for the study of pulmonary microenvironment and the load of yeast forms. BAL of immunocompromised patients with HIV shows numerous macrophages with intracellular yeast forms. BAL has a sensitivity of around 50% in acute histoplasmosis. When combined with histoplasma antigen testing on BAL fluid the sensitivity increases to 97% [35].

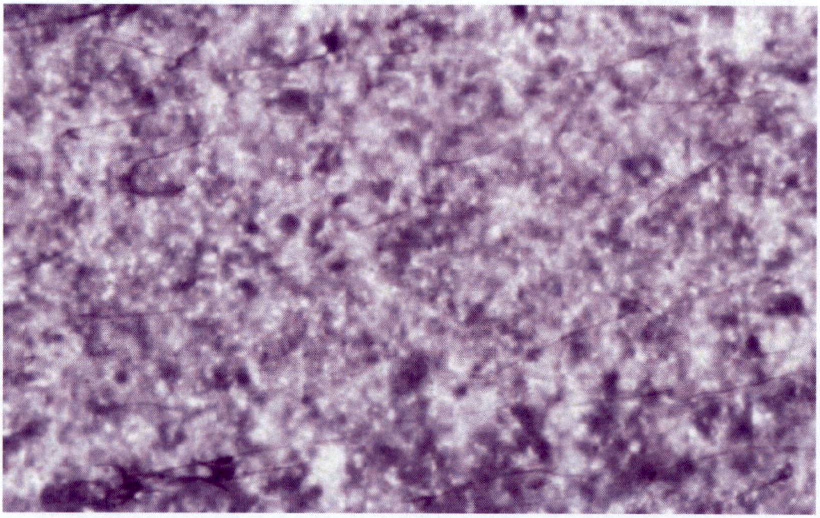

A

Figure 6. (Continued)

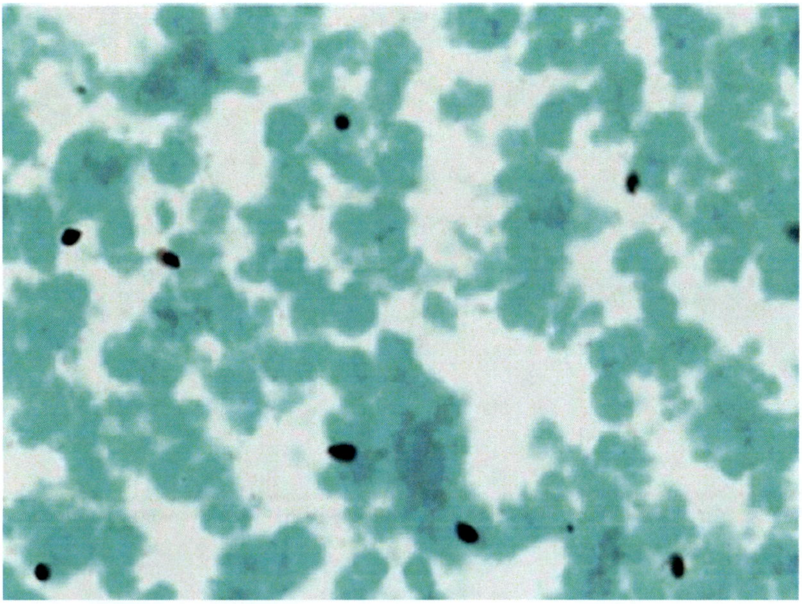

B

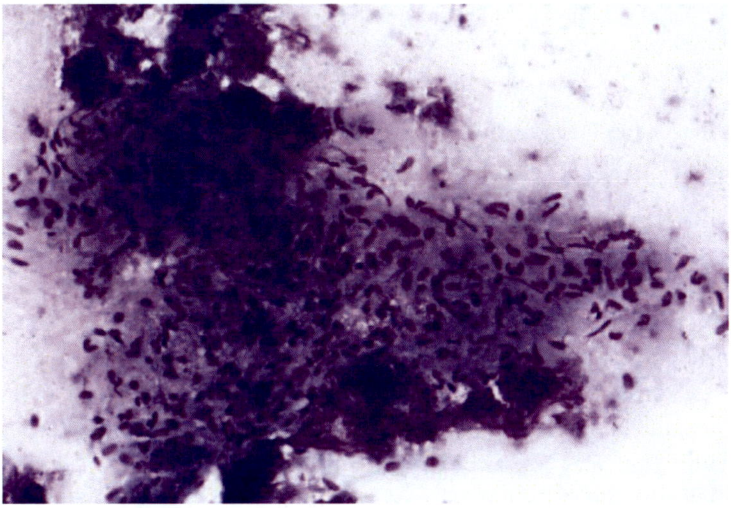

C

Figure 6. (Continued)

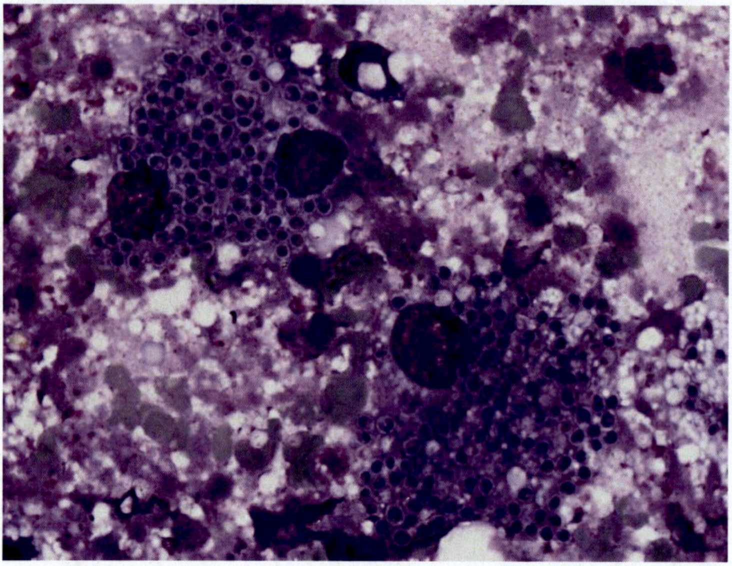

D

Figure 6. Fine needle aspiration smears showing (A) bland acellular necrosis without neutrophilic infiltrate (Romanowsky stain 400x). (B) Numerous scattered fungal profiles identified in necrotic areas on Grocott' s stain (GMS 1000X). (C) Granulomas without identifiable yeast forms (Romanowsky stain 400x). (D) Numerous intracellular yeast forms of H. Capsulatum in immunosuppressed patient (Romanowsky stain 1000x). Courtesy of open-source article [32].

Diagnosis of Histoplasma requires a multifaceted approach to clinical and radiologic findings with supportive laboratory evidence. Gold standard methods for diagnosis include isolation of H. capsulatum on culture or identification of yeast on histopathology. Biopsy and FNAC provide relatively rapid diagnostic results compared to culture which allows for rapid diagnosis in ill patients. Serologic tests are also available which are sensitive and easily interpretable for clinical use. Molecular methods may be the next frontier in Histoplasma diagnostics. The optimal diagnostic method depends on the time point in the natural course of the disease, the clinical specimen being sampled, and the patient's immune status.

Conclusion

Non-culture-based methods which provide early, and rapid detection of histoplasmosis is essential to establish a suitable antifungal therapy to reduce morbidity and mortality. Histoplasma antigen assays are the most sensitive tests but its unavailability in many parts of the world and cross reactivity with other fungi is a major obstacle to early diagnosis. Histopathology continues to be a rapid and cost-effective tool of providing a presumptive or definitive diagnosis of an invasive fungal infection. It is important to be familiar with the morphology and staining properties of Histoplasma to distinguish it from other fungi and intracellular pathogens to prevent misidentification for diagnostic purposes. Molecular assays are useful in culture negative cases but are expensive and not widely available. A combination of culture and non-culture-based studies is required for timely diagnosis of histoplasmosis and identify dual infections in immunocompromised patients with HIV and transplant recipients.

References

[1] Guarner J, Brandt M E. (2011). Histopathologic diagnosis of fungal infections in the 21st century. *Clin. Microbiol. Rev.*, 24(2):247-80.

[2] Kauffman C A. (2007) Histoplasmosis: a clinical and laboratory update. *Clin. Microbiol. Rev.*, 20(1):115-32.

[3] Azar M M, Hage C A. (2017) Laboratory Diagnostics for Histoplasmosis. J. *Clin. Microbiol.*, 55(6):1612-1620.

[4] Goodwin R A, Loyd J E, Des Prez R M. (1981). Histoplasmosis in normal hosts. *Medicine*, 60(4):231–266.

[5] Darling, S. T. (1906). A protozoan general infection producing pseudotubercles in the lungs and focal necroses in the liver, spleen, and lymph nodes. *JAMA*, 46(17):1283-1285.

[6] Allendörfer R, Brunner G D, Deepe G S Jr. (1999). Complex requirements for nascent and memory immunity in pulmonary histoplasmosis. *J. Immunol.*, 162(12):7389-96.

[7] Garrido L, Mata-Essayag S, Hartung de Capriles C, Eugenia Landaeta M, Pacheco I, Fuentes Z. (2006) Pulmonary histoplasmosis: unusual histopathologic findings. *Pathol. Res. Pract.*, 202(5):373-8.

[8] Gurney J W, Conces D J. (1996). Pulmonary histoplasmosis. *Radiology*, 199(2):297-306.

[9] Rakislova N, Hurtado J C, Palhares A E M, Ferreira L, Freire M, Lacerda M, Monteiro W, Navarro M, Casas I, Teixeira M M, Castillo P, Rodrigo-Calvo M T,

Marimon L, Guerrero J, Varo R, Delgado V, Quintó L, Marco F, Letang E, Vila J, Bassat Q, Menéndez C, Ordi J, Martínez M J. (2021). High prevalence and mortality due to Histoplasma capsulatum in the Brazilian Amazon: An autopsy study. *PLoS Negl. Trop. Dis.*,15(4): e0009286.

[10] Wheat L J, Wass J, Norton J, Kohler R B, French M L. (1984). Cavitary histoplasmosis occurring during two large urban outbreaks. Analysis of clinical, epidemiologic, roentgenographic, and laboratory features. *Medicine (Baltimore)*, 63(4):201-9.

[11] Wheat L J, Slama T G, Eitzen H E, Kohler R B, French M L, Biesecker J L. (1981). A large urban outbreak of histoplasmosis: clinical features. *Ann. Intern. Med.*, 94(3):331-7.

[12] Mukhopadhyay S, Farver C F, Vaszar L T, Dempsey O J, Popper H H, Mani H, Capelozzi V L, Fukuoka J, Kerr K M, Zeren E H, Iyer V K, Tanaka T, Narde I, Nomikos A, Gumurdulu D, Arava S, Zander DS, Tazelaar HD. (2012). Causes of pulmonary granulomas: a retrospective study of 500 cases from seven countries. *J. Clin. Pathol.*, 65(1):51-7.

[13] Al-Harbi A, Al-Otaibi S, Abdulrahman A, Al-Jahdali F, Al-Harbi F, Bamefleh H, Gamdi M, Al-Jahdali H. (2017). Lung granuloma: A clinicopathologic study of 158 cases. *Ann. Thorac. Med.*, 12(4):278-281.

[14] Demkowicz R, Procop GW. (2021) Clinical Significance and Histologic Characterization of Histoplasma Granulomas. *Am. J. Clin. Pathol.*, 15;155(4):581-587.

[15] Wheat L J, Smith E J, Sathapatayavongs B, Batteiger B, Filo R S, Leapman S B, French M V. (1983). Histoplasmosis in Renal Allograft Recipients: Two Large Urban Outbreaks. *Arch. Intern. Med.*, 143(4):703–707.

[16] Kauffman C A, Israel K S, Smith J W, White A C, Schwarz J, Brooks GF. (1978). Histoplasmosis in immunosuppressed patients. *Am. J. Med.*, 64(6):923-932.

[17] Davis AM, Pierson R N, Loyd J E. (2001) Mediastinal fibrosis. *Semin. Respir. Infect.*, 16(2):119-130.

[18] Jain S, Koirala J, Castro-Pavia F. (2004). Isolated gastrointestinal histoplasmosis: case report and review of the literature. *South Med. J.*, 97(2):172-174.

[19] Bhinder J, Mori A, Cao W, Malieckal A. (2018). A Case of Isolated Gastrointestinal Histoplasmosis. *Cureus*, 10(7): e2951.

[20] Lamps L W, Molina C P, West A B, Haggitt R C, Scott M A. (2000) The Pathologic Spectrum of Gastrointestinal and Hepatic Histoplasmosis. *American Journal of Clinical Pathology*, 113(1): 64–72.

[21] Muhanna A, Nimri F M, Almomani Z A, Momani L A, Likhitsup. (2021) Granulomatous hepatitis secondary to Histoplasmosis in an immunocompetent patient. *Cureus*, 13(9): e17631

[22] Folk G A, Nelson B L. (2017) Oral Histoplasmosis. *Head Neck Pathol.*,11(4):513-516.

[23] Paixão M, Miot H A, Avancini J, Belda Júnior W. (2015) Primary cutaneous histoplasmosis developed in the penis of an immunocompetent patient. *An. Bras. Dermatol*, 90(2):255-7.

[24] Shine M M, Shah M M, Hanna C A, Bevis K S. (2013) Vulvar histoplasmosis as a rare cause of genital ulceration. *Obstet. Gynecol,* 122(2):449-452.

[25] Larbcharoensub N, Boonsakan P, Aroonroch R, Rochanawutanon M, Nitiyanant P, Phongkitkarun S, Poonvutikul S, Watcharananan SP, Ngarmukos C (2011) Adrenal histoplasmosis: a case series and review of the literature. *Southeast Asian. J. Trop. Med. Public Health*, 42(4):920-925.

[26] Mata-Essayag S, Colella M T, Roselló A, de Capriles C H, Landaeta M E, de Salazar CP, Magaldi S, Olaizola C, Calatroni M I, Garrido L. (2008). Histoplasmosis: a study of 158 cases in Venezuela, 2000-2005. *Medicine (Baltimore)*, 87(4):193-202.

[27] Riddell J 4th, Kauffman C A, Smith J A, Assi M, Blue S, Buitrago M I, Deresinski S, Wright P W, Drevets D A, Norris S A, Vikram H R, Carson P J, Vergidis P, Carpenter J, Seidenfeld S M, Wheat L J. (2014). Histoplasma capsulatum endocarditis: multicenter case series with review of current diagnostic techniques and treatment. *Medicine (Baltimore)*, 93(5):186-193.

[28] Wheat J, Myint T, Guo Y, Kemmer P, Hage C, Terry C, Azar MM, Riddell J, Ender P, Chen S, Shehab K, Cleveland K, Esguerra E, Johnson J, Wright P, Douglas V, Vergidis P, Ooi W, Baddley J, Bamberger D, Khairy R, Vikram HR, Jenny-Avital E, Sivasubramanian G, Bowlware K, Pahud B, Sarria J, Tsai T, Assi M, Mocherla S, Prakash V, Allen D, Passaretti C, Huprikar S, Anderson A. (2018) "Central nervous system histoplasmosis: Multicenter retrospective study on clinical features, diagnostic approach and outcome of treatment." *Medicine*, 97(13): e0245.

[29] Wheat L J, Batteiger B E, Sathapatayavongs B. (1990). Histoplasma capsulatum infections of the central nervous system. A clinical review. *Medicine (Baltimore)*, 69(4):244-260.

[30] Schestatsky P, Chedid M F, Amaral O B, Unis G, Oliveira F M, Severo LC. (2006). Isolated central nervous system histoplasmosis in immunocompetent hosts: a series of 11 cases. *Scand. J. Infect. Dis.*, 38(1):43-48.

[31] Nyalakonda H, Albuerne M, Suazo Hernandez LP, Sarria JC. (2016). Central Nervous System Histoplasmosis in Acquired Immunodeficiency Syndrome. *Am. J. Med. Sci.*, 351(2):177-186.

[32] Gailey M P, Klutts J S, Jensen C S. (2013) Fine-needle aspiration of histoplasmosis in the era of endoscopic ultrasound and endobronchial ultrasound: cytomorphologic features and correlation with clinical laboratory testing. *Cancer Cytopathol.*, 121(9):508-517.

[33] Gupta N, Arora S K, Rajwanshi A, Nijhawan R, Srinivasan R. (2010) Histoplasmosis: cytodiagnosis and review of literature with special emphasis on differential diagnosis on cytomorphology. *Cytopathology*,21(4):240-244.

[34] Kapatia G, Saha A, Rohilla M, Gupta P, Gupta N, Srinivasan R, Rajwanshi A, Dey P. (2020) Clinical and Morphological Spectrum of Histoplasmosis on Cytology Along with the Review of Literature. *Acta Cytol.*, 64(6):532-538.

[35] Hage C A, Davis T E, Fuller D, Egan L, Witt JR 3rd, Wheat L J, Knox K S. (2010). Diagnosis of histoplasmosis by antigen detection in BAL fluid. *Chest*, 137(3):623–628.

Chapter 7

Pulmonary Complications of Histoplasmosis

Rohan Kumar Ochani[1,*]
Hafsa Nazir Jatoi[2]
Asim Shaikh[3]
Iqbal Ratnani[4]
and Salim Surani[5]

[1]Department of Internal Medicine, SUNY Upstate Medical University, Syracuse, New York, USA
[2]Department of Internal Medicine, Dow University of Health Sciences, Karachi, Pakistan
[3]Department of Medicine, Aga Khan University Hospital, Karachi, Pakistan
[4]Department of Anesthesiology and Critical Care, Methodist DeBakey Heart and Vascular Center, Houston Methodist Hospital, Houston, Texas USA
[5]Adjunct Clinical Professor, Department of Medicine and Pharmacology, Texas A&M University, Corpus Christi, Texas, USA, Research Collaborator, Mayo Clinic, Rochester, Minnesota, USA

Abstract

Histoplasmosis is one of the most common endemic mycoses in the United States, caused by the organism Histoplasma Capsulatum. The classic type is characterized by pulmonary disease. The African type, on the other hand, has extrapulmonary manifestations such as ulcers and bone lesions. Histoplasma first enters the body of a human host as conidia inhaled from the soil into the bronchioles and alveoli. When alveolar macrophages invade the yeasts, the inhaled conidia convert into yeast in the body, resulting in the pathogenesis of Histoplasmosis. Histoplasma

* Corresponding Author's Email: rohanochani@gmail.com.

In: Histoplasmosis
Editors: Salim Surani, Syed Anjum Khan and Reena Shah
ISBN: 979-8-89113-129-3

can infect skin, bones, lymph nodes, spleen, muscles, liver, oral cavity, and mucosa, but it primarily affects the pulmonary system. Early Histoplasmosis diagnosis is lifesaving because it allows for prompt treatment and reduces the risk of serious complications. Histopathology, culture, and cytology are common Histoplasma diagnostic tests. Isolation of the intracellular form of the yeast on culture is the gold standard test for Histoplasma. The symptoms include dyspnea, a nonproductive cough, chest pain, and diffuse lung involvement. Extrapulmonary symptoms include fever, chills, malaise, hepatosplenomegaly, lymphadenopathy, bone marrow suppression (pancytopenia), and elevated liver function tests. According to current practice guidelines, the management of Histoplasmosis should be based on the specific clinical manifestations and severity. In all cases, the two most used antifungal agents are azoles and amphotericin B. Furthermore, for those who are unable to tolerate first-line agents, the relatively limited research availability on second and third-line agents becomes a significant barrier.

Keywords: histoplasmosis, pulmonary histoplasmosis, extrapulmonary histoplasmosis, cavitary histoplasmosis, CNS histoplasmosis

Introduction

Histoplasmosis is an invasive fungal disease typically found affecting the people of Mississippi, Ohio, and the Southwestern United States. This disease is one of the most prevalent endemic mycoses in the US and is caused by an organism named *Histoplasma Capsulatum.* The classical type usually presents with pulmonary disease. However, the African type presents with extrapulmonary manifestations, including ulcers and bone lesions [1, 2]. This disease was described in the early 1900s by Dr. Samuel Darling when he noted the presence of an intracellular organism in the lung during an autopsy. Darling discovered *Histoplasma Capsulatum*, a plasmodium-like organism that invaded the cytoplasm of histiocyte-like cells and was enveloped by a capsule. Histoplasma was correctly identified as a fungus and demonstrated to be dimorphic fungi two decades later in the 1930s [3].

Histoplasma is typically found in soil that consists of bird or bat droppings and is, therefore, most prevalent in areas with high bird or bat populations. In most cases, the infection is commonly acquired by inhaling microconidia, and most people with Histoplasmosis usually have mild or no symptoms. However, this condition can lead to severe effects and can even become fatal in some cases. Diagnosis is typically made via a combination of symptoms, physical examination, and various laboratory tests. This condition is usually treated by antifungal medications; however, in case of increased severity, patients may require hospitalization [1, 3].

Pulmonary Histoplasmosis

Acute Pulmonary Histoplasmosis

Only one-tenth of the patients infected with Histoplasmosis present with symptoms of acute pulmonary Histoplasmosis. The symptoms initially consist of fever, chills, malaise shortness of breath, cough, and retrosternal chest pain, which may eventually lead to acute respiratory distress syndrome [3, 4]. The condition is typically treated as viral or bacterial pneumonia due to the reduced commonality of this disease than other common conditions; therefore, diagnosing pulmonary Histoplasmosis in patients with a potential exposure unable to be treated via the antimicrobials given requires a high index of clinical suspicion and judgment. Imaging in the case of acute pulmonary Histoplasmosis shows diffuse patchy opacities in the lung, as well as hilar or mediastinal adenopathy in immunocompetent patients. In immunocompromised patients, this can lead to a severe disease forming a miliary pattern. Laboratory testing shows pancytopenia in disseminated disease and a narrow-based budding ovoid Histoplasma yeast [3-6].

Subacute Pulmonary Histoplasmosis

Subacute pulmonary Histoplasmosis is characterized by milder respiratory and constitutional symptoms that develop over several months because of exposure to a lower inoculum. Patients initially presenting with signs and symptoms consistent with Histoplasmosis may be missed as they can have several different organ involvements, including colon, adrenals, and bone marrow, before the involvement of lungs, delaying the pulmonary imaging [3, 7].

Chronic Cavitary Pulmonary Histoplasmosis

Chronic cavitary pulmonary Histoplasmosis can develop after acute pulmonary Histoplasmosis. It can also be seen in patients who are smokers and may have chronic obstructive pulmonary disease. The symptoms consist of fever, productive cough, night sweats, weight loss, malaise, and shortness of breath, imitating the symptoms of pulmonary tuberculosis, leading to an anti-tuberculous treatment and, therefore, a delayed diagnosis of pulmonary Histoplasmosis [3, 8-9].

Initially, patchy infiltrates are seen on chest imaging, which then progresses into dense consolidation with radio-translucent pockets, frequently involving the apical and apical-posterior segments of the lungs. This leads to the development of large cavities and fibrosis. Pleural thickening and calcification of mediastinal and hilar lymph nodes are also observed. Eventually, this can progress and involve the entire lobe and lung, causing its necrosis, a phenomenon termed a "marching cavity" [3, 8-9].

Extrapulmonary Histoplasmosis

A small portion of patients with Histoplasmosis may include organ systems other than the pulmonary. It can cause rheumatologic manifestations where patients may have arthralgias, arthritis, erythema nodosum, and erythema multiforme [10]. This combination of signs and symptoms can also lead to difficulty differentiating the condition from sarcoidosis. Rarely, pericarditis can also be seen in patients with acute pulmonary Histoplasmosis, presenting as chest pain, shortness of breath, and enlargement of the mediastinal lymph nodes, in addition to progression to cardiomegaly and pericardial effusion [4, 11].

Histoplasmosis can also involve the central nervous system, when disseminated, may include chronic meningitis, focal brain or spinal cord lesions, encephalitis, and hydrocephalus. The involvement of the CNS system is usually seen in immunocompromised patients. However, one-third of the cases are seen in immunocompetent patients. The symptoms include confusion, headache, and impaired cognition, and when a CT scan or an MRI is conducted, it may reveal ring-enhanced focal mass lesions [12].

Epidemiology and Prevalence

Prevalence within the USA

Histoplasmosis, being one of the most common endemic mycoses, is found almost everywhere. However, it is mostly found in North and Central America. Histoplasma primarily inhabits the central and eastern United States, particularly the Ohio and Mississippi River Valleys, where 60-90% of the people living near these valleys have been at least exposed once to Histoplasma during their lifetime. Sporadic histoplasmosis cases in humans and animals in Alaska, California, and Florida, on the other hand, suggest that Histoplasma can survive in other environments given suitable environmental conditions [13, 14].

A study calculated the incidence of Histoplasmosis to 3.4 cases per 100,000 population in the US, while the rate was highest in the Midwest with an incidence of 6.1 cases per 100,000. Furthermore, chronic obstructive pulmonary disease was the most common comorbid condition, while diabetes mellitus was the second-most common [15, 16].

According to a descriptive analysis done between the years 2011-2014, a total of over 3400 cases were reported from 12 states, where 62% were white, 10% were black, and the remaining 26% were of unknown ethnicity. The data for symptoms was reported in 4 states, where cough was the most commonly reported symptom (67%), followed by shortness of breath (64%) and fever (56%). Furthermore, nine states provided the data for laboratory data of 1929 patients with any positive histoplasmosis test result, only 33% were positive for antigen test, 55% were positive for antibody test, and 13% were positive for culture result. Of 33% positive antigen tests, 83% of those had tests done on the urine specimen, and 23% were performed on serum. While of 55% positive antibody tests, 59% were done via immunodiffusion test, and 81% were done via complement fixation test [15-18].

Prevalence Outside the USA

Africa

The prevalence of Histoplasmosis is relatively low outside the US when compared to the US; however, it is found in various parts of the world, including Western, Southern, Eastern, and Central Africa. The African variant of the illness is caused by *Histoplasma capsulatum var. Duboisii (Hcd)* typically presents with extrapulmonary manifestations like bone lesions and ulcers. The classical form is caused by *Histoplasma capsulatum var. Capsulatum (Hcc),* typically presenting with the classic pulmonary presentation.

The greatest attributable risk factor causing disseminated Histoplasmosis is being immunocompromised, particularly in individuals with HIV/AIDs; therefore, in the late 1980s, Histoplasmosis was defined as an AIDS-defining illness. However, despite the apparent rising cases, the prevalence of Histoplasmosis is low in Africa due to multiple reasons, including poor clinician awareness, suboptimal diagnostic techniques, and a lower index of clinical suspicion, to name a few [2].

However, with the data provided by Oladele and colleagues, in the period of six decades from 1952-2017, 470 cases of Histoplasmosis were identified. The highest (n = 173; 38%) was in Western Africa, followed by 150 (32%) cases in Southern Africa, where most cases were found to have the classical form of *Histoplasma capsulatum var. Capsulatum (Hcc).* Most of these cases stemmed from 5 African countries due to the lack of access to diagnostic abilities in the rest of Africa [19]. Another recent review from 1993 to 2019 by Develoux et al. demonstrated a total of 94 cases, where about one-third of cases were found to be in individuals less than 18 years of age [20].

Recently, a detailed cross-sectional study conducted in 2022 showed that the prevalence of Histoplasmosis in patients with an advanced HIV disease, specifically in Nigeria, is almost 7.7%. A total of 988 participants were included with symptoms suggestive of either tuberculosis or Histoplasmosis, where 76 participants in total had Histoplasma antigenuria, most (51.3%) participants were in the 41–60-year range, and 47.3% were in the less than 40-year range [21].

India

Southeast Asia, specifically India, also receives its share of histoplasmosis cases in relation to Africa. According to a review conducted in India, a total of 316 cases were identified, where 43 cases had a pre-diagnosed HIV infection, 111 cases had adrenal involvement, and only 4 of the cases had a pulmonary involvement. The highest number of cases (89) were identified in the Tamil Nadu region in India, followed by 72 cases in Uttar Pradesh, India. This, again, is also not an accurate estimation due to the lack of reported data and the localized occurrence of the disease [22].

Vietnam

According to a review conducted by Duong et al., over 2 million fungal infections were identified in Vietnam in 2020, of which only 166 cases of Histoplasmosis were recorded annually. This was generally seen in HIV patients, as identified as an AIDS-defining illness, where it was restricted only to an advanced disease of CD4 count < 100 cells/µl, and not seen in patients with a CD4 count between 100 and 200 cells/µl [23].

Pathogenesis

Histoplasma's pathogenesis depends on many factors, especially factors like immune status, size of the inoculum, and virulence of the infecting strain. Histoplasmosis in immunocompetent individuals typically remains benign and nonharmful; however, in patients who have conditions making them immunosuppressed can cause the spread of the disease, making it extremely hazardous [24].

There are some general criteria for a pathogenic organism to cause a disease which includes:

- The ability to invade or bypass host barriers to reach internal tissues.
- The ability to grow at or above the host temperature.
- The ability to evade or withstand the immune system.
- The diverse enzymatic repertoire is used to acquire nutrients by hydrolyzing and consuming human tissue components.

Entry

Initially, when Histoplasma enters the body of a human host, it enters as conidia being inhaled from the soil into the bronchioles and alveoli. The inhaled conidia then convert into yeast in the body, eventually causing the pathogenesis of Histoplasmosis, when the alveolar macrophages invade the yeasts. Initial binding of the Histoplasma antigen with macrophage is done via the CD18 family of adhesion binding proteins (LFA-1 (CD11a), CR3 (CD11b), and p150, 95) [25-27].

These alveolar macrophages then multiply into several numbers and are invaded by other alveolar and inflammatory macrophages in the lung.

Repeating this pattern causes infection to spread via lymphatics to the lymph nodes and other organs comprising many mononuclear phagocytes. The development of specific cell-mediated immunity triggers the primary infection, which leads to M activation and infection resolution, a hallmark of host defense against Histoplasma. However, a deficiency of T-cell-mediated immunity causes this fungus to disseminate by delaying the clearance of the organism and may also reactivate the latent infection from the formed granulomas [25, 27].

Histoplasma can go through multiple pathways. One is the classical pathway where the fungus cell replicates frequently and intensely, leading to host cell death which gets presented to T-cell activating the cell-mediated immunity. However, different routes have been utilized and explored in the pathogenesis of Histoplasma, where Histoplasma can bind macrophages via mammalian B2 integrins or binding dendritic cells. Another possible expansion is by avoiding the host oxidative burst and travels through traditional opsono-phagocytosis resulting in the production of a cascade of toxic reactive molecules which can damage membranes, enzymes, and nucleic acids, such as superoxide anion, hydrogen peroxide, and hydroxyl radical [28].

Replication and Iron Utilization

Once the fungus enters the host, it gets incorporated within a membrane-bound vacuole, which then undergoes phagolysosomal fusion modifying the environment and reducing the pH to less than 4. This pH change leads to the fungus getting exposed to various lysosomal enzymes, specifically hydrolases, when activated at low pH. Although viable yeasts do survive, some may be destroyed by heat when treated with either cycloheximide, a protein synthesis inhibitor, or amphotericin B, an antifungal antibiotic that targets the membrane ergosterol [28].

To survive inside the host cell, the essential nutrient required is competed between the mammalian host and nearly all pathogens, including Histoplasma. Most of the iron in the host is not freely available but rather bound to transferrin; therefore, this iron may not be utilized appropriately or at all at physiologic iron levels of maturation at 20-75%. At least three different mechanisms of action have been devised and proposed in iron acquisition toward the infectivity of Histoplasmosis in the host organism [28, 29].

First, the fungal releases several hydrophobes, which may include various secreted chelating agents. These small-secreted chelating agents get attached to ferric iron and then compete for iron with host transferrin, potentially obtaining iron from other sources in the host.

Second, the concept of ferric reduction has been proposed where constraints of iron may cause Histoplasma to utilize ferric reductase. This enzyme can use reduced glutathione as the cofactor and holotransferrin, ferrisiderophores, and hemin as substrates to form ferrous iron, which then finally leads to withdrawing the ferrous iron from the host or extracellular iron-binding compounds.

Third, the last mechanism put forward is the acidic pH-dependent release of transferrin-bound iron. Transferrin has two sites for ferric to be bound, which sequentially release iron when the pH reduces below neutral or to an acidic level making it available for the fungus to use. However, the pH does not need to be too low as that would lead to activation of the lysosomal-based enzymes, which target destroying the fungus. Therefore, the fungus should balance that the pH is low enough to release the iron from transferrin but not low enough for the lysosomal enzymes to be activated, inadvertently destroying the fungus [28, 29].

Organs Affected by Histoplasma

Histoplasma can affect multiple sites, including skin, bones, lymph nodes, spleen, muscles, liver, oral cavity, and mucosa [30]; however, it primarily affects the pulmonary system as the inhaled particles can adhere to the respiratory tract and reach the lungs [24]. The most common extrapulmonary site is the hilar lymph nodes and the skin, where it presents as erythema nodosum [30].

Pulmonary System

Pulmonary Histoplasmosis develops when the mold form of the fungus is inhaled into the lungs, where it transforms into the yeast form (tissue-invasive form) [31]. Initially, the fungus resides within macrophages and later spreads via the lymphatic system to reach organs of the reticuloendothelial system [32]. The infection presents with fever, cough, weight loss, lymphadenopathy, and abdominal pain. These cardinal signs are also seen with pulmonary TB, bronchiectasis, or pneumonia; hence, patients with Histoplasmosis are commonly misdiagnosed [30]. Failure in prompt diagnosis may lead to an increase in mortality and morbidity due to increasing cavitations.

Reticuloendothelial System and Bone Marrow

Disseminated *Histoplasma Capsulatum* can spread hematogenously into the reticuloendothelial system before the development of a cellular immune response (initial 2 weeks) [31]. Evidence regarding liver involvement without primary lung infection is rare, but it is recommended that clinicians remain vigilant regarding the possibility of such a presentation for prompt diagnosis and management [32]. With liver involvement, the infection can present with vomiting, nausea, elevated LFTs, jaundice, portal hypertension, and ascites and can lead to the formation of hepatic granulomas [32, 33].

The fungus interacts with the Hematopoietic stem cells (HSCs) via TLR2, TLR4, and Dectin-1. This leads to a rise in cytokine production and release; the fungus also alters the proliferation of HSC and induces their apoptosis. This directly affects hematopoiesis and leads to anemia as well as pancytopenia and hence, modulation of the immune response in the host [34]. Through the same mechanism of interaction, the fungus also affects the mesenchymal stromal cells (MSCs), particularly reducing their differentiation potential [35].

Central Nervous System

CNS involvement occurs in up to 5 to 10% of disseminated histoplasmosis cases [12]. Affected individuals are reported to have lymphocytic or neutrophilic pleocytosis. The common brain changes include meningeal enhancement, ventricular enlargement, brain infarcts, white matter alterations, low-density cerebellar changes, subdural hematoma, and mass focal lesions [12]. Spinal cord involvement can include protrusion of the intervertebral disc, compression of the cord, or bone lesions. The common presenting complaints of these patients include headache, confusion, and altered mental status [12].

Diagnosis

Early diagnosis of Histoplasmosis is lifesaving as it allows prompt management of the condition and reduces the risk of any serious complication. Standard diagnostic tests for Histoplasma include histopathology, culture, and cytology [33].

The gold standard test for *Histoplasma* is the isolation of the intracellular form of the yeast on culture [36]. Most of the cases are now diagnosed via direct cytopathological examination of bronchoalveolar lavage (BAL) due to their rapidity and sensitivity. Histoplasma antigen may also be used for diagnosis using a urine sample or BAL for rapid diagnosis [36].

Histopathology

Tissue samples for biopsy may be obtained from any affected organ of the body, including lymph nodes, liver, bone marrow, skin, or mucous membranes. The presence of *H. capsulatum* yeast in sample tissue confirms the presence of the yeast, but it does not necessarily indicate active infection [36]. The yeast cells, measuring up to 2 to 4μm, may be seen as ovoid cells with cell walls, residing within macrophages or rarely in the extracellular space. The fungus may demonstrate narrow-based budding. Methenamine silver stain or periodic acid-Schiff stains may be used to visualize the tissue samples via microscopy as they significantly highlight the yeast cell wall. The pathology is visualized as an incomplete granulomatous reaction or fibrosis [36].

Culture

Culture specimens with yeast isolates are again obtained from the organs involved in the disease, such as the liver, bone marrow, mucous, skin lesions, BAL fluid, and sputum. The acquired specimen must be grown on a medium with suitable conditions to allow fungal growth and multiplication, such as Sabouraud agar. The temperature of the medium is maintained at 25 to 30°C, allowing the fungus's white mold form to be visualized. The mycelial phase may take up to 8 weeks. During this time, based on the growth of the fungus, it may appear as septated hyphae, smooth microconidia, or trabeculate macroconidia. Cultures at 37°C will reveal the yeast form of the dimorphic fungus and will appear small and round with narrow-based budding. This conversion was previously used as a method to confirm the presence of a dimorphic fungus, but the use of DNA probes in identification has now widely replaced it. The sensitivity of this test is based on the severity of the infection; disseminated histoplasmosis culture has a higher sensitivity than acute pulmonary Histoplasmosis. Blood cultures may also be used in the identification of the fungus, but conventional cultures have lower sensitivity compared to the lysis centrifugation tubes from blood cultures; however, the latter is no longer being used despite its high sensitivity [36, 37].

Antigen Detection

A definitive diagnosis of Histoplasmosis requires culture or biopsy. Still, a plausible diagnosis may also be made using antigen detection tests as they are considered more effective at reaching a diagnosis of Histoplasmosis. These become more important in the case of acute disease when antibodies to the fungus are not detectable. A particularly effective method in disseminated disease is the radioimmunoassay (RIA) for fungus polysaccharide antigens in urine and serum specimens using rabbit serum [37]. Additionally, two ELISA tests, sandwich-ELISA and Inhibition-ELISA have also been introduced but are less sensitive than RIA. These tests are rapid and have a high sensitivity for diagnosis [37].

Furthermore, after repeated evaluations, the modified version of the EIA, MiraVista assay, is now available but requires testing at a central laboratory. It provides highly sensitive results, especially for patients with HIV [36]. In a multicenter study, the sensitivity was reported as highest for disseminated infection of the fungus and then for chronic disease. Additional diagnostics are also developing, such as IMMY ALPHA Histoplasma EIA, which was approved by the FDA for use on urine samples at local laboratories in 2007. Its sensitivity, however, was lower than the MiraVista EIA assay. Hence, after further developments, IMMY, an analyte-specific reagent (ASR) antigen EIA has a high sensitivity but still not as high as MiraVista EIA's. Antigen detection tests, however, have possible cross-reactions with other fungal antigens, including Blastomycoses dermatitis and *Paracoccidioides brasiliensis*, limiting their use [36].

Antibody Detection

Antibodies in peripheral blood are only suitable for diagnosis of early acute infection after 4 to 8 weeks; hence it is mainly used for chronic cases of Histoplasmosis. This is the major detection test due to its rapid response time [37]. The routine assays used include complement fixation (CF), immunodiffusion (ID), and enzyme immunoassay (EIA) considering their high accuracy and convenience. This test, however, is not specific to H. *capsulatum* as Histoplasma-like antigens may appear in patients with other fungal infections such as *Blastomycosis, Coccidiomycosis, Paracoccidiomycosis, Aspergillosis, Candidiasis,* and *Cryptococcosis* [37].

Histoplasma mycelial culture is used to obtain an antigenic extract called histoplasmin (HMIN) which is then used to detect antibodies. The C, M, and H antigens in HMIN are useful in detecting antibodies to galactomannan, catalase, and β-glucosidase, respectively. Since C-antigen is not specific to Histoplasmosis, the test mainly relies on the presence of anti-M and anti-H antibodies [36].

The CF assay detects antibodies in the individual's serum depending on the extent of complement fixation to antigen-antibody complexes formed involving the patient's antibodies and histoplasmin antigens. The person is reported to have an acute infection if the antibody titer rise is at least 4 folds [36].

The ID assay identifies the patient's antibodies which precipitate upon exposure to histoplasmin antigens on agar gel. The H band confirms acute infection and is seen with an M band. The M-band remains positive in most patients for a long time; hence, it is unsuitable for differentiating between acute, chronic, and resolved infection. The newly approved EIA test identifies IgG and IgM antibodies [36, 38].

The CF method is considered more sensitive than the ID method of assay but is less specific. The EIA is twice as sensitive than either CF or ID [36]. Research by Richer et al. suggests that the sensitivity of antibody tests can be improved by combining it with Mvista EIA as it can provide the best diagnostic yield in case of acute pulmonary Histoplasmosis as the results show that 77 out of 80 positive results were obtained when using the combination and appears to be the most useful in immunocompromised individuals [39].

Molecular tests: Molecular testing is far more rapid and specific than the previously mentioned diagnostic tests; however, currently, there is no FDA-approved molecular test available for *Histoplasma Capsulatum,* which could be immediately applied to clinical samples. The laboratory-developed PCR techniques, such as real-time and nested PCR, have different molecular targets, but with the need for a PCR assay for immediate use by clinicians, there is ongoing research into the development of newer polymerase chain reaction (PCR) techniques.

Clinical Manifestations

The clinical manifestations of histoplasmosis range from an asymptomatic state to a severe infection like diffuse pneumonitis. These depend in part on the immunity of the individual and the level of exposure. The disease is initially contained with the formation of caseating or non-caseating granulomas. In the case of an immune-compromised patient, however, the fungus cannot be contained within granulomas as the patient lacks IFN-gamma, TNF-alpha, and IL-17, which are necessary cytokines for granuloma formation [1].

Asymptomatic cases, in immunocompetent individuals, are incidentally diagnosed using CT scans highlighting enlargement of mediastinal or hilar lymph nodes and as pulmonary calcified or non-calcified nodules [33].

Acute Pulmonary Histoplasmosis

In the case of an immunocompetent host with high-level exposure, the patient will present with respiratory symptoms within 2 weeks of exposure. Acute symptomatic disease occurs in children and young adults [40].

These symptoms include dyspnea, non-productive cough, chest pain as well as diffuse involvement of the lungs. Patients also present with extrapulmonary symptoms, including fever, chills, malaise, hepatosplenomegaly, lymphadenopathy, bone marrow suppression with pancytopenia and anemia, and elevated LFTs. In critical cases, respiratory failure may lead to the death of the patient if prompt management is not provided [1, 33].

Acute pulmonary Histoplasmosis may also lead to mediastinal lymphadenitis and granuloma formation. This presents as severe sharp chest pain anteriorly, aggravating during inspiration, and frequently mistaken for pleuritic chest pain. Most cases resolve in 10 days, but some may lead to complications that are rare but may include compression of the trachea and esophagus, especially in children [33]. The patients may also develop acute respiratory distress syndrome due to severe hypoxia [1, 33].

Chronic Cavitary Pulmonary Histoplasmosis

Risk factors of chronic pulmonary Histoplasmosis include male sex, old age, history of COPD, and immunosuppression [33]. Up to 40% of chronic pulmonary Histoplasmosis presents with cavitations, mostly in the upper lobes of the lung bilaterally. These cavitary lesions contain inflammatory cytokines which progressively destroy the lung causing volume loss and pleural thickening [33]. The hilar lymph nodes frequently undergo calcification. Additionally, there is a vascular compromise, tissue necrosis, and fibrosis [33].

The recurrence rate of chronic cavitary pulmonary Histoplasmosis is 20%, mostly in immunocompromised individuals [1]. The disease has a slow course but may lead to mortality if not managed promptly and is frequently misdiagnosed as reactivated TB due to a similar presentation of chronic cough, dyspnea, chest pain, fatigue, fever, and night sweats [33].

Progressive Disseminated Histoplasmosis

The risk factors for Progressive Disseminated Histoplasmosis (PDH) include hematologic malignancy, steroid administration, solid-organ transplant, AIDS, and age older than 65 years or in infancy [40].

Patients with PDH present with worsening symptoms such as fever, weight loss, hepatosplenomegaly, hematologic disorders, and respiratory distress [1]. Chest X-rays reveal diffuse reticulonodular, interstitial, or miliary infiltrate in up to 70% of the patients. PDH can be classified as mild, moderate, or severe, depending on the symptoms. Immunocompromised individuals are mostly faced with severe complications such as hemophagohistiocytosis which, if left untreated, have a 100% mortality rate [1].

PDH is mostly seen in the pediatric population or immunocompromised adults who have weak cell-mediated immunity [40]. In infants, PDH can present as fever, hepatosplenomegaly, growth retardation, and cytopenia due to hematologic abnormalities, gastrointestinal ulcers, interstitial pneumonitis, and adrenal gland involvement; however, if sufficient and prompt therapy is provided, the mortality rate is reduced from 100% to less than 20% [40].

Pulmonary Complications of Histoplasmosis

Acute

Acute pulmonary Histoplasmosis may rarely progress to granulomatous mediastinitis, which refers to the enlargement and necrosis of multiple mediastinal lymph nodes [40]. This further complicates disease presentation when enlarged lymph nodes obstruct the adjacent structures in the thorax. This can lead to tracheal retraction and hence post-obstructive pneumonia, hypoxemia, and bronchiectasis [1].

The postinfectious phase of the disease can cause extrapulmonary complications such as erythema nodosum, erythema multiforme, and reactive arthritis [40].

Chronic

Chronic Histoplasmosis can also lead to some rare but serious complications, including mediastinal fibrosis, histoplasmoma, and broncholithiasis [41]. Mediastinal fibrosis is due to a chronic fibrotic response and can progress to encompass surrounding thoracic structures such as pulmonary arteries, veins, and superior vena cava (SVC) [42]. Obstruction of SVC may lead to superior vena cava syndrome, obstruction of pulmonary veins may present as a mitral stenosis-like syndrome, and obstruction of the pulmonary artery may lead to congestive heart failure [42].

Management of Histoplasmosis

Pharmaceutical Therapy

Current practice guidelines indicate that the specific clinical manifestations and severity should determine the management of Histoplasmosis [43]. In all cases, however, the two main antifungal agents of choice remain azoles and amphotericin B [44]. It should be noted that echinocandins are not recommended as they failed to demonstrate efficacy against Histoplasmosis [45]. Management of acute pulmonary Histoplasmosis is further influenced by the severity of clinical symptoms experienced by infected individuals. In mild to moderate illness cases, if symptoms persist for less than four weeks, no treatment is indicated [44]. However, for mild to moderate cases lasting greater than 4 weeks, the first line agent of choice remains Itraconazole, with an initial loading dose of 200 milligrams every 8 hours for 72 hours, followed by 200 milligrams up to twice daily for a maximum of 12 weeks or less, depending on the resolution in symptom severity [46].

However, recommendations differ when symptom severity elevates to signify the acute pulmonary infection as moderately severe to severe and diffuse. In these cases, combination therapy employing both amphotericin B and Itraconazole is recommended. Firstly, amphotericin B is administered intravenously, with dosage depending on the type of formulation chosen, such as liposomal, lipid complex, or deoxycholate, for a period of up to two weeks. This is followed by itraconazole therapy using the same treatment algorithm as recommended for mild to moderate disease, with a 200-milligram loading dose for three days followed by 12-week therapy with up to two oral doses daily [47]. Corticosteroids such as methylprednisolone are adjunctively administered for concurrent respiratory complications and have demonstrated efficacy in the reduction of pulmonary distress and hypoxemia [48].

When patients develop a chronic cavitary pulmonary infection, itraconazole is recommended with similar loading dosages as for acute infection. However, the total length of treatment is increased to a minimum of 12 months [8]. However, in some cases, patients with chronic infection can develop other manifestations of pulmonary disease, including mediastinal fibrosis, granuloma formation, broncholithiasis, as well as pulmonary nodules. Of these, only mediastinal granulomas are treated with pharmaceutical therapy, with recommendations remaining the same as that for treatment for acute mild disease. The other conditions are not targeted with pharmaceutical therapy. Instead, interventional management with stenting of obstructed vessels is recommended for fibrosis, while broncholiths are simply removed with bronchoscopy [49, 50].

Multiple azoles, namely: itraconazole, voriconazole, posaconazole, isavuconazole and fluconazole, have shown in vitro efficacy against histoplasmosis. While, theoretically, all can be administered, physicians should remain cognizant of the fact that randomized controlled trials demonstrating undeniable efficacy have only been conducted on two azole drugs: Itraconazole and fluconazole, and amphotericin B [51, 52].

Efficacy and Safety of Therapy

While Itraconazole remains the most efficacious within the cohort of all azoles with activity against Histoplasmosis, with a curative rate of >80% [53], it requires high steady-state serum concentrations for maximum effectiveness. Oral delivery of Itraconazole is largely understood to be safe and tolerable, with most side effects being reversible and mild and extremely low hepatic toxicity [54]. It is known to cause headaches, dizziness, and gastrointestinal effects [55]. However, serious cardiovascular adverse events have been associated with its use, most commonly heart failure with preserved ejection fraction and, rarely, resistant hypertension [56].

Fluconazole, on the other hand, is recommended only in patients that cannot tolerate Itraconazole or in those that experience difficulty in sustaining adequate blood levels. It has a significantly lower curative rate (<60%) [57] and often leads to rapid resistance development in patients with concurrent HIV infection [58]. While it is also tolerated well, it should be noted that in addition to developing mild adverse effects like Itraconazole, fluconazole can also cause xerosis, alopecia, and fatigue. In addition, greater than half of individuals who experience adverse effects require a change in pharmaceutical management strategy, either via changes in dosages or via switching to an alternative drug altogether, especially with chronic therapy [59].

An important consideration is the teratogenic nature of azoles, especially in the first trimester. Modified management strategies are therefore required in pregnant individuals, with amphotericin B as the first line agent administered under the care of an infectious disease expert [60, 61].

Ultimately, amphotericin B, the initial drug of choice in severe acute clinical manifestations, has considerable associated adverse events that need to be evaluated carefully. Firstly, the deoxycholate formulation has the potential to induce gastrointestinal disturbances, fever, rigors, hypoxia, hypertension as well as hypotension. However, its primary adverse effect, owing to chronic use and elevated dosages, is renal injury. Evidence shows that sodium loading prior to administration can reduce its nephrotoxic potential [62].

In addition, amphotericin B use has also been commonly associated with electrolyte imbalances, including hypokalemia and hypomagnesemia. It can also lower erythropoietin concentrations. A rare but debilitating adverse event is the development of demyelinating encephalopathy in certain select individuals, namely those who have received a bone marrow transplant with concomitant total body irradiation or those currently being administered cyclosporine [63, 64].

Future Recommendations, Novel Evidence, and Advancements

The management of Histoplasmosis is well understood and agreed upon in the medical literature. This is demonstrated by the most recent practice guidelines being as old as 16 years old (2007) [52]. However, in the United States, mortality can be as high as 16% in immunocompetent individuals, and it can escalate to almost 25% in immunocompromised individuals, and the advent of modern antiretroviral therapy seems to have not played a role in reducing mortality [65].

Therefore, the role of other aspects, apart from management strategies, in reducing Histoplasmosis associated mortality has been brought into question. One study [66] evaluated the role of social characteristics in worsening mortality and found that individuals with limited insurance coverage regarding antiretroviral therapy, case management, and mental health services were at higher risk, as supported by other evidence [67] However, conflicting evidence has also been reported, with no increase in Histoplasmosis associated mortality in those with a history of psychiatric illness and substance use [65]. Large-scale studies evaluating the role of specific socio-economic parameters in impacting outcomes are needed.

Moreover, Histoplasmosis can often present with nonspecific symptoms, including high fever and cough [68], or with non-classic symptoms, such as isolated fever, in the absence of concomitant symptoms [69]. Therefore, it is unsurprising that diagnosis is often delayed, on average, by 40 days, with about 4 missed opportunities in >80% of infected individuals, and current diagnostic methods have been blamed [70]. There is a need for the development of additional diagnostic procedures that are rapid or minimize the role of administration of a battery of multiple diagnostic procedures, as it currently stands. Very recently, some additional non-classic tests have been identified and used successfully in a rarity of cases, such as metagenomic next generation sequencing [69], blood smears [71, 72], and bone marrow sampling [73].

Furthermore, a few recent case reports have alluded to an unusual relationship between the SARS-CoV-2 virus (COVID-19) and Histoplasmosis. It appears that in some cases, in patients with COVID-19, Histoplasmosis can mimic primary bronchogenic carcinoma [74] or disseminate in those requiring mechanical ventilation [75]. Exhaustive clinical research is needed before any causal link can be established.

Finally, it is surprising that even though azoles are widely considered the first line of treatment in most patients, only two agents have been evaluated in clinical trials. While it is extensive in vitro evidence, it is important to consider that in many cases, azole tolerability is a concern and that the alternative agent of choice, amphotericin B, also poses numerous risks with its comprehensive list of drug-drug interactions and additional serious side effects. The role of other agents, such as posaconazole, should also be further evaluated as it has already proven to be effective as salvage therapy [76].

Conclusion

Pulmonary manifestations of histoplasmosis only develop in a select subset of patients who are often immunocompromised, with most immunocompetent patients remaining asymptomatic with eventual infection resolution. In those who experience acute pulmonary symptoms, resolution typically occurs within 4 weeks and when this occurs, treatment is not mandated. However, when symptoms last for more than 4 weeks, or development of subacute or chronic infection is suspected, the role of treatment becomes urgent and significant. Management in such cases is guided by the severity of symptoms and often involves medium to long term conjunctive therapy with azoles and amphotericin B, with simultaneous corticosteroid administration for worsening respiratory or circulatory sequelae. Even though treatment success rates are high (>80%) with first line agents, one of the primary concerns remains diagnostic ease. Diagnostic delays, due to variability in and the non-specific nature of presenting symptoms, coupled with misdiagnosis of tuberculosis in infected patients contribute to the morbidity and mortality in infected individuals. In addition, in those who cannot tolerate first line agents, the relatively low research availability on second- and third-line agents becomes a significant hindrance. Therefore, even though clinical practice guidelines may have remained unchanged for over a decade, large scale studies in infected individuals evaluating the role of drugs that have shown high efficacy in invitro studies, as well as the search for rapid diagnostic tests with high sensitivities, should not be halted.

References

[1] Akram SM, Koirala J. Histoplasmosis. [Updated 2022 Aug 8]. In: StatPearls [Internet]. Treasure Island (FL): *StatPearls Publishing*; 2022 Jan-. Available from: https://www.ncbi.nlm.nih.gov/books/NBK448185/.

[2] Bongomin F, Ekeng BE, Kibone W, Nsenga L, Olum R, Itam-Eyo A, Kuate MPN, Pebolo FP, Davies AA, Manga M, Ocansey B, Kwizera R, Baluku JB. Invasive Fungal Diseases in Africa: A Critical Literature Review. *J Fungi (Basel).* 2022;8(12):1236. doi: 10.3390/jof8121236. PMID: 36547569; PMCID: PMC9853333.

[3] Araúz AB, Papineni P. Histoplasmosis. *Infect Dis Clin North Am.* 2021;35(2):471-491. doi: 10.1016/j.idc.2021.03.011. PMID: 34016287.

[4] Poplin V, Smith C, Milsap D, Zabel L, Bahr NC. Diagnosis of Pulmonary Infections Due to Endemic Fungi. *Diagnostics (Basel).* 2021;11(5):856. doi: 10.3390/diagnostics11050856. PMID: 34068825; PMCID: PMC8151383.

[5] Azar MM, Hage CA. Clinical Perspectives in the Diagnosis and Management of Histoplasmosis. *Clin Chest Med.* 2017;38(3):403-415. doi: 10.1016/j.ccm.2017.04.004. Epub 2017 May 17. PMID: 28797485.

[6] Cataño J, Porras J. Pulmonary Histoplasmosis. *Am J Trop Med Hyg.* 2023;108(2):239-240. doi: 10.4269/ajtmh.22-0541. PMID: 36623482.

[7] Choi SJ, Choi HS, Chun JY, Kim CJ, Lee MJ, Kim M, Choe GY. Subacute progressive disseminated histoplasmosis in immunocompetent patient. *Korean J Intern Med.* 2016;31(5):999-1002. doi: 10.3904/kjim.2015.069. PMID: 26898594; PMCID: PMC5016276.

[8] Baker J, Kosmidis C, Rozaliyani A, Wahyuningsih R, Denning DW. Chronic Pulmonary Histoplasmosis-A Scoping Literature Review. *Open Forum Infect Dis.* 2020;7(5):ofaa119. doi: 10.1093/ofid/ofaa119. PMID: 32411810; PMCID: PMC7210804.

[9] Goodwin RA Jr, Snell JD, Hubbard WW, Terry RT. Early chronic pulmonary histoplasmosis. *Am Rev Respir Dis.* 1966;93(1):47-61. doi: 10.1164/arrd.1966.93.1.47. PMID: 5901386.

[10] Sizemore TC. Rheumatologic manifestations of histoplasmosis: a review. *Rheumatol Int.* 2013;33(12):2963-5. doi: 10.1007/s00296-013-2816-y. PMID: 23835880.

[11] Wheat LJ, Stein L, Corya BC, Wass JL, Norton JA, Grider K, Slama TG, French ML, Kohler RB. Pericarditis as a manifestation of histoplasmosis during two large urban outbreaks. *Medicine (Baltimore).* 1983;62(2):110-9. doi: 10.1097/00005792-198303000-00004. PMID: 6827979.

[12] Wheat J, Myint T, Guo Y, Kemmer P, Hage C, Terry C, Azar MM, Riddell J, Ender P, Chen S, Shehab K, Cleveland K, Esguerra E, Johnson J, Wright P, Douglas V, Vergidis P, Ooi W, Baddley J, Bamberger D, Khairy R, Vikram HR, Jenny-Avital E, Sivasubramanian G, Bowlware K, Pahud B, Sarria J, Tsai T, Assi M, Mocherla S, Prakash V, Allen D, Passaretti C, Huprikar S, Anderson A. Central nervous system histoplasmosis: Multicenter retrospective study on clinical features,

diagnostic approach and outcome of treatment. *Medicine (Baltimore).* 2018;97(13):e0245. doi: 10.1097/MD.0000000000010245.

[13] Gómez LF, Torres IP, Jiménez-A MDP, McEwen JG, de Bedout C, Peláez CA, Acevedo JM, Taylor ML, Arango M. Detection of Histoplasma capsulatum in Organic Fertilizers by Hc100 Nested Polymerase Chain Reaction and Its Correlation with the Physicochemical and Microbiological Characteristics of the Samples. *Am J Trop Med Hyg.* 2018;98:1303–1312.

[14] Ashraf N, Kubat RC, Poplin V, Adenis AA, Denning DW, Wright L, McCotter O, Schwartz IS, Jackson BR, Chiller T, Bahr NC. Re-drawing the Maps for Endemic Mycoses. *Mycopathologia.* 2020;185:843–865.

[15] Armstrong PA, Jackson BR, Haselow D, Fields V, Ireland M, Austin C, Signs K, Fialkowski V, Patel R, Ellis P, Iwen PC, Pedati C, Gibbons-Burgener S, Anderson J, Dobbs T, Davidson S, McIntyre M, Warren K, Midla J, Luong N, Benedict K. Multistate Epidemiology of Histoplasmosis, United States, 2011–2014. *Emerging Infectious Diseases.* 2018;24(3):425-431. doi:10.3201/eid2403.171258.

[16] Cano MV, Hajjeh RA. The epidemiology of histoplasmosis: a review. *Semin Respir Infect.* 2001;16:109–18.

[17] Bahr NC, Antinori S, Wheat LJ, Sarosi GA. Histoplasmosis infections worldwide: thinking outside of the Ohio River valley. *Curr Trop Med Rep.* 2015;2:70–80.

[18] Manos NE, Ferebee SH, Kerschbaum WF. Geographic variation in the prevalence of histoplasmin sensitivity. *Dis Chest.* 1956;29:649–68.

[19] Oladele RO, Ayanlowo OO, Richardson MD, Denning DW. Histoplasmosis in Africa: An emerging or a neglected disease? *PLoS Negl Trop Dis* 2018;12: e0006046. doi: 10.1371/journal.pntd.0006046.

[20] Develoux M, Amona FM, Hennequin C. Histoplasmosis Caused by Histoplasma capsulatum var. duboisii: A Comprehensive Review of Cases From 1993 to 2019. *Clin Infect Dis Off Publ Infect Dis Soc Am.* 2021;73:e543–e549. doi: 10.1093/cid/ciaa1304.

[21] Oladele RO, Osaigbovo II, Akanmu AS, Adekanmbi OA, Ekeng BE, Mohammed Y, Alex-Wele MA, Okolo MO, Ayanbeku ST, Unigwe US, Akase IE, Dan-Jumbo A, Isralski D, Denning DW, Pasqualotto AC, Chiller T. Prevalence of Histoplasmosis among Persons with Advanced HIV Disease, Nigeria. *Emerg Infect Dis.* 2022;28(11):2261-2269. doi: 10.3201/eid2811.220542. PMID: 36286009; PMCID: PMC9622240.

[22] Ray A, Aayilliath K A, Banerjee S, Chakrabarti A, Denning DW. Burden of Serious Fungal Infections in India. *Open Forum Infect Dis.* 2022;9(12):ofac603. doi: 10.1093/ofid/ofac603. PMID: 36589484; PMCID: PMC9792086.

[23] Duong TN, Le MH, Beardsley J, Denning DW, Le NH, Nguyen BT. Updated estimation of the burden of fungal disease in Vietnam. *Mycoses.* 2022. doi: 10.1111/myc.13559. PMID: 36564981.

[24] Valdez AF, Miranda DZ, Guimarães AJ, Nimrichter L, Nosanchuk JD. Pathogenicity & virulence of *Histoplasma capsulatum* - A multifaceted organism adapted to intracellular environments. *Virulence.* 2022;13(1):1900-1919. doi: 10.1080/21505594.2022.2137987. PMID: 36266777; PMCID: PMC9621017.

[25] Newman SL, Gootee L, Hilty J, Morris RE. Human macrophages do not require phagosome acidification to mediate fungistatic/fungicidal activity against Histoplasma capsulatum. *J Immunol.* 2006;176(3):1806-13. doi: 10.4049/jimmunol.176.3.1806. PMID: 16424211.

[26] Pitangui NS, Sardi JC, Silva JF, Benaducci T, Moraes da Silva RA, Rodríguez-Arellanes G, Taylor ML, Mendes-Giannini MJ, Fusco-Almeida AM. Adhesion of Histoplasma capsulatum to pneumocytes and biofilm formation on an abiotic surface. *Biofouling.* 2012;28(7):711-8. doi: 10.1080/08927014.2012.703659. PMID: 22784100.

[27] Newman SL. Macrophages in host defense against Histoplasma capsulatum. *Trends Microbiol.* 1999;7(2):67-71. doi: 10.1016/s0966-842x(98)01431-0. PMID: 10081083.

[28] Woods JP. Histoplasma capsulatum molecular genetics, pathogenesis, and responsiveness to its environment. *Fungal Genet Biol.* 2002;35(2):81-97. doi: 10.1006/fgbi.2001.1311. PMID: 11848673.

[29] Woods JP. Knocking on the right door and making a comfortable home: Histoplasma capsulatum intracellular pathogenesis. *Curr Opin Microbiol.* 2003;6(4):327-31. doi: 10.1016/s1369-5274(03)00080-8. PMID: 12941399.

[30] Ekeng BE, Edem K, Akintan P, Oladele RO. Histoplasmosis in African children: clinical features, diagnosis, and treatment. *Ther Adv Infect Dis.* 2022; 9:20499361211068592.

[31] Pathogensis and clinical manifestation of disseminated histoplasmosis. *UpToDate.* Available at: https://www.uptodate.com/contents/pathogenesis-and-clinical-manifestations-of-disseminated-histoplasmosis#H5 [accessed: 24 Dec 2022].

[32] Sayeed M, Benzamin M, Nahar L, Rana M, Aishy AS. Hepatic Histoplasmosis: An Update. *J Clin Transl Hepatol.* 2022;10(4):726-729. doi:10.14218/JCTH.2020.00080.

[33] Hage CA, Wheat LJ, Loyd J, Allen SD, Blue D, Knox KS. Pulmonary histoplasmosis. *Semin Respir Crit Care Med.* 2008;29(2):151-165. doi:10.1055/s-2008-1063854.

[34] Rodríguez-Echeverri C, Gómez BL, González Á. *Histoplasma capsulatum* Activates Hematopoietic Stem Cells and Their Progenitors through a Mechanism Dependent on TLR2, TLR4, and Dectin-1. *J Fungi (Basel).* 2022;8(10):1108.. doi:10.3390/jof8101108.

[35] Rodríguez-Echeverri C, Gómez BL, González Á. Histoplasma capsulatum modulates the immune response, affects proliferation and differentiation, and induces apoptosis of mesenchymal stromal cells [published online ahead of print, 2022 Oct 11]. *Mycoses.* 2022;10.1111/myc.13537. doi:10.1111/myc.13537.

[36] Azar MM, Hage CA. Laboratory Diagnostics for Histoplasmosis. *J Clin Microbiol.* 2017;55(6):1612-1620. doi:10.1128/JCM.02430-16.

[37] Guimarães AJ, Nosanchuk JD, Zancopé-Oliveira RM. DIAGNOSIS OF HISTOPLASMOSIS. *Braz J Microbiol.* 2006;37(1):1-13. doi:10.1590/S1517-83822006000100001.

[38] Wheat LJ, Kohler RB, French ML, Garten M, Kleiman M, Zimmerman SE, Schlech W, Ho J, White A, Brahmi Z. Immunoglobulin M and G histoplasmal antibody

response in histoplasmosis. *Am Rev Respir Dis.* 1983;128(1):65-70. doi:10.1164/arrd.1983.128.1.65.

[39] Richer SM, Smedema ML, Durkin MM, Herman KM, Hage CA, Fuller D, Wheat LJ. Improved Diagnosis of Acute Pulmonary Histoplasmosis by Combining Antigen and Antibody Detection. *Clin Infect Dis.* 2016;62(7):896-902. doi:10.1093/cid/ciw007.

[40] Adderson E. Histoplasmosis. *Pediatr Infect Dis J.* 2006;25(1):73-74. doi:10.1097/01.inf.0000196922.46347.66.

[41] Linder KA, Kauffman CA. Histoplasmosis: Epidemiology, diagnosis, and clinical manifestations. *Curr Fungal Infect Rep.* 2019;13(3):120-8.

[42] Matthew C. Washam and Lara A. Danziger-Isakov. *Nelson Textbook of Pediatrics*, Histoplasmosis *(Histoplasma capsulatum)*. Chapter 265, 1650-1652.e1.

[43] Wheat J, Sarosi G, McKinsey D, Hamill R, Bradsher R, Johnson P, Loyd J, Kauffman C. Practice Guidelines for the Management of Patients with Histoplasmosis. *Clin Infect Dis.* 2000;30(4):688-95.

[44] Mazi PB, Arnold SR, Baddley JW, Bahr NC, Beekmann SE, McCarty TP, Polgreen PM, Rauseo AM, Spec A. Management of Histoplasmosis by Infectious Disease Physicians. *Open Forum Infect Dis.* 2022;9(7):ofac313.

[45] Hage CA, Ribes JA, Wengenack NL, Baddour LM, Assi M, McKinsey DS, Hammoud K, Alapat D, Babady NE, Parker M, Fuller D, Noor A, Davis TE, Rodgers M, Connolly PA, El Haddad B, Wheat LJ. A multicenter evaluation of tests for diagnosis of histoplasmosis. *Clin Infect Dis.* 2011;53(5):448-54.

[46] Hecht FM, Wheat J, Korzun AH, Hafner R, Skahan KJ, Larsen R, Limjoco MT, Simpson M, Schneider D, Keefer MC, Clark R, Lai KK, Jacobson JM, Squires K, Bartlett JA, Powderly W. Itraconazole maintenance treatment for histoplasmosis in AIDS: a prospective, multicenter trial. *J Acquir Immune Defic Syndr Hum Retrovirol.* 1997;16(2):100-7.

[47] Kauffman CA. Histoplasmosis: a clinical and laboratory update. *Clin Microbiol Rev.* 2007;20(1):115-32.

[48] Klein M, Khan M, Salinas JL, Sanchez R. Disseminated pulmonary histoplasmosis in immunocompetent patients: a common epidemiological exposure. *BMJ Case Rep.* 2019;12(3).

[49] Bhagavan BS, Rao DR, Weinberg T. Histoplasmosis producing broncholithiasis. *Arch Pathol.* 1971;91(6):577-9.

[50] Mocherla S, Wheat LJ. Treatment of histoplasmosis. *Semin Respir Infect.* 2001;16(2):141-8.

[51] Hendrix MJ, Larson L, Rauseo AM, Rutjanawech S, Franklin AD, Powderly WG, Spec A. Voriconazole Versus Itraconazole for the Initial and Step-down Treatment of Histoplasmosis: A Retrospective Cohort. *Clin Infect Dis.* 2021;73(11):e3727-e32.

[52] Wheat LJ, Freifeld AG, Kleiman MB, Baddley JW, McKinsey DS, Loyd JE, Kauffman CA, Infectious Diseases Society of America. Clinical practice guidelines for the management of patients with histoplasmosis: 2007 update by the Infectious Diseases Society of America. *Clin Infect Dis.* 2007;45(7):807-25.

[53] Dismukes WE, Bradsher RW Jr, Cloud GC, Kauffman CA, Chapman SW, George RB, Stevens DA, Girard WM, Saag MS, Bowles-Patton C. Itraconazole therapy for

blastomycosis and histoplasmosis. NIAID Mycoses Study Group. *Am J Med.* 1992;93(5):489-97.
[54] Gupta AK, Chwetzoff E, Del Rosso J, Baran R. Hepatic safety of itraconazole. *J Cutan Med Surg.* 2002;6(3):210-3.
[55] Haria M, Bryson HM, Goa KL. Itraconazole. A reappraisal of its pharmacological properties and therapeutic use in the management of superficial fungal infections. *Drugs.* 1996;51(4):585-620.
[56] Denolle T, Azizi M, Massart C, Zennaro MC. [Itraconazole: a new drug-related cause of hypertension]. *Ann Cardiol Angeiol (Paris).* 2014;63(3):213-5.
[57] McKinsey DS, Kauffman CA, Pappas PG, Cloud GA, Girard WM, Sharkey PK, Hamill RJ, Thomas CJ, Dismukes WE. Fluconazole therapy for histoplasmosis. The National Institute of Allergy and Infectious Diseases Mycoses Study Group. *Clin Infect Dis.* 1996;23(5):996-1001.
[58] Wheat LJ, Connolly P, Smedema M, Brizendine E, Hafner R. Emergence of resistance to fluconazole as a cause of failure during treatment of histoplasmosis in patients with acquired immunodeficiency disease syndrome. *Clin Infect Dis.* 2001;33(11):1910-3.
[59] Davis MR, Nguyen MH, Donnelley MA, Thompson Iii GR. Tolerability of long-term fluconazole therapy. *J Antimicrob Chemother.* 2019;74(3):768-71.
[60] Giavini E, Menegola E. Are azole fungicides a teratogenic risk for human conceptus? *Toxicol Lett.* 2010;198(2):106-11.
[61] Pilmis B, Jullien V, Sobel J, Lecuit M, Lortholary O, Charlier C. Antifungal drugs during pregnancy: an updated review. *J Antimicrob Chemother.* 2015;70(1):14-22.
[62] Laniado-Laborín R, Cabrales-Vargas MN. Amphotericin B: side effects and toxicity. *Rev Iberoam Micol.* 2009;26(4):223-7.
[63] Luo S, Wen H, Zhou M, Wu C, Hong D. Case report: Reversible encephalopathy associated with liposomal amphotericin B in a patient with cryptococcal meningitis. *Front Neurol.* 2022;13:1019137.
[64] Usami E, Kimura M, Kanematsu T, Yoshida S, Mori T, Nakashima K, Matsuoka T, Yoshimura T, Mori H, Sugiyama T, Teramachi H. Evaluation of hypokalemia and potassium supplementation during administration of liposomal-amphotericin B. *Exp Ther Med.* 2014;7(4):941-6.
[65] Cherabie J, Mazi P, Rauseo AM, Ayres C, Larson L, Rutjanawech S, O'Halloran J, Presti R, Powderly WG, Spec A. Long-Term Mortality after Histoplasma Infection in People with HIV. *J Fungi (Basel).* 2021;7(5).
[66] Hevey MA, Presti RM, O'Halloran JA, Larson L, Raval K, Powderly WG, Spec A. Mortality After Cryptococcal Infection in the Modern Antiretroviral Therapy Era. *J Acquir Immune Defic Syndr.* 2019;82(1):81-7.
[67] Weiser J, Beer L, Frazier EL, Patel R, Dempsey A, Hauck H, Skarbinski J. Service Delivery and Patient Outcomes in Ryan White HIV/AIDS Program-Funded and -Nonfunded Health Care Facilities in the United States. *JAMA Intern Med.* 2015;175(10):1650-9.
[68] Aidé MA. Chapter 4--histoplasmosis. *J Bras Pneumol.* 2009;35(11):1145-51.

[69] Wang N, Zhao C, Tang C, Wang L. Case Report and Literature Review: Disseminated Histoplasmosis Infection Diagnosed by Metagenomic Next-Generation Sequencing. *Infect Drug Resist.* 2022;15:4507-14.

[70] Miller AC, Arakkal AT, Koeneman SH, Cavanaugh JE, Thompson GR, Baddley JW, Polgreen PM. Frequency and Duration of, and Risk Factors for, Diagnostic Delays Associated with Histoplasmosis. *J Fungi (Basel).* 2022;8(5).

[71] Santos Júnior CJD, Rocha TJM, Souza AKP. Disseminated histoplasmosis diagnosed through blood smear. *Rev Soc Bras Med Trop.* 2022;55.

[72] Suárez EU, Atencia CJ, Quintero-Valencia C. Disseminated histoplasmosis in peripheral blood smear. *Med Clin (Barc).* 2022;158(3):148.

[73] Mussá NY, Ismail S, Carvalho D. Disseminated histoplasmosis diagnosed in a bone marrow sample. *Hematol Transfus Cell Ther.* 2022;44(1):138-9.

[74] D'Ambrosio PD, Costa AN, Scordamaglio PR, Terra RM. Endobronchial histoplasmosis mimicking primary bronchogenic carcinoma during the COVID-19 pandemic. *J Bras Pneumol.* 2022;48(2):e20210048.

[75] Perez Del Nogal G, Mata A, Ernest P, Salinas I. Disseminated histoplasmosis in an immunocompetent patient with COVID-19 pneumonia. *BMJ Case Rep.* 2022;15(1).

[76] Restrepo A, Tobón A, Clark B, Graham DR, Corcoran G, Bradsher RW, Goldman M, Pankey G, Moore T, Negroni R, Graybill JR. Salvage treatment of histoplasmosis with posaconazole. *J Infect.* 2007;54(4):319-27.

Chapter 8

Gastrointestinal Manifestations in Histoplasmosis

Gowthami Sai Kogilathota Jagirdhar[1,*]
Andres Perez[2]
Syed Anjum Khan[3]
and Salim Surani[4]
[1]Department of Medicine, Saint Michael's Medical Center, Newark, New Jersey, USA
[2]Department of Medicine, Saint Francis health system, Tulsa, Oklahoma, USA
[3]Department of Critical Care, Mayo Clinic Health System, Mankato, Minnesota, USA
[4]Department of Medicine & Pharmacy, Texas A&M University, Texas, USA

Abstract

Histoplasmosis presents as either a self-limited respiratory infection or an asymptomatic disease caused by *Histoplasma Capsulatum.* Its gastrointestinal (GI) manifestations are not under the radar for clinicians as it is usually asymptomatic or presents with vague abdominal pain in most patients. GI manifestations occur only in 3 to 12% of patients with disseminated Histoplasmosis, with the colon commonly involved followed by the small bowel. However, about 70% of patients with disseminated Histoplasmosis during autopsy have GI involvement. Due to the macro and micro characteristics, it can easily be misdiagnosed as Inflammatory bowel disease (IBD). These patients can be started on immunosuppressive therapy, which can be devastating. This review aims to unite the most updated information so that physicians know how to recognize the infection early. Histoplasmosis can be fatal in immunocompromised patients. They are more prone to histoplasmosis

* Corresponding Author's Email: gowthamireddykj@gmail.com.

In: Histoplasmosis
Editors: Salim Surani, Syed Anjum Khan and Reena Shah
ISBN: 979-8-89113-129-3

dissemination and infection of the gastrointestinal system. We performed a literature review in the PubMed database, including the terms "gastrointestinal," "GI," and "histoplasmosis" for the latest updates on the gastrointestinal manifestations of Histoplasmosis, including its epidemiology, pathogenesis, clinical presentation, treatment, and prognosis. Most of the studies included retrospective studies. There was also important information obtained from case reports. By the end of this chapter, clinicians should be able to recognize the various gastrointestinal manifestations of Histoplasmosis, its complications, and differential diagnosis.

Keywords: histoplasmosis, gastrointestinal, fungal infection, disseminated histoplasmosis, histoplasma capsulatum

Introduction

Histoplasma Capsulatum gets into the system by inhalation of fungal spores [1]. Around 90% of the population in North America's Ohio and Mississippi river valleys are exposed to it during their lifetime, per Centers for Disease Control and Prevention (CDC). Surveillance data from 12 states in the United States by Armstrong et al. from 2011 to 2014 found 3409 histoplasmosis cases [2]. Infection occurs through the spread of disease from the respiratory tract to the lymph nodes and dissemination to the other organs, including the gastrointestinal tract. Gastrointestinal infection occurs in immunocompetent and immunocompromised patients [3]. Most patients with disseminated Histoplasmosis with gastrointestinal involvement are asymptomatic or have vague signs and symptoms. The symptomatic disease occurs in patients with Human immunodeficiency virus/acquired immunodeficiency syndrome (HIV/AIDS) [4], with diarrhea being the most common manifestation. Patients often develop severe unremitting diarrhea that can lead to malabsorption, weight loss, and cachexia. Abdominal pain and tenderness can also be present.

Gastrointestinal involvement commonly occurs in patients with disseminated Histoplasmosis though isolated gastrointestinal involvement is also reported in the literature. Infection is more common in immunocompromised populations, such as patients with HIV not receiving antiretroviral therapy. Severe pulmonary infections, hematogenous and disseminated presentations occur in HIV patients with CD4 counts $<150/\mu L$. In the survey by Armstrong et al., more than half of the patients with available data were hospitalized with a hospital length of seven days, and death was reported in 7% of the patients [2].

Etiology and Pathogenesis

When soil is altered by excavation or construction, the spores become airborne and are inhaled; after reaching the alveoli, they convert to the yeast form, which is the invasive tissue form [5]. Neutrophils, macrophages, lymphocytes, and natural killer cells are attracted in response to the infection. The yeasts ingested by macrophages multiply inside them in the pre-immune phase of the illness. They spread to the reticuloendothelial system through the lymphatics. In immunocompetent patients, once cell-mediated immunity develops, cytokines eliminate the infection [5, 6]. The macrophages kill or prevent the organism from growing by forming a calcified granuloma around it [3]. A cell-mediated immune response is key for the recovery from Histoplasmosis, either by killing the organism or forming a calcified granuloma. Failing to mount a cell-mediated immunity is one of the main reasons for disseminated Histoplasmosis [7]. As in other granuloma-inducing infections, granuloma formation is required to contain fungal growth, prevent systemic dissemination, and protect the organs from widespread inflammatory tissue damage [8]. Failure to activate macrophage fungicidal capacity is likely the critical defect in *Histoplasma Capsulatum* in patients with disseminated Histoplasmosis. In an animal model study, in mice with severe combined immunodeficiency, administration of Interleukin 12 increased Interferon-gamma, tumor necrosis factor-alpha, and nitric oxide, resulting in decreased colony counts of *Histoplasma Capsulatum*. Therefore, patients on IFN gamma and TNF alpha inhibitors express severe forms of the disease [9]. Immunosuppressed patients, particularly those with aberrant cell-mediated immunity, are more prone to develop reactivation of dormant infection. Reactivation of old foci contained in the liver or progressive dissemination from a primary site in the lung reaching the liver.

Colonic Histoplasmosis

Gastrointestinal Histoplasmosis is an uncommon entity with protean manifestations. It can be misdiagnosed as Ulcerative Colitis, Crohn's disease, or malignancy, leading to inappropriate therapies or surgical interventions [10]. It occurs most commonly in immunocompromised patients and transplant patients. According to a study by Rashi et al., the various complaints included loose stools, diarrhea, altered bowel habits, and gastrointestinal bleeding [11]. Colonic Histoplasmosis is the infection of the colon with Histoplasma. This occurs commonly through the spread of inhaled bacteria through the lymph nodes into the colon. Host phagocytes carry the infection from lymph nodes to various organs, including the colon. The primary determining factor for the dissemination of the infection is the host's inflammatory response. This predicts the ability of Histoplasma to evade the immune system. It also predicts the development of latent histoplasmosis and determines the severity of symptoms and clinical presentation. Since disseminated histoplasmosis can have a non-specific presentation, disseminated infection can escape diagnosis, thereby progressing to chronic or latent histoplasmosis, which can reactivate later.

Epidemiology

Lamps et al. studied the incidence of gastrointestinal and hepatic Histoplasmosis et al. on 52 immunocompromised and immunocompetent patients with disseminated histoplasmosis presentation. Forty-three percent of the patients were presented with gastrointestinal symptoms instead of pulmonary manifestations. Thirty-one percent of patients had gastrointestinal lesions [12]. In a 15-year study on Histoplasmosis in French Guiana, 38.5% of samples involved the gastrointestinal tract. The colon was involved in 70% and the small intestine in 18% of the specimens [13, 14]. (Figueroa et al). Assi et al. identified 152 cases of Histoplasmosis after a solid organ transplant [15]. Less commonly, the oral mucosa [16], esophagus [17], stomach, rectum, appendix, pancreas, gallbladder, and anal region were involved [18].

Clinical Characteristics

According to Lamps et al., the most common sites for the involvement of the gastrointestinal tract are the small bowel (79%) and large bowel (55%) [12]. The most common site of involvement is the right colon, rectum, and descending colon [19]. Since Histoplasma spreads through the lymphatics, any lymphoid tissue from the mouth to the anus can be involved. The terminal ileal mucosa is most involved since it has Peyer's patches [10]. Figure 1 shows the various gastrointestinal manifestations of histoplasmosis.

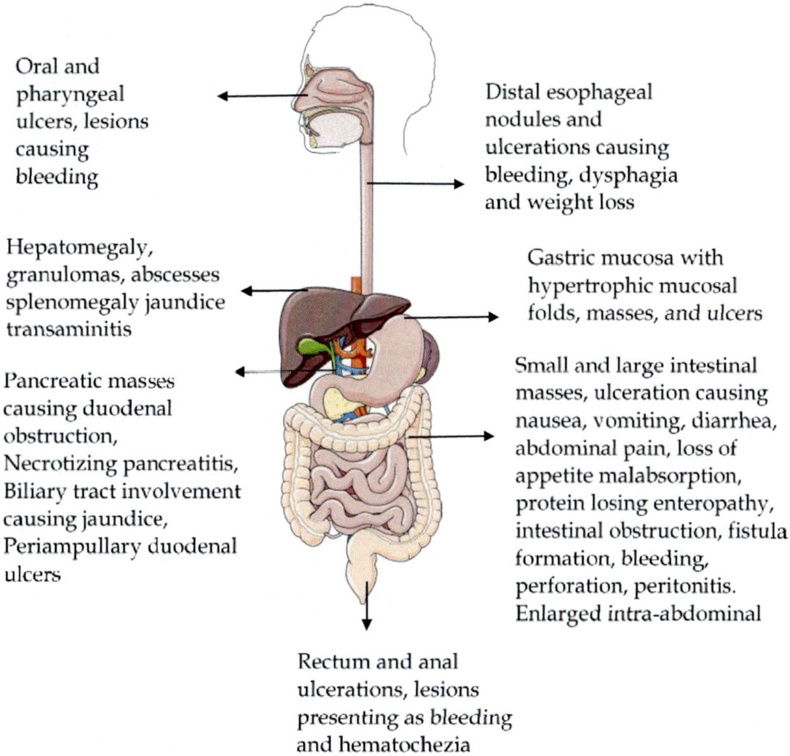

Figure 1. Gastrointestinal manifestations of histoplasmosis.

In a study by Lamps et al. on gastrointestinal and hepatic Histoplasmosis samples, fever was the most common presenting symptom. Other accompanying symptoms include diarrhea, weight loss, bleeding, abdominal pain, difficulty swallowing, nausea, and vomiting. These symptoms can sometimes be non-specific, and diagnosis can be missed [12]. In a study on four patients with Histoplasmosis by Zhu et al., hepatosplenomegaly and lymphadenopathy were the most common signs. Nonspecific symptoms such as irregular fevers, weight loss, abdominal pain, and distension were the most common symptoms [20]. Oral and pharyngeal mucosa involvement with ulcers and distal esophageal nodules and ulcerations that are erythematous and friable are described [10]. This involvement can cause dysphagia and esophageal and oral bleeding. Yvamoto et al. describe a patient who presented with progressive dysphagia and vomiting post-feeding with severe weight loss [17]. Histoplasma lesions and shallow ulcers that are painful and lined by a pseudo membrane in the gingiva and palate are described by Nakamura et al. [16]. Gastric mucosal involvement is rare and presents as erythema, ulcers, gastric masses, and hypertrophic mucosal folds. The lesions can rarely become large and mimic cancer.

Gastrointestinal bleeding can occur due to ulceration of the bowels and perforation leading to peritonitis. Immunocompromised and AIDS patients often present with GI lesions that bleed. Patients also presented with chronic large bowel obstruction from annular or polypoid lesions. These manifestations are seen in severe prolonged immunodeficiency [12]. Early satiety, decreased appetite, and weight loss from disseminated Histoplasmosis can often be confused with colon cancer or peritoneal carcinomatosis [21].

Rectal Histoplasmosis can present as a painful perianal and anal lesion or ulcerations mimicking malignancy on examination and imaging [22]. This presentation is often seen in AIDS patients. It mimics Crohn's disease in presentation. Hematochezia and rectal bleeding were also noted in some patients [15, 23]. Protein-losing enteropathy and hypogammaglobulinemia are other manifestations that are documented in the literature [24]. Enlargement of the paraaortic, celiac and mesenteric lymph nodes can be identified on imaging, along with the thickening of the bowels [10, 23, 25]. In a study by Assi et al., solid organ transplant recipients had a high risk of acquiring the infection within the first year of diagnosis. They also had severe, disseminated infections requiring intensive care unit management [15].

Pathology and Diagnosis

Standard staining techniques for the fungus include Grocott methenamine silver (GMS) and Periodic Acid Schiff (PAS) stains. Occasionally Ziehl-Neelsen staining is also positive. The fungus appears with a pseudo capsule that does not stain due to protoplasm retracting during fixation. Biopsy specimens of Histoplasma are obtained by colonoscopy, laparotomy, or biopsy. The most common colonic lesions from Histoplasmosis are ulcers. Gross gastrointestinal lesions in Histoplasmosis can also include erosions, nodules, polyps, strictures, perforations, bleeding, obstructive masses, and normal colonic mucosa [12, 13, 20, 26, 27]. On pathology, the lesions colon cancer observed are diffuse lymphohistiocytic infiltration of the lamina propria with fungi in the macrophages. Intracellular clusters of small narrow-based budding yeast, often with a halo, are seen. Ulceration and lymphohistiocytic nodules are other common pathology findings. Some specimens with minimal inflammatory reaction have also been documented. Rarely well-formed granulomas are described in literature [12].

The histopathological appearance of colonic Histoplasmosis often mimics colon cancer. Other common infections that look grossly similar to Histoplasmosis and appear like colon cancer include *Chlamydia Trachomatis* (Lymphogranuloma venereum), *Basidiobolus Ranarum*, and *Treponema Pallidum.* Pathology specimens of *Leishmania donovani, Talaromyces Marneffei*, Malakoplakia, *Pneumocystis Carinii, and Candida Glabrata* can mimic Histoplasmosis [19]. Leishmania parasite stains are negative on GMS and positive on Giemsa staining. Talaromyces can be differentiated by the presence of sausage cells with centrally located cross walls or transverse septum due to fission. It is positive on GMS and PAS stains like Histoplasmosis. Malakoplakia can be seen as granular histiocytes with targetoid concretions. *Pneumocystis Carinii* lacks budding and is extracellular. *Candida Glabrata* fungus is positive on gram stain, is predominantly extracellular, and has a neutrophilic response in contrast to Histoplasma, which elicits a histiocytic or lymphogranulocytic response [28]. Candida also has pseudo hyphae and greater size variability compared to Histoplasma. Blastomyces and cryptococcus can be differentiated by their morphology. In addition, pathology of the lymph nodes often shows necrotizing granulomas with Histoplasma in the macrophages. According to a retrospective multicentric study conducted by Nacher et al., there was a comparison between histopathology, direct examination, and culture 139 patients were diagnosed by a single technique, 132 by 2, and 77 by direct analysis, pathology, and culture. The patients more likely to have 2 or 3 positive methods were those with cutaneous and oral lesions" [29].

Differential Diagnosis

Gastrointestinal Histoplasmosis can have similar presentation and symptomatology to Inflammatory bowel disease [30], appendicitis, malignancy, intestinal tuberculosis, and sarcoidosis leading to incorrect treatments, including immunosuppressive therapy and unnecessary procedures [10, 12, 31]. Other gastrointestinal, fungal, and bacterial infections can have a similar presentation to Histoplasmosis. Gastric, small, and large bowel obstruction can occur in patients, rarely mimicking a neoplasm [13, 32, 33]. Disseminated Histoplasmosis should be differentiated from conditions with systemic febrile illness or infection, disseminated malignancies, and autoimmune disorders. A normal-appearing gastrointestinal mucosa or mild inflammatory reaction grossly and microscopically can still be associated with infection, particularly in immunocompromised adults and children.

Hepatic Histoplasmosis

Histoplasma Capsulatum can affect patients by getting into the respiratory tract. The most common presentation of disseminated histoplasmosis is hepatic involvement. In such patients, early diagnosis is essential for timely treatment [3]. Hepatic Histoplasmosis presents in children and adults, in immunocompetent and immunocompromised patients, and in endemic or non-endemic areas [3]. Liver involvement is the least common gastrointestinal manifestation of patients infected with histoplasmosis [7]. Various conditions can predispose to disseminated Histoplasmosis, i.e., AIDS, immunosuppressive medications like glucocorticoids, antirejection therapies in solid organ transplant or TNF alpha inhibitors, primary immunodeficiency, and extremes of age [5].

Epidemiology

Lamps et al., in their study on 56 specimens of disseminated Histoplasmosis from endemic and nonendemic areas, found liver lesions in 10% of the patients and combined liver and gastrointestinal lesions in 43% of the patients. (2000) Hepatomegaly and splenomegaly are frequent in disseminated histoplasmosis and are seen in 30-100% of patients [10].

Clinical Characteristics

The severity of the disease varies according to the intensity of the exposure and the host's immunity response [34]. In immunocompromised patients, the infection progressively disseminates to other organs leading to nonspecific syndromes [13]. According to Lamps et al., the typical hepatic presenting symptoms include hepatomegaly, jaundice, and elevated serum transaminases. Right upper quadrant pain in patients with cholestatic hepatitis from disseminated Histoplasmosis might be confused with biliary colic. [12]. There is a case report by Hjermstad from a 50-year-old woman on adalimumab for rheumatoid arthritis who presented with right upper quadrant pain, fever, jaundice, and dyspnea. Endoscopic retrograde cholangiopancreatography suggested Mirizzi syndrome, but successful sphincterotomy did not improve jaundice over subsequent days. Bronchoscopy and liver biopsy revealed budding yeast and grew H. Capsulatum [35]. Another report of a 66-year-old female patient on methotrexate and adalimumab for rheumatoid arthritis presented with a fever of unknown origin. Further extensive workup showed granulomatous inflammation with ovoid 2-4 micrometers narrow-based budding fungal organisms on Methenamine-Silver staining suggestive of Histoplasmosis. Serum titers with antigen enzyme Immunoassay (EIA) detection tests were also positive based on biopsy results [5].

Differential Diagnosis

Hepatic Histoplasmosis can mimic various other infectious processes (infiltrative or non-infiltrative diseases) presenting in a hepatocellular and cholestatic pattern. According to a study by Harrington et al., hepatic granulomas are present in 2.4% to 10% of the liver tissue specimens examined in general hospitals. Granulomas are seen in sarcoidosis and tuberculosis as well [36]. Depending on the clinical situation, it can also have an extended differential, but special attention should be paid to immunocompromised patients. In a study conducted by Rihanna et al., common differential entities were sarcoidosis, primary biliary cirrhosis, tuberculosis, fungal infections, Q fever, brucellosis, or it might be idiopathic [5]. Symptoms of hepatic Histoplasmosis can also mimic other infectious hepatitis. Figure 2 shows the differential diagnosis that can present similar to gastrointestinal histoplasmosis.

Pathology and Diagnostic Tests

In the study by Lamps et al., lymphohistiocytic portal inflammation in the lamina propria with fungus identified intracellularly in the portal and sinusoidal macrophages was commonly identified [12]. Sinusoidal Kupffer cell hyperplasia was present [13]. Well-formed hepatic granulomas occurred in less than 20% of the liver pathology specimens. Hepatomegaly and congested livers from yeast-laden macrophages within the sinusoids were commonly noted. Rarely discrete granulomas were seen in the portal and lobular regions of the liver [37]. Immunocompromised adults and young children with Histoplasmosis can have a normal-appearing or mild inflammatory reaction on hepatic parenchyma both grossly and microscopically and yet have the infection.

Clinicians should keep a high level of suspicion for Histoplasmosis in any immunosuppressed patient who presents with unexplained fever, hepatosplenomegaly, generalized lymphadenopathy, pancytopenia, abnormal liver function tests, or bilateral pulmonary infiltrates [38]. It can be diagnosed using antigen detection, cultures, serology, or direct microscopy. Laboratory values are variable and nonspecific. Transaminase levels can be elevated above the upper limit of normal [3]. Elevated alkaline phosphatase is also seen; according to a retrospective review by Assi et al., in a single-center study of 111 patients, liver enzymes were elevated in 27% of the patients [15]. Liver biopsy is often obtained with serum and urine antigen studies [3]. Additionally, biopsies of lesions using methenamine silver or periodic acid-Schiff stains can visualize H. capsulatum yeast [39]. Urine histoplasmosis antigen detection was the most sensitive diagnostic method for Histoplasmosis in a study conducted by Assi et al. [15]. The early lesions in the tissue specimen contain many macrophages and lymphocytes, with epithelioid cells and multinucleated giant cells. Histology can show central caseation and occasionally calcification. The characteristic finding can be areas of caseous necrosis with a surrounding fibrous capsule which is the host reaction to prevent the organism's spread [3].

Asymptomatic pylephlebitis in a liver transplant patient with infiltration of Histoplasma in the portal vein and hepatic granulomas is described in the literature [40]. Granulomatous hepatitis presenting with fever of unknown origin and abnormal liver function tests in a patient on immunosuppressive therapy with infliximab is reported [5] According to a multicenter retrospective study, fifty-six specimens from 52 patients with gastrointestinal and hepatic Histoplasmosis between 1946 and 1998 were retrieved. Of the 36 patients with hepatic involvement, grossly anatomic findings were enlarged livers, 17 (47%); 14(39%) had mottled or markedly congested livers, and only 6(17%) had discrete, grossly apparent hepatic lesions. Microscopically most affected livers contained lymphohistiocytic portal inflammation in 14(39%) of the specimens. Sinusoidal Kupffer cell hyperplasia was present in 12(33%) of the cases. Discrete granulomas were seen in 7(19%), and (8)22% had hepatic sinusoidal congestion [12].

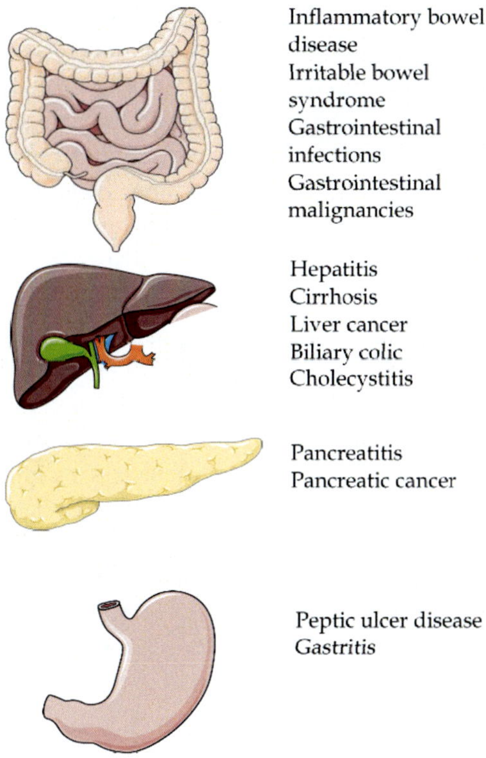

Figure 2. Differential diagnosis for various gastrointestinal manifestations of histoplasmosis.

Pancreaticobiliary Histoplasmosis

Lamps et al. described disseminated Histoplasmosis, of which three patients had pancreatic and biliary histoplasmosis manifestations [12]. Asif et al. describe a patient with necrotizing pancreatitis who died [41]. Autopsy findings identified disseminated Histoplasmosis on testing. Pancreatic masses from Histoplasmosis can cause duodenal obstruction [42-44]. Biliary obstruction with jaundice and duodenal ulcers in the periampullary region [43] is described in the literature. Most of the patients had disseminated histoplasmosis manifestations and nonspecific and vague symptoms. Pathological findings on pancreatic biopsy included lymphohistiocytic inflammation and fungi-laden macrophages within the fibrous septa of the pancreas. Gallbladder findings were similar to that seen in the colon, with lymphohistiocytic infiltration in the mucosa and submucosa of the gallbladder. Interestingly in a study conducted by Lamps et al., gastrointestinal, and hepatic Histoplasmosis was noted to be different between immunocompromised patients, children younger than 18 months of age, and immunocompetent adult patients. Immunocompromised adults and young children were more likely to have many organisms ($P < 0.03$). Young children were more likely to have grossly visible lymphoid hyperplasia of the bowel ($P < 0.01$). Immunocompromised adult patients were more likely to have normal mucosa in the bowel ($P < 0.05$). There was no statistical difference regarding large obstructive masses in the intestine and grossly apparent liver lesions, comparing immunocompromised and young children with immunocompetent patients. Of note, the number of patients included in each group was small. Granulomas were present in immunocompetent and immunocompromised adults but not in young Children, although this association was not statistically significant. Viral and bacterial coinfections were more common in immunocompromised adults, whereas bacterial infections were more common in immunocompetent patients [12].

Treatment

The most commonly agents used for the treatment of histoplasmosis are amphotericin B and Itraconazole. For moderately severe to severe disease, amphotericin B (3 mg/kg/day) is suggested for 1-2 weeks, followed by oral Itraconazole (200 mg thrice daily for three days and then 200 mg twice daily for a total of at least 12 months [3, 17, 23]. Itraconazole can be used in mild to moderate diseases. HIV patients with CD4 count less than<150 cells/mm3, those living in endemic areas, or occupational exposure to histoplasmosis require itraconazole daily prophylaxis of 200 mg daily. Lifelong suppressive therapy with Itraconazole (200 mg daily) may be required in immunosuppressed patients if immunosuppression cannot be reversed. Antigen levels in urine can be used to monitor patient response to therapy; antigen levels decline by the end of 12 weeks; most of the decline was seen more in serum than in urine. If there is an increase in antigen concentration, this should raise the concern of relapse or treatment failure, and further evaluation of the adequacy of treatment is indicated [3, 5]. There are no available guidelines on the management of complications from obstructive gastrointestinal Histoplasmosis. A multidisciplinary approach and close surveillance are needed when managing these patients.

Prognosis

The mortality rate due to untreated disseminated Histoplasmosis, which includes hepatic Histoplasmosis, is 80%; however, it can be reduced to less than 25% with antifungal therapy. The mortality rate among AIDS patients with severe disease is 50%, compared with 2% among those with mild disease [34]. 28% of 152 solid organ transplant patients with Histoplasmosis had severe infections requiring intensive care unit admission. In a retrospective study of colonic Histoplasmosis by Sharma et al. in India on five patients. 2 patients died within a few days of diagnosis due to late diagnosis and complications from the infection. This reinstates the importance of early diagnosis, aggressive treatment, and the high fatality of untreated cases [11]. In a retrospective study by Assi et al., mortality was 10% of patients despite starting treatment. The highest rate of deaths was noted in the first month after diagnosis. The authors also noted a relapse rate of 6% [15].

Prophylaxis

In patients with AIDS and CD4 £150 cells/µL, there is limited data to suggest the administration of prophylactic Itraconazole. However, in areas where Histoplasmosis is hyperendemic (>1 case/100 patients-years), such as certain parts of South America and French Guiana, some providers administer Itraconazole as a prophylactic measure (200 mg daily). In the scenario of individuals who live or visit areas where Histoplasmosis is endemic, they could avoid exposure to H. Capsulatum. Those with CD4 counts <150 cells/µL should avoid activities associated with an increased risk of Histoplasmosis, i.e., working with surface soil; cleaning chicken coops; problematic areas contaminated with bird or bat droppings; cleaning, remodeling, or demolishing old buildings; and exploring caves [45].

Conclusion

Symptoms of Histoplasmosis are often respiratory, as it is predominantly confined to the lungs; however, once it disseminates extracellularly, it goes to organs like the gastrointestinal tract. Clinicians should have a high index of suspicion for timely diagnosis and treatment. They should be aware of the various differential diagnoses of Histoplasma. Often testing for Histoplasmosis by routine tests is negative, stressing the importance of a high index of suspicion. This is a life-threatening condition that requires a multidisciplinary team approach and treatment in a timely manner.

Acknowledgements

Figures were drawn by using pictures from Servier Medical Art. Servier Medical Art by Servier is licensed under a Creative Commons Attribution 3.0 Unported License (https://creativecommons.org/licenses/by/3.0/)

References

[1] Panuganti, S., Varala, S., Damarla, S. V., and Prasad, J. (2022 Jul 1). A rare case of disseminated cutaneous histoplasmosis. *Indian J Dermatol Venereol Leprol*, [Internet]. [cited 2023 Feb 25], 88(4), 533–6. Available from: https://www.ijdvl.com/a-rare-case-of-disseminated-cutaneous-histoplasmosis/.

[2] Armstrong, P. A., Jackson, B. R., Haselow, D., Fields, V., Ireland, M., Austin, C., Signs, K., Fialkowski, V., Patel, R., Ellis, P., Iwen, P. C., Pedati, C., Gibbons-Burgener, S., Anderson, J., Dobbs, T., Davidson, S., McIntyre, M., Warren, K., Midla, J., Luong, N., and Benedict, K. (2018 Mar 1). Multistate Epidemiology of Histoplasmosis, United States, 2011–20141. *Emerg Infect Dis*, [Internet]. [cited 2023 Feb 21];24(3):425. Available from: /pmc/articles/PMC5823339/.

[3] Sayeed, M., Benzamin, M., Nahar, L., Rana, M., and Aishy, A. S. (2022 Aug 8). Hepatic Histoplasmosis: An Update. *J Clin Transl Hepatol*, [Internet]. [cited 2023 Feb 21], 10(4), 726. Available from: /pmc/articles/PMC9396312/.

[4] Linder, K. A., and Kauffman, C. A. (2019 Sep 15). Histoplasmosis: Epidemiology, Diagnosis, and Clinical Manifestations. *Curr Fungal Infect Rep*, [Internet]. [cited 2023 Feb 25], 13(3), 120–8. Available from: https://link.springer.com/article/10.1007/s12281-019-00341-x.

[5] Rihana, N. A., Kandula, M., Velez, A., Dahal, K., and O'Neill, E. B. (2014). Histoplasmosis Presenting as Granulomatous Hepatitis: Case Report and Review of

the Literature. *Case Rep Med*, [Internet]. [cited 2023 Feb 11], 2014. Available from: /pmc/articles/PMC4070324/.

[6] Jiang, Y., Guo, J., Tang, X., Wang, X., Hao, D., and Yang, H. (2022 May 20). The Immunological Roles of Olfactory Ensheathing Cells in the Treatment of Spinal Cord Injury. Front Immunol., 13, 2350.

[7] Muhanna, A., Nimri, F. M., Almomani, Z. A., al Momani, L., and Likhitsup, A., (2021 Sep 1). Granulomatous Hepatitis Secondary to Histoplasmosis in an Immunocompetent Patient. *Cureus*, [Internet]. [cited 2023 Feb 7], 13(9), Available from: https://pubmed.ncbi.nlm.nih.gov/34513533/.

[8] Heninger, E., Hogan, L. H., Karman, J., Macvilay, S., Hill, B., Woods, J. P., and Sandor, M. (2006 Sep 9). Characterization of the Histoplasma capsulatum-Induced Granuloma. *J Immunol*, [Internet]. [cited 2023 Feb 9], 177(5), 3303. Available from: /pmc/articles/PMC2748851/.

[9] Zhou, P., Sieve, M. C., Tewari, R. P., and Seder, R. A. (1997). Interleukin-12 modulates the protective immune response in SCID mice infected with Histoplasma capsulatum. *Infect Immun*, [Internet]. [cited 2023 Feb 9], 65(3), 936–42. Available from: https://pubmed.ncbi.nlm.nih.gov/9038300/.

[10] Kahi, C. J., Wheat, L. J., Allen, S. D., and Sarosi, G. A. (2005 Jan). Gastrointestinal histoplasmosis. *Am J Gastroenterol*, [Internet]. [cited 2023 Feb 21], 100(1), 220–31. Available from: https://pubmed.ncbi.nlm.nih.gov/15654803/.

[11] Sharma, R., Lipi, L., Gajendra, S., Mohapatra, I., Goel, R. K., Duggal, R., Mishra, S. R., and Gautam, D. (2017 Oct 1). Gastrointestinal Histoplasmosis: A Case Series. *Int J Surg Pathol*, [Internet]. [cited 2023 Feb 21], 25(7), 592–8. Available from: https://pubmed.ncbi.nlm.nih.gov/28530163/.

[12] Lamps, L. W., Molina, C. P., West, A. B., Haggitt, R. C., and Scott, M. A. (2000). The Pathologic Spectrum of Gastrointestinal and Hepatic Histoplasmosis. *Am J Clin Pathol*, [Internet]. [cited 2023 Jan 28], 113, 64–72. Available from: https://academic.oup.com/ajcp/article/113/1/64/1757611.

[13] Drak Alsibai, K., Couppié, P., Blanchet, D., Adenis, A., Epelboin, L., Blaizot, R., Louvel, D., Djossou, F., Demar, M., and Nacher, M. (2020 Oct 29). Cytological and Histopathological Spectrum of Histoplasmosis: 15 Years of Experience in French Guiana. *Front Cell Infect Microbiol.*, 10, 662.

[14] Samji, N. S., Verma, R., Mohammed, S. Y., Khan, F., and Ismail, M. K. (2021 Nov 19). Disseminated Histoplasmosis Involving Soft Palate, Duodenum, Sigmoid Colon and Bone Marrow in a Patient With Isolated CD4+ T-Lymphocytopenia. *Cureus* [Internet]. [cited 2023 Feb 21], 13(11). Available from: https://pubmed.ncbi.nlm.nih.gov/34938625/.

[15] Assi, M. A., Sandid, M. S., Baddour, L. M., Roberts, G. D., and Walker, R. C. (2007 May). Systemic histoplasmosis: A 15-year retrospective institutional review of 111 patients. *Medicine*, [Internet]. [cited 2023 Feb 21], 86(3), 162–9. Available from: https://journals.lww.com/md-journal/Fulltext/2007/05000/Systemic_Histoplasmosis__A_15_Year_Retrospective.4.aspx.

[16] Nakamura, A., Tawara, I., Ino, K., Matsumoto, T., Hayashi, A., Imai, H., Muraosa, Y., Kamei, K., and Katayama, N., (2020 Mar 1). Achievement of long-term

remission of disseminated histoplasmosis in an AIDS patient. *Med Mycol Case Rep.*, 27, 25–8.

[17] Yvamoto, E. Y., Hemerly, M. C., Baba, E. R., Guimraes, Hourneaux, and De Moura, E. (2023). A case of esophageal histoplasmosis mimicking carcinoma on endoscopy. *Revista espanola de enfermedades digestivas*, [Internet]. [cited 2023 Feb 21], Available from: https://pubmed.ncbi.nlm.nih.gov/36688438/.

[18] Gomez, B. L., Figueroa, J. I., Hamilton, A. J., Ortiz, B. L., Robledo, M. A., Restrepo, A., and Hay, R. J. (1997). Development of a novel antigen detection test for histoplasmosis. *J Clin Microbiol*, [Internet]. [cited 2023 Feb 24], 35(10), 2618. Available from: /pmc/articles/PMC230021/?report=abstract.

[19] Westerhoff, M. (2022 Feb 1). Histologic features of colonic infections. Pathologe [Internet]. [cited 2023 Feb 21], 43(1), 16. Available from: /pmc/articles/PMC8588779/

[20] Zhu, L. L., Wang, J., Wang, Z. J., Wang, Y. P., and Yang, J. L. (2016 Apr 4). Intestinal histoplasmosis in immunocompetent adults. *World J Gastroenterol*, [Internet]. [cited 2023 Feb 21];22(15):4027. Available from: /pmc/articles/PMC4823253/.

[21] Romano, R. C., Soape, M. M., Thirumala, S., and Ghandour, E. (2015 Jun 1). Disseminated histoplasmosis mimicking metastatic disease of the colon and omentum: Report of a case and literature review. *Arab Journal of Gastroenterology.*, 16(2), 66–8.

[22] Wheelwright, M., Yousaf, H., Plummer, R., Cartwright, D., Gaertner, W., and Amin, K. (2019). Perianal Histoplasmosis Presenting as a Mass Suspicious for Malignancy: A Case Report with Review of Gastrointestinal Manifestations of Histoplasmosis. *Am J Case Rep*, [Internet]. [cited 2023 Feb 21], 20, 1740. Available from: /pmc/articles/PMC6892389/.

[23] Zhong, Q., Ordaya, E. E., Fernandez, S. D., Lescalleet, K., Larson, D., Pritt, B., and Berbari, E. (2022 Jan 1). Disseminated histoplasmosis and hemophagocytic lymphohistiocytosis in a patient receiving TNF-alpha inhibitor therapy. *IDCases*, [Internet]. [cited 2023 Feb 21];29. Available from: /pmc/articles/PMC9418189/.

[24] Kok, J., Chen, S. C. A., Anderson, L., Berglund, L., Sleiman, S., Moss, A., Bourke, M., Fulcher, D., and Gilroy, N. (2010 May). Protein-losing enteropathy and hypogammaglobulinaemia as first manifestations of disseminated histoplasmosis coincident with Nocardia infection. *J Med Microbiol*, [Internet]. [cited 2023 Feb 21];59(Pt 5):610–3. Available from: https://pubmed.ncbi.nlm.nih.gov/20133412/.

[25] Flavio Sangiorgi, Riccardo Torelli, Federica Castri, Valentina Siciliano, Roberto Cauda, Massimo Fantoni, Maurizio Sanguinetti, and Francesco Taccari. (2007 Jun). Colonic histoplasmosis. *J Travel Med*, [Internet]. [cited 2023 Feb 21], 3(6), 459–60. Available from: https://academic.oup.com/jtm/advance-article/doi/10.1093/jtm/taad007/6987080.

[26] Kauffman, C. A. (2007 Jan). Histoplasmosis: a clinical and laboratory update. *Clin Microbiol Rev*, [Internet]. [cited 2023 Feb 21], 20(1), 115–32. Available from: https://pubmed.ncbi.nlm.nih.gov/17223625/.

[27] Lee, J. T., Dixon, M. R., Murrell, Z., Konyalian, V., Agbunag, R., Rostami, S., French, S., and Kumar, R. R. (2022 Nov 28). Colonic Histoplasmosis Presenting as

Colon Cancer in the Nonimmunocotnpromised Patient: Report of a Case and Review of the Literature. https://doi.org/101177/000313480407001105 [Internet]. [cited 2023 Feb 21], 70(11), 959–63. Available from: https://journals.sagepub.com/doi/abs/10.1177/000313480407001105?journalCode=asua.

[28] Rajeshwari, M., Xess, I., Sharma, M. C., and Jain, D. (2017). Acid-Fastness of Histoplasma in Surgical Pathology Practice. *J Pathol Transl Med*, [Internet]. [cited 2023 Feb 21], 51(5), 482–7. Available from: http://www.jpatholtm.org/journal/view.php?doi=10.4132/jptm.2017.07.11.

[29] Nacher, M., Valdes, A., Adenis, A., Blaizot, R., Abboud, P., Demar, M., Djossou, F., Epelboin, L., Misslin, C., Ntab, B., Drak, Alsibai, K., and Couppié, P. (2021 Nov 1). Review of diagnostic methods and results for HIV-associated disseminated histoplasmosis: Pathologists are not sufficiently involved. *Tropical Medicine & International Health*, [Internet]. [cited 2023 Jan 29], 26(11), 1462–9. Available from: https://onlinelibrary.wiley.com/doi/full/10.1111/tmi.13663.

[30] Miller, A. C., Arakkal, A. T., Koeneman, S. H., Cavanaugh, J. E., Thompson, G. R., Baddley, J. W., and Polgreen, P. M. (2022 May 1). Frequency and Duration of, and Risk Factors for, Diagnostic Delays Associated with Histoplasmosis. *Journal of Fungi*, [Internet]. [cited 2023 Feb 21], 8(5), 438. Available from: https://www.mdpi.com/2309-608X/8/5/438/htm.

[31] Hamada, Y., Tanaka, K., Horiki, N., Baba, Y., and Takei, Y. (2020 Apr 1). Colonic histoplasmosis resembling early colon cancer. *Gastrointest Endosc*, [Internet]. [cited 2023 Feb 21], 91(4), 951–2. Available from: http://www.giejournal.org/article/S0016510719324046/fulltext.

[32] Montalvo, R., Pomalaza, G., Sandoval, M., and Quispe, J. (2020 Jun 1). Disseminated Histoplasmosis and Miliary Tuberculosis Imitating Colon Cancer in Patient with HIV Who Refuses to Antirretroviral Treatment. *Mycopathologia*, [Internet]. [cited 2023 Feb 21], 185(3), 583–6. Available from: https://pubmed.ncbi.nlm.nih.gov/32385592/.

[33] Peterson, K. J., Rose, M. R., Davitt, C., and Ludwig, K. A. (2022 Dec 1). Disseminated Histoplasmosis: An Unusual Cause of Bowel Obstruction. *WMJ*, [Internet]. [cited 2023 Feb 21], 121(4), e66–70. Available from: https://europepmc.org/article/med/36637849.

[34] Aidé, M. A. (2009). Chapter 4: histoplasmosis. *Jornal Brasileiro de Pneumologia*, [Internet]. [cited 2023 Feb 9], 35(11), 1145–51. Available from: http://www.scielo.br/j/jbpneu/a/VCd59gPVhLgGDbJ7KSsCbzm/?lang=en.

[35] Hjermstad, B., Snover, D., and Debes, J. D. (2022 Jun 15). Case Report: Histoplasma Hepatitis Presenting as Common Bile Duct Obstruction. *Am J Trop Med Hyg*, [Internet]. [cited 2023 Jan 29], 106(6), 1627–8. Available from: https://www.ajtmh.org/view/journals/tpmd/106/6/article-p1627.xml.

[36] Harrington, P. T., Gutiérrez, J. J., Ramirez-Ronda, C. H., Quiñones-Soto, R., Bermúdez, R. H., and Chaffey, J. (1982 May 1). Granulomatous Hepatitis. *Rev Infect*, Dis [Internet]. [cited 2023 Feb 24], 4(3), 638–55. Available from: https://academic.oup.com/cid/article/4/3/638/378665.

[37] Paul, S., Sepehr, G. J., Weinstein, B., and Roper, J. (2014 Nov 18). Co-occurrence of idiopathic granulomatous hepatitis and primary biliary cirrhosis. *Dig Dis Sci*, [Internet]. [cited 2023 Feb 25], 59(11), 2831–5. Available from: https://pubmed.ncbi.nlm.nih.gov/25108519/.

[38] McKinsey, D. S., Smith, D. L., Driks, M. R., and O'Connor, M. C. (1994). Histoplasmosis in Missouri: historical review and current clinical concepts. *Mo Med*, [Internet]. [cited 2023 Jan 29], 91(1), 27–32. Available from: https://pubmed.ncbi.nlm.nih.gov/8121370/.

[39] Gandhi, D., Gandhi, T., Wolfe, A., Kichloo, A., Singh, J., Batts, K. P., and Patel, L. (2021 Aug 1). Disseminated histoplasmosis leading to end stage liver failure in immunocompetent patient: case report and review of literature. *Radiol Case Rep*, [Internet]. [cited 2023 Feb 25], 16(8), 2214. Available from: /pmc/articles/PMC8213978/.

[40] Phoompoung, P., Chayakulkeeree, M., Ngamskulrungroj, P., and Pongpaibul, A. (2019 Feb 15). Asymptomatic Histoplasma Pylephlebitis in an Orthotopic Liver Transplant Recipient: A Case Report and Literature Review. *Mycopathologia*, [Internet]. [cited 2023 Feb 21], 184(1), 177–80. Available from: https://pubmed.ncbi.nlm.nih.gov/29789991/.

[41] Asif, A. A., Roy, M., and Ahmad, S. (2020 Dec 19). Fulminant Pancreatitis Due to Disseminated Histoplasmosis: Case Report and Literature Review. *Cureus*, [Internet]. [cited 2023 Feb 21], 12(12). Available from: https://pubmed.ncbi.nlm.nih.gov/33364138/.

[42] Choudhury, A. K., Mishra, A. K., Gautam, D. K., Tilak, R., Tilak, V., and Gambhir, I. S. Chakrabarti, S. S. (2020). Case Report: Histoplasmosis Accompanying Disseminated Tuberculosis in an Immunocompetent Adolescent Boy. *Am J Trop Med Hyg*, [Internet]. [cited 2023 Feb 24], 102(2), 352. Available from: /pmc/articles/PMC7008309/.

[43] Agrawal, V., Brinda, B. J., and Farag, S. S. (2020 Feb 12). Histoplasma capsulatum Infection in an Allogeneic Hematopoietic Stem Cell Transplant Patient Receiving Voriconazole Prophylaxis. *Case Rep Hematol*, [Internet]. [cited 2023 Feb 24];2020:1–5. Available from: /pmc/articles/PMC7039042/.

[44] Abu, A. l., Rub, F., Whitt, K., and Tombazzi, C. (2009 Jul 1). Disseminated histoplasmosis presenting with biliary obstruction and duodenal ulcer. *Tenn Med*, [Internet]. [cited 2023 Feb 24], 102(7), 45–6. Available from: https://europepmc.org/article/med/19634648.

[45] What's New in the Guidelines | NIH [Internet]. [cited 2023 Feb 9]. Available from: https://clinicalinfo.hiv.gov/en/guidelines/hiv-clinical-guidelines-adult-and-adolescent-opportunistic-infections/whats-new.

Chapter 9

Histoplasmosis in Human Immunodeficiency Virus Patients

Divya E. Abraham[1]
Sajiny John[2]
Salim Surani[3,4]
Reena Shah[5]
and Rahul Kashyap[1,4,6,*]

[1]Department of Research, GCSRT, Harvard Medical School, Postgraduate Medical Education, Boston, Masssachussetts, USA
[2]Clinical Research Coordinator, Department of Cardiology, Icahn School of Medicine, Mount Sinai, New York, USA
[3]Adjunct Clinical Professor, Department of Medicine & Pharmacology, Texas A&M University, Texas, USA
[4]Department of Anesthesiology and Critical Care, Mayo Clinic, Rochester, Minnesota, USA
[5]Department of Medicine, Aga Khan University Hospital, Nairobi, Kenya
[6]Department of Research, York Hospital, WellSpan Health, York, Pennsylvania, USA

Abstract

In the U.S., Histoplasmosis caused by H. capsulatum is estimated to have around 15,000 new infections and 9000 deaths among people living with Human Immunodeficiency Virus (HIV)-PLHIV. It has been estimated that about half a million people acquire an infection per year and 100,000 develop disseminated one· An adequate diagnostic test with high sensitivity & specificity needs to be considered. The treatment of the

[*] Corresponding Author's Email: kashyapmd@gmail.com- Yes that is correct. Please Divya Abraham as Divya E. Abraham

In: Histoplasmosis
Editors: Salim Surani, Syed Anjum Khan and Reena Shah
ISBN: 979-8-89113-129-3

infection, along with co-infection with T.B. and Histoplasmosis, Pneumocystis jirovecii (PJ) and Histoplasmosis and HIV needs to be managed appropriately. WHO's priority to have access to rapid testing and availability of treatment drugs for Histoplasmosis is notable.

Keywords: histoplasmosis, HIV, AIDS, PLHIV, diagnosis, treatment, antigen, EIA, itraconazole, amphotericin

Introduction

Histoplasmosis is a thermally dimorphic worldwide distributed fungi Histoplasma capsulatum var. capsulatum is distributed globally and is endemic to some states in United States of America (USA) such as Ohio, Mississippi River Valley & most Latin American countries. [1] H. Capsulatum var. dubosii is rare and is found mainly in Africa. The clinical presentation ranges from asymptomatic to subacute, acute, and chronic pulmonary infections to fatal, endemic-prone, PDH (Progressive Disseminated Histoplasmosis). [2] PDH is more common in immunosuppressed patients especially HIV-positive ones, leading to mortality in 30-50% when treated and 100% among untreated. A CD 4 <150 cells/mm3 is associated with an increased risk of PDH risk while a CD 4 >300 usually limits disease to the respiratory tract. [3] A reduction in cellular immunity can also reactivate a quiescent focal infection (especially in nonendemic areas). In the U.S., Histoplasmosis caused by H. capsulatum is estimated to have around 15,000 new infections and 9000 deaths among people living with HIV (PLHIV). [4, 5, 6] It has been estimated that about half a million people acquire an infection per year and 100,000 develop disseminated one. [5] However, the actual global burden of Histoplasmosis is unknown due to the facts that - notification is not mandatory, challenging nonspecific clinical symptoms (confused with T.B.) that lead to misdiagnosis, underdiagnosis, limited global access to diagnostic assays, laboratory diagnosis, treatments as well as their high expenses. [6, 7]

Diagnosis

In 2020, WHO published the first global guidelines for diagnosing and managing Disseminated Histoplasmosis in PLHIV. The guidelines are - (1)

diagnosis- lab assay to detect circulating Histoplasma antigens (2) treatment – moderately severe/severe disease - Induction therapy with liposomal amphotericin, followed by maintenance therapy with itraconazole for 12 months; the duration of maintenance can be reduced if the patient is clinically stable and immune status has improved; (3) In patients with Histoplasma and no CNS involvement – initiation of antiretroviral therapy (ART) as soon as possible; and (4) treatment of co-infection with Histoplasmosis and tuberculosis (T.B.), treatment of T.B. should be first initiated. [8]

PLHIV in endemic areas, when CD 4 falls to ≤ 150cellc/microL and the presence of clinical symptoms (fever/weight loss, cough, dyspnea, skin or mucous membrane lesions, nausea, vomiting, abdomen pain, hepatosplenomegaly, lymphadenopathy, pancytopenia & other dependent on the organ system involved) need to be assessed for Histoplasmosis. Prompt diagnostic testing is necessary. [9] Our first approach may be to send serum & urine for Histoplasma antigen as well as fungal blood cultures via lysis – the centrifugation technique. Confirmation of the diagnosis needs identification of H.capsulatum by staining or culture. In a patient with disseminated Histoplasmosis, a peripheral blood smear shows organisms engulfing WBCs, and a histopathological exam of the biopsy specimen from involved tissues often demonstrates the 2-4 μm in diameter budding yeast cells. Though a positive antigen test strongly supports the diagnosis, there has been cross-reactivity with other endemic fungi (e.g., blastomycosis, coccidioidomycosis, paracoccidioidomycosis). Guideline Development Group recommended antigen tests, microscopic analysis of buffy coat, histopathological analysis, culture & antibody, or DNA detection in patients with a different presentation than disseminated disease. [8, 10]

Antigen Test

The detection of H. antigen in the serum and urine is the most sensitive test and the best initial diagnostic work up, especially in disseminated histoplasmosis. [11, 12, 13] It is a rapid and an excellent diagnostic test for PLHIV with an acute infection but may be insensitive to chronic forms of pulmonary infection. H antigen testing can also be performed on specimens of BAL or CSF (bronchoalveolar lavage or cerebrospinal, fluid respectively). Positive results may be seen in both or only one (Serum or urine). One study showed a diagnosis of disseminated Histoplasmosis in advanced HIV in urine (97%), blood/serum (83%) and CSF (67%). [14] Another study in PLHIV and histoplasmosis, showed using a newer quantitative assay, H antigen was detected in 100% urine samples and 92% serum samples. [1] A meta-analysis showed antigen- detecting assay in PLHIV pooled Sensitivity 95% /specificity 97%. [8, 13] Antigen detection can be universally available and implemented in low-level labs (level 1 & 2).

Histoplasma antigen can be diagnosed by enzyme immunoassay (EIA). [16] Two assays based on enzyme-linked immunosorbent assay (ELISA) have shown good diagnostic performance and have been commercialized, although availability is limited.

MiraVista Diagnostics (2008), improved sensitivity of their test by introducing a 2nd generation H antigen EIA testing- that needed pretreatment of the serum, thus eliminating interference caused by immune complex formation. [17] A 3rd generation MVista Quantitative Laboratory Develop Test (LDT), (2007), MVista® Quantitative Histoplasma antigen EIA has not been FDA cleared, but it can be performed only at MiraVista Diagnostics. A multicenter study that incorporated the pretreatment serum into the assay reported a sensitivity of serum 94.2% and urine 100%. [13] Thus, always both urine and serum need to be tested. MVista EIA can also detect the antigen in BAL and CSF. Still, cross-reactivity occurs in 80% of patients with Talaromyces marneffei and Paracoccidioides brasiliensis infections [15] due to similar cell wall galactomannan class, [18] 10% of the patients with coccidioidomycosis, [20, 19] and in <5% with aspergillosis [20] but no cross reactivity with cryptococcosis. [21] Turnover time usually $\leq$ 24hrs. 2. ImmunoMycologics (IMMY; Norman, Oklahoma) 2007, produced a FDA cleared polyclonal- based H. antigen EIA in vitro device (IVD) to detect the antigen in urine. IMMY in 2013 replaced the IVD with a non -FDA approved monoclonal antibody-based H antigen assay using analyte-specific reagents (ASR). Recently, IMMY released the Histoplasma GM ELISA test that has superior performance and reproducibility rate, but the tests can only be done on urine samples. [22] A study reported IMMY ASR sensitivity of 72% and specificity of 98%. [23] Another reported sensitivity & specificity range 95-98%. Turnover time is < 2.15 hours. A meta-analysis done in Latin America showed MVista H antigen LDT sensitivity of 95% and specificity of 97%. [24] Though MVista LDT shows persistent antigenuria (>12 weeks during successful treatment), more than IMMY ASR, the drawback is its availability only at MiraVista Diagnostics. Thus, despite the high degree of cross-reactivity, antigen detection assay is widely used especially in endemic areas. Its usage in non-endemic areas is limited due to low-cost effectiveness.

A new diagnostic methodology and immunochromatographic assay have been developed that can be used at the point of care "like a pregnancy test" as turnaround time is less than an hour and can be performed via lateral flow devices (LFD), requiring minimal lab equipment. Thus, these are beneficial in low- and middle-income countries. [25, 26] MVista recently came up with a dipstick sandwich immunochromatographic assay based on recognition of H. Capsulatum's G.M. antigen in PLHIV that shows high sensitivity/ specificity (96/90%), and it seems promising. [27]

Culture Testing and Histopathology/Direct Microscopy

Culture: Culture of the blood, respiratory samples and any available tissue or fluid specimen can be performed (e.g., B. Marrow aspirates, lymph node aspirates, Skin tissue biopsy). The gold standard is the isolation of H. capsulatum via culture (sensitivity of 89.5%) and /or visualization of the yeast cells by cytology/histopathology (sensitivity 73.8%) using specific strains. [28] Though cultures may take 4-6 weeks to grow, and sensitivity depends on disease burden and type of specimen, it remains the gold standard. H. capsulatum also known as a fastidious fungus takes 4 weeks to grow and requires Biosafety level (BSL3) containment measures. [29] At 77-86°F (25-30°C), it grows as a white cottony mycelium that evolves to brown (the invasive form of the disease). This mycelial form is the most dangerous, as spores inhaled can cause the infection and represent the tuberculate macroconidia. [30] Some lab contamination with Sepedonium species has been noted. At our body temperature, 98.6°F (37°C), the mycelial phase converts to the yeast form (pathogenic from of the disease), that are thick-walled ovoid forms with a narrow base at the smaller end.

The main limitation of culture is the long turnover time needed to reach a definitive diagnosis and it also needs further confirmation by other methods. Earlier, internal transcribed spacer (ITS) of ribosomal DNA sequencing and later, a single-stranded DNA probe, were considered as powerful tools, but both were time-consuming. [31] Recently, matric-assisted laser desorption/ionization-time of flight mass spectrometry (MALDI-ToF MS) has emerged to identify H strains. [32] The results seem promising as it can recognize different varieties (var.capsulatum, var.duboisii)and pathogen forms (yeast and mold), thus reducing response time and the risk of culture manipulation.

Histopathology/Direct Microscopy

One can examine tissues /body fluids for the fungi via specific stains (e.g., Giemsa stain for B. Marrow aspirates, methenamine silver stain for tissue specimens). Some other stains are Wright, PAS or May-Grünwald-Giemsa stains. Direct microscopy can also be performed on routine peripheral blood smear or buffy coat preparations, with Wright staining to visualize the organism within macrophages. This is an inexpensive and rapid identification method although sensitivity is very low (<10%). Granulomas/clusters with budding yeasts, seen in body fluids, in extrapulmonary sites, is diagnostic and consistent with disseminated disease, although occasionally confused with C. glabrata, Talaromyces marneffei, or Leishmania's amastigote form. H.capsulatum appears to be at 2-4µm while var.duboisii, an oval fungi is 8-15µm. [28] However, histopathologic examination of tissues using special stains requires additional facilities, pathologist, delay diagnosis, and low sensitivity/specificity. One should combine blood culture with peripheral smear direct microscopy, to increase diagnostic yield. An 88% sensitivity was reported in a study of 36 PLHIV and suspected disseminated disease.

Serology

Serologic tests are of limited value in the initial diagnosis of Histoplasmosis since results may be delayed for up to two weeks. Serology testing is the detection of antibodies via various methods - complement fixation (C.F.), immunodiffusion (I.D.), and MVista® IgG, IgM EIA [34] and Western blot. [35] In AIDS patients the production of antibodies is impaired, and a combined C.F and I.D., yields a diagnostic value of about 70-92%, in advanced HIV & Histoplasmosis. [25, 31] Some nonreactivity has been described. I.D. has less sensitivity but more specificity than C.F. [36]

DNA based detection method: The identification of organisms isolated from culture via PCR is the only established role for molecular methods. [33] These tests are simple, have a short turnaround time, are highly specific and have real-time PCR formats (qPCR), that allow nonspecific DNA binding dyes or fluorescent-labeled probes. Most PCR tests target specific multicopy regions of rDNA or single copy Hcp100 gene and are performed via conventional/nested or qPCR formats. It requires standardization, availability, & adequate DNA in the invasive sample. When there is no clear suspicion of Histoplasmosis, a pan-fungal or broad-range PCRs is used, especially in non-endemic areas, since universal primers can detect any fungal DNA in the sample. A meta-analysis evaluating results from 5 studies in PLHIV in Latin America reported a sensitivity of 95.4% and specificity of 98.7% but were inadequate to recommend PCR. [24] Non-PCR-based methods like Loop-mediated isothermal amplification (LAMP) uses DNA polymerase with high displacement strand activity and a set of specifically designed primers to amplify targeted DNA from a sample. [22]

Newer Techniques

Next-Generation Sequencing (NGS) from samples are compared against reference databases, enabling their specific genus & species identification, especially used in chronic meningitis. The identification of H.capsulatum in body fluids is done via host and fungal biomarkers. Further advances require refinements to antibody detection platforms and antigen detection by POC methods. [28]

Diagnosis of Meningitis

Culture or pathology of CSF shows lymphocytic pleocytosis, elevated protein, and low glucose, but fungal strains are usually negative and positive culture is marginally seen. A retrospective multicenter study that tested culture or pathology of CSF, brain, meninges, or spinal cord, reported positive in only 37.7% (26 of 69, 71.4% HIV patients). [37] H. antigen detection in CSF or antibody against H capsulatum is seen in more than half of patients. CSF volumes of 10-20 mL must be cultured to achieve the highest sensitivity. Patients sometimes may have negative culture, pathology, antigen, and antibody in CSF findings but positive results from other sites. [37] If all tests are negative, a presumptive diagnosis of Histoplasma meningitis is needed for prompt treatment, if patients with disseminated Histoplasmosis have no other attributable cause. Repeat antigen and antibody testing and culture or CNS tissue culture and histopathology may be needed to establish a definite diagnosis. Another study checking M.Vista IgG or IgM antibody was positive in 82.2% (37 of 45), and either antigen or antibody was positive in 98% (48 of 49) patients. [36] Sensitivity for antibody detection was slightly higher by C.F. (50%) than I.D. (44%). The specificity of antigen detection in CSF was 96.6% (140 of 145) and IgG or IgM antibody detection was 92.8% (142 of 153). [37]

Treatment

Treatment is indicated for all AIDS patients with Histoplasmosis. If untreated, acute-disseminated infection is progressive with a 100% fatality rate. Treatments should focus on the administration of effective antifungal therapy and starting HIV medication.

Dose, duration: The occurrence of meningitis by Histoplasmosis and its treatment is challenging. In an experimental mice study, fluconazole compared to itraconazole with amphotericin B, was less effective despite greater CSF penetration. [38-40] The recommended treatment of Histoplasmosis Meningitis is 4-6 weeks of Liposomal amphotericin B followed by itraconazole for at least 1yr. The dose of itraconazole is 200 mg twice daily, adjusted not to exceed 10 mcg/ml. Deoxycholate amphotericin B has increased toxicity risk so liposomal is preferred.

Liposomal amphotericin B should be used, especially in hospitalized patients, as it improves mean survival time to 11 mts. Amphotericin B is transitioned to oral itraconazole, when the patient is afebrile/significant improvement, as it requires no monitoring of Blood pressure or ventilatory support or IV fluids. Itraconazole is the treatment of choice in patients with non-life-threatening manifestations of Histoplasmosis. Posaconazole is preferred if itraconazole cannot be administered. [40-46]

When to Stop Treatment

Patients receiving antiretroviral therapy, may discontinue itraconazole after one year of therapy to achieve more immune reconstitution and HIV viral load suppression. At one year, CSF should be evaluated, including large-volume culture and Histoplasma antigen determination at the time of discontinuation. CSF cell profile and chemistry should be within normal limits and antigen and culture should be negative. Urine and serum antigen, if positive initially, should be repeated at 3–6-month intervals, if clinical findings are concerning for recurrence, or HIV viremia and CD4 counts suggest recurrence or antiretroviral therapy is no longer effective.

Relapse

One of the main predictors for relapse of Histoplasmosis is nonadherence to treatment. The relapsed patient has a higher risk of CNS Histoplasmosis and relapses are higher in patients who had CNS Histoplasmosis initially, than in patients without CNS involvement. [41]

Treatment of Co-infection in AIDS Patients

1. Medical management of T.B. and histoplasmosis co-infection
   One of the challenges faced is determining patients with co-infection, due to a similar presentation, as both opportunistic infections can have pulmonary, nodal, or miliary involvement. The diagnosis, treatment & prognosis is challenging, when both infections occur at the same time. When a patient fails to respond well to appropriate therapy, we must consider the probability of a co-infection. Due to the high drug-to-drug interaction between rifampin and itraconazole, an alternative treatment must be considered. [47-52]

   Fluoroquinolones, especially moxifloxacin [51, 52] is a drug that is used for multidrug-resistant T.B. and as per a retrospective review of HIV-infected patients, who had been treated for both T.B. and Histoplasmosis (1992-2011 at the Hospital La María albeit), showed that moxifloxacin did not interact with itraconazole. Thus, proving an effective satisfactory response for treating coinfected with T.B. & Histoplasmosis.51 According to current recommendations, if an alternative drug is used in place of rifampin, the therapy needs to be extended by 12-18 months.53 Drug-Drug interaction is still a concern, as ART drugs, depending on the type can either increase or decrease the concentration of itraconazole in the blood. Hence it is imperative to conduct routine itraconazole blood concentration checks for the duration of treatment. [54]
2. Medical management of pneumocystis jirovecii (PJ) and histoplasmosis co-infection

   As mentioned earlier, poor treatment response in AIDS patients with Histoplasmosis is indicative of a concomitant opportunistic infection. The treatment, in these cases, is similar to treating patients with an individual opportunistic infection. Therefore, they should be treated with intravenous antibiotics and Trimethoprim/ sulfamethoxazole, to cover PJ when suspected, in addition to, either itraconazole or amphotericin B depending on the severity of histoplasmosis. [55]

Monitoring Treatment Response

Histoplasma antigen monitoring is recommended during treatment. The decline of Histoplasma antigen was noted within 2 weeks of therapy in the serum, and in the urine the decline was even slower. This decline was more evidently seen in patients on amphotericin compared to itraconazole. [40] Monitoring for the antigen - starts at treatment initiation, at the end of amphotericin phase, at 3, 6 and 12 months, and when considering discontinuation of therapy. Monitoring should continue at 6–12-month intervals even in cases where the therapy is not working anymore or any evidence of recurrence. [40, 42] If an elevation of antigen or clinical worsening during or after treatment is noted then the concentration of itraconazole, treatment adherence treatment, IRIS or a different opportunistic infection should be investigated for. Lifelong suppressive therapy with 200 mg of itraconazole daily is recommended in refractory cases - if histoplasmosis relapsed despite proper therapy or when immunosuppression does not reverse. [41] A good alternative is Posaconazole if itraconazole cannot be used. [46]

Special Considerations and Timing for Starting Antiretroviral Therapy

According to the guidelines for the prevention and treatment of opportunistic infections in adults and adolescents with HIV, it is recommended that antiretroviral treatment be initiated at the start of the antifungal therapy itself, even though there is a risk of immune reconstitution. Inflammation in tissues involved in the infection (pulmonary, lymphadenopathy, skin lesions, and CNS sites) and worsening of clinical findings may occur as a response to an effective antiretroviral therapy. [46]

Management of Immune Reconstitution Inflammatory Syndrome (IRIS)

In people living with HIV, the incidence of Histoplasmosis associated IRIS was low, but significant morbidity was observed, according to a retrospective multicenter study conducted from 1997 to 2017 in French Guinea. In another study comprising of 22 patients, IRIS was seen four times more in females compared to males, and the time to IRIS was 11 days after starting antiretroviral therapy. [47] IRIS features include: (1) AIDS with CD4 count (pretreatment levels) less than 100 cells/microL. [49, 48] (2) a positive virologic and immunological response to ART. [50] (3) absence of resistance to antiretroviral therapy, drug allergy or other adverse drug reactions, a concomitant non-fungal infection, noncompliance by patients, or drug-to-drug interactions or malabsorption that reduce drug levels, after other causes for worsening is evaluated. (4) clinical manifestations that are consistent with an inflammatory condition. [51] (5) a temporal association between the initiation of ART and onset of clinical features of illness. [52]

Histoplasmosis therapy is initiated, and ART is continued in patients who manifest IRIS at the time of diagnosis. For patients who were not on ART, a 2-week delay is recommended. [54] In patients with severe symptoms, already on amphotericin B or itraconazole, it may be appropriate to treat with corticosteroids, even though its role in the management of IRIS is unclear. [49, 54]

Preventing Exposure

In endemic areas, patients with AIDS cannot completely avoid exposure to Histoplasmosis. There are multiple ways of exposure to Histoplasmosis - creating dust when working with surface soil; cleaning chicken coops that have contaminated droppings; disturbing areas that were contaminated with bird or bat droppings; cleaning, remodeling, or demolishing old buildings; and spelunking. AIDS patients with CD4 counts <150 cells/mm^3 should avoid activities that may put them at an increased risk of exposure to Histoplasmosis.

Preventing Disease

Prophylactic therapy is important, especially in patients with low CD4 cell count, and depends on the incidence of Histoplasmosis. In areas with an incidence of Histoplasmosis of >10 cases per 100 patient years, itraconazole at a dose of 200 mg daily was found to be effective in patients with CD4 cell counts <150 cells/mm.^{3} [47] In patients with advanced HIV and living in areas that are highly endemic for Histoplasmosis, prophylactic therapy with itraconazole only reduced the frequency of Histoplasmosis and did not affect the mortality of the disease. [49] In the United States, only during outbreaks do we see an incidence of Histoplasmosis of >10 cases/100. In some Latin American countries, on the other hand, the incidence may be above 10%.

However, the cost of the therapy might be high and hence less affordable to the public. This can be mitigated by discontinuing prophylaxis in patients who are on antiretroviral therapy and have a CD4 cell count ≥150 cells/mm^3 for 6 months and should be restarted if the count falls <150 cells/mm^3. [49]

In 2019, the WHO included Histoplasma antigen tests in the second edition of the EDL (Lists of Essential In Vitro Diagnostics) and representatives from most of Latin America made "The Manaus Declaration" on Histoplasmosis in the Americas and the Caribbean, "By 2025, every country should have access to rapid testing for Histoplasmosis (antigen or PCR/molecular)" [37] and "By 2025, every country should have availability of itraconazole and both standard and lipid formulation of amphotericin B in the public sector."

Conclusion

Histoplasmosis resides globally but are noted more in some U.S. states. The diagnosis, treatment and prognosis are challenging. Co-infection and low specificity & sensitivity makes matters worse. WHO has made a priority to have access to rapid testing and availability of treatment drugs for Histoplasmosis.

References

[1] Wheat L.J., Azar M.M., Bahr N.C., Spec A, Relich R.F., Hage C. Histoplasmosis. *Infectious Disease Clinics of North America.* 2016;30(1):207-227. DOI: 10.1016/j.idc.2015.10.009

[2] Bongomin F., Kwizera R., Denning D.W. Getting Histoplasmosis on the map of international recommendations for patients with advanced HIV disease. *Journal of Fungi.* 2019;5(3). DOI: 10.3390/jof503008

[3] Myint T., Leedy N., Villacorta Cari E., Wheat L.J. HIV-Associated Histoplasmosis: Current Perspectives. *HIV AIDS (Auckl).* 2020;12:113-125. Published 2020 Mar 19. doi:10.2147/HIV.S185631

[4] Medina N., Rodriguez-Tudela J.L., Aguirre L., Salazar L.R., Gamboa O., Bonilla O., Pérez J.C., Arathoon E., Denning D.W, Alastruey-Izquierdo A. Incidence of Histoplasmosis in a Cohort of People with HIV: From Estimations to Reality. *Microorganisms.* 2021; 9(12):2596. https://doi.org/10.3390/microorganisms 9122596

[5] Bongomin F., Kwizera R., Denning D.W. Getting Histoplasmosis on the map of international recommendations for patients with advanced HIV disease. *Journal of Fungi.* 2019;5(3). DOI: 10.3390/jof5030080

[6] Adenis, A.A., Valdes, A., Cropet, C., McCotter, O.Z., Derado, G., Couppie, P., Chiller, T., Nacher, M. Burden of HIV-associated Histoplasmosis compared with tuberculosis in Latin America: A modelling study. *Lancet Infect. Dis* 2018, 18, 1150–1159.

[7] Ashraf, N., Kubat, R.C., Poplin, V., Adenis, A.A., Denning, D.W., Wright, L., McCotter, O., Schwartz, I.S., Jackson, B.R., Chiller, T., et al. Re-drawing the Maps for Endemic Mycoses. *Mycopathologia* 2020, 185, 843–865.

[8] *PAHO/WHO Guidelines for Diagnosing and Managing Disseminated Histoplasmosis among People Living with HIV.*

[9] Adamian C.M.C., de Lima Mota M.A., Martins A.A.F., Aragão M.C., Carvalho M.S., Meneses G.C., Silva Júnior G.B.D., Leitão T.D.M.J.S., De Francesco Daher E. Progressive Disseminated Histoplasmosis in HIV-positive patients. *Int J STD AIDS.* 2022;33(6):544-553. doi:10.1177/09564624221076605

[10] Leitão T., Oliveira Filho A.M.P., Sousa Filho J.E.P., Tavares B.M., Mesquita J.R.L., Farias L., Mota R.S., Nacher M., Damasceno L.S. Accuracy of Buffy Coat in the Diagnosis of Disseminated Histoplasmosis in AIDS-Patients in an Endemic Area of Brazil. *J. Fungi.* 2019;5:47. doi: 10.3390/jof5020047.

[11] Baddley J.W., Sankara I.R., Rodriquez J.M., Pappas P.G., Many W.J. Jr. Histoplasmosis in HIV-infected patients in a southern regional medical center: poor prognosis in the era of highly active antiretroviral therapy. *Diagn Microbiol Infect Dis.* 2008;62(2):151-156. doi:10.1016/j.diagmicrobio.2008.05.006

[12] Hage C.A., Ribes J.A., Wengenack N.L., Baddour L.M., Assi M., McKinsey D.S., Hammoud K., Alapat D., Babady N.E., Parker M., Fuller D., Noor A., Davis T.E., Rodgers M., Connolly P.A., El Haddad B., Wheat L.J. A multicenter evaluation of tests for diagnosis of Histoplasmosis [published correction appears in Clin Infect

Dis. 2012 Feb 1;54(3):454]. *Clin Infect Dis.* 2011;53(5):448-454. doi:10.1093/cid/cir435

[13] Caceres D.H., Knuth M, Derado G, Lindsley M.D. Diagnosis of Progressive Disseminated Histoplasmosis in Advanced HIV: A Meta-Analysis of Assay Analytical Performance. *J Fungi (Basel).* 2019;5(3):76. Published 2019 Aug 18. doi:10.3390/jof5030076

[14] Wheat L.J., Connolly-Stringfield P.A., Baker R.L., Curfman M.F., Eads M.E., Israel K.S., Norris S.A., Webb D.H., Zeckel M.L. Disseminated Histoplasmosis in the acquired immune deficiency syndrome: clinical findings, diagnosis and treatment, & review of the literature. *Medicine (Baltimore).* 1990;69(6):361–374. doi: 10.1097/ 00005792-199011000-00004

[15] Connolly P.A., Durkin M.M., Lemonte A.M., Hackett E.J., Wheat L.J.. Detection of Histoplasma antigen by a quantitative enzyme immunoassay. *Clin Vaccine Immunol.* 2007;14(12):1587-1591.

[16] Durkin M.M., Connolly P.A., Wheat L.J.. Comparison of radioimmunoassay and enzyme-linked immunoassay methods for detection of Histoplasma capsulatum var. capsulatum antigen. *J Clin Microbiol.* 1997;35(9):2252–2255. doi:10. 1128/JCM.35.9.2252- 2255.1997

[17] Swartzentruber S., LeMonte A., Witt J., Fuller D., Davis T., Hage C., Connolly P., Durkin M., Wheat L.J. Improved detection of Histoplasma antigenemia following dissociation of immune complexes. *Clin Vaccine Immunol.* 2009;16(3):320–322. doi:10.1128/CVI.00409-08

[18] Azuma I., Kanetsuna F., Tanaka Y., Yamamura Y., Carbonell L.M.. Chemical and immunological properties of galactomannans obtained from Histoplasma duboisii, Histoplasma capsulatum, Paracoccidioides brasiliensis and Blasomyces dermatitidis. *Mycopathol Mycol Appl.* 1974;54(1):111–125. doi:10.1007/BF02055979

[19] Durkin M., Connolly P., Kuberski T., Myers R., Kubak B.M., Bruckner D., Pegues D, Wheat L.J. Diagnosis of coccidioidomycosis with use of the Coccidioides antigen enzyme immunoassay. *Clin Infect Dis.* 2008;47(8):e69–e73. doi:10.1086/593299

[20] Durkin M., Estok L., Hospenthal D., Crum-Cianflone N., Swartzentruber S., Hackett E., Wheat L.J. Detection of Coccidioides antigenemia following dissociation of immune complexes. *Clin Vaccine Immunol.* 2009;16(10):1453–1456. doi:10.1128/CVI.00227-09

[21] Bahr N.C., Sarosi G.A., Meya D.B., Bohjanen P.R., Richer S.M., Swartzentruber S., Halupnick R., Jarrett D., Wheat L.J., Boulware D.R. Seroprevalence of Histoplasmosis in Kampala, Uganda. *Med Mycol.* 2016;54(3):295–300. doi:10.1093/mmy/myv081

[22] Cloud .JL., Bauman S.K., Neary B.P., Ludwig K.G., Ashwood E.R. Performance characteristics of a polyclonal enzyme immunoassay for the quantitation of Histoplasma antigen in human urine samples. *Am J Clin Pathol.* 2007;128(1):18–22. Epub 2007 Jan 07. 10.1309/Q7879TYDW5D93QK7

[23] Zhang C., Lei G.S., Lee C.H., Hage C.A. Evaluation of two new enzyme immunoassay reagents for diagnosis of Histoplasmosis in a cohort of clinically characterized patients. *Med Mycol.* 2015;53 (8):868–873. doi:10.1093/mmy/myv062

[24] Caceres D.H., Knuth M., Derado G., Lindsley M.D., Diagnosis of progressive disseminated Histoplasmosis in advanced HIV: a meta-analysis of assay analytical performance. *J Fungi (Basel).* 2019;5(3):76

[25] Kozel T.R., Burnham-Marusich A.R. Point-of-care testing for infectious diseases: Past, present, & future. *Journal of Clinical Microbiology.* 2017;55(8):2313-2320. DOI: 10.1128/JCM.00476-17

[26] Prattes J., Heldt S., Eigl S., Hoenigl M. Point of care testing for the diagnosis of fungal infections: Are we there yet? *Current Fungal Infection Reports.* 2016;10:43-50. DOI: 10.1007/s12281-016-0254-5

[27] Cáceres D.H., Gómez B.L., Tobon A.M., Chiller T.M., Lindsley M.D. Evaluation of a Histoplasma antigen lateral flow assay for the rapid diagnosis of progressive disseminated histoplasmosis in Colombian patients with AIDS. *Mycoses.* 2020;63(2):139-144. DOI: 10.1111/myc.13023

[28] Buitrago, M.J., Valero, C. Laboratory Diagnosis of Histoplasmosis: An Update. In: Bongomin, F., editor. *Histoplasma and Histoplasmosis [Internet].* London: IntechOpen; 2020

[29] Wheat L.J., Azar M.M., Bahr N.C., Spec A, Relich R.F., Hage C. Histoplasmosis. *Infectious Disease Clinics of North America.* 2016;30(1):207-227. DOI: 10.1016/j.idc.2015.10.009

[30] Fleming DO., Hunt D.L., *Biological Safety, Principles and Practices.* 4th ed. Washington: ASM Press; 2006. DOI: 10.1590/S0036-46652001000600013

[31] Gómez B.L., Molecular diagnosis of endemic and invasive mycoses: Advances and challenges. Revista Iberoamericana de Micología[Iberoamerican Journal of Mycology]. 2014;31(1):35-41. DOI: 10.1016/j.riam.2013.09.009

[32] Valero C., Buitrago M.J., Gago S., Quiles-Melero I., García-Rodríguez J. A matrix-assisted laser desorption/ionization time of flight mass spectrometry reference database for the identification of Histoplasma capsulatum. *Medical Mycology.* 2018;56(3):307-314. DOI: 10.1093/mmy/myx047

[33] Azar M.M., Hage C.A., Laboratory diagnostics for Histoplasmosis. *J Clin Microbiol.* 2017;55(6):1612–1620. doi:10.1128/JCM.02430-16

[34] Richer S.M., Smedema M.L., Durkin M.M., Herman K.M., Hage C.A., Fuller D., Wheat L.J. Improved diagnosis of acute pulmonary Histoplasmosis by combining antigen and antibody detection. *Clin Infect Dis.* 2016;62(7):896–902. doi:10.1093/cid/
ciw007

[35] Almeida M.A., Damasceno L.S., Pizzini C.V., Muniz M.M., Almeida-paes R, Zancope-oliveira R.M. Role of Western blot assay for the diagnosis of Histoplasmosis in AIDS patients from a National Institute of Infectious Diseases in Rio de Janeiro, Brazil. *Mycoses.* 2019;62(3):261–267. doi:10.1111/myc.12877

[36] Arango-Bustamante K., Restrepo A., Cano L.E., de Bedout C., Tobón A.M., González A. Diagnostic value of culture and serological tests in the diagnosis of

Histoplasmosis in HIV and non-HIV Colombian patients. *Am J Trop Med Hyg.* 2013;89(5):937-942. doi:10.4269/ajtmh.13-0117

[37] Caceres D.H., Adenis A., Souza J.V.B., Gomez B., Santana K.C., Pasqualotto A.C., Ravasi G., Perez F., Chiller T., Lacerda M., Nacher M., The International Histoplasmosis Advocacy Group. The Manaus Declaration: Current Situation of Histoplasmosis in the Americas, Report of the II Regional Meeting of the International Histoplasmosis Advocacy Group. *Current Fungal Infection Reports.* 2019;13(4):244. doi:10.1007/s12281-019-00365-3

[38] Wheat J., Myint T., Guo Y., Kemmer P., Hage C., Terry C., Azar M.M., Riddell J., Ender P., Chen S., Shehab K, Cleveland K., Esguerra E., Johnson J., Wright P., Douglas V., Vergidis P., Ooi W., Baddley J., Bamberger D., Khairy R., Vikram H.R., Jenny-Avital E., Sivasubramanian G., Bowlware K., Pahud B., Sarria J., Tsai T., Assi M., Mocherla S., Prakash V., Allen D., Passaretti C., Huprikar S., Anderson A. Central nervous system Histoplasmosis: Multicenter retrospective study on clinical features, diagnostic approach and outcome of treatment [published correction appears in Medicine (Baltimore). 2018 Apr;97(16):e0537]. *Medicine* (Baltimore). 2018;97(13): e0245. doi:10.1097/MD.0000000000010245

[39] Bloch K.C,. Myint T., Raymond-Guillen L., Hage C.A., Davis T.E., Wright P.W., Chow F.C., Woc-Colburn L., Khairy R.N., Street A.C., Yamamoto T., Albers A., Wheat L.J. Improvement in Diagnosis of Histoplasma Meningitis by Combined Testing for Histoplasma Antigen and Immunoglobulin G and Immunoglobulin M Anti-Histoplasma Antibody in Cerebrospinal Fluid. *Clin Infect Dis.* 2018;66(1):89-94. doi:10.1093/cid/cix706

[40] Haynes R.R., Connolly P.A., Durkin M.M., LeMonte A.M., Smedema M.L., Brizendine E., Wheat L.J. Antifungal therapy for central nervous system Histoplasmosis, using a newly developed intracranial model of infection. *J Infect Dis.* 2002; 185 (12): 1830-2. Doi: 10.1086/340825

[41] Myint T., Anderson A.M., Sanchez A., Farabi A., Hage C., Baddley J.W., Jhaveri M., Greenberg R.N., Bamberger D.M., Rodgers M., Crawford T.N., Wheat L.J. Histoplasmosis in patients with human immunodeficiency virus/acquired immunodeficiency syndrome (HIV/AIDS). *Medicine (Baltimore).* 2014; 93 (1): 11-18. Doi: 10.1097/MD.0000000000000016

[42] Hage C.A., Azar M.M., Bahr N, Lloyd J, Wheat L.J., Histoplasmosis: Up-to-date evidence-based approach to diagnosis and management. *Semin Respir Crit Care Med.* 2015: 36 (5):729-45. doi: 10.1055/s-0035-1562899

[43] Shelburne S.A., Montes M, Hamill R.J., Immune reconstitution inflammatory syndrome: more answers, more questions. *J Antimicrob Chemother.* 2006; 57(2):167–170. doi:10.1093/jac/dki444

[44] Novak R.M., Richardson J.T., Buchacz K., Chmiel J.S., Durham M.D., Palella F.J., Wendrow A., Wood K., Young B., Brooks J.T. HIV Outpatient Study (HOPS) Investigators. Immune reconstitution inflammatory syndrome: incidence and implications for mortality. *AIDS.* 2012;26(6):721–730. doi:10.1097/QAD.0b013e3283511e91

[45] Meintjes G., Scriven J., Marais S. Management of the immune reconstitution inflammatory syndrome. *Curr HIV/AIDS Rep.* 2012;9(3):238–250. doi:10.1007/s11904-012-0129-5

[46] Krishna Bobbili, Sami Akram, Vidya Sundareshan, Vidhya Prakash, Isha Tyagi, Sana Waqar, Scott Bergman, Janak Koirala. Comparison of posaconazole and itraconazole for treatment of Histoplasmosis. *Open forum infectious diseases.* 2016;3(1):1646. doi: 10.1093/ofid/ofw172.1346

[47] Myint T., Leedy N., Cari E.V. and Wheat L.J., HIV-associated Histoplasmosis: Current perspectives. *HIV AIDS (Auckl).* 2020; 12: 113-125. doi: 10.2147/HIV.S185631

[48] Mitchell Goldman, Robert Zackin, Carl J. Fichtenbaum, Daniel J. Skiest, Susan L. Koletar, Richard Hafner, L. Joseph Wheat, Peter M. Nyangweso, Constantin T. Yiannoutsos, Carol T. Schnizlein-Bick, Susan Owens, Judith A. Aberg, AIDS Clinical Trials Group A5038 Study Group. Safety of discontinuation of maintenance therapy for disseminated Histoplasmosis after immunologic response to antiretroviral therapy. *Clin Infect Dis.* 2004;38(10):1485–1489. doi:10.1086/420749

[49] McKinsey D.S., Wheat L.J., Cloud G.A., Pierce M., Black J.R., Bamberger D.M., Goldman M., Thomas C.J., Gutsch H.M., Moskovitz B., Dismukes W.E., Kauffman C.A. Itraconazole prophylaxis for fungal infections in patients with advanced human immunodeficiency virus infection: randomized, placebo-controlled, double-blind study. National Institute of Allergy and Infectious Diseases Mycoses Study Group. *Clin Infect Dis.* 1999;28(5):1049–1056. doi:10.1086/cid.1999.28.issue-5

[50] Agudelo C.A., Restrepo C.A., Molina D.A., Tobón A.M., Kauffman C.A., Murillo C., Restrepo A. Tuberculosis and Histoplasmosis co-infection in AIDS patient. *Am J Trop Med Hyg.* 2012;87(6):1094-1098. doi: 10.4269/ajtmh.2012.12-0292.

[51] Dorman S.E., Johnson J.L., Goldberg S, Muzanye G, Padayatchi N, Bozeman L, Heilig C.M., Bernardo J, Choudhri S, Grosset J.H., Guy E, Guyadeen P, Leus M.C., Maltas G, Menzies D, Nuermberger E.L., Villarino M, Vernon A, Chaisson R.E., Tuberculosis Trials Consortium Substitution of moxifloxacin for isoniazid during intensive phase treatment of pulmonary tuberculosis. *Am J Respir Crit Care Med.* 2009;180:273–280.

[52] Conde M.B., Efron A, Loredo C, De Souza G.R., Graça N.P., Cezar M.C., Ram M, Chaudhary M.A., Bishai W.R., Kritski A.L., Chaisson R.E., Moxifloxacin in the initial therapy of tuberculosis: a randomized, phase 2 trial. *Lancet.* 2009;373:1183–1189.

[53] Centers for Disease Control and Prevention Treatment of tuberculosis, American Thoracic Society, CDC, and Infectious Diseases Society of America. *MMWR Morb Mortal Wkly Rep.* 2003;52:1–80.

[54] Caceres D.H., Valdes A. Histoplasmosis and Tuberculosis co-occurence in people with advanced HIV. *J Fungi (Basel).* 2019;5(3):73. doi: 10.3390/jo5030073.

[55] Wahab A, Chaudhary S, Khan M and Smith S.J. Concurrent Pneumocystis jirovecii and pulmonary Histoplasmosis in an undiagnosed HIV patient. *BMJ Case Rep.* 2018;2018:bcr2017223422. doi: 10.1136/bcr-2017-223422

Chapter 10

Histoplasma Capsulatum Endocarditis

Anwar Khedr[1,*]
Aalaa Eissa[2]
Hussam Hennawi[3]
Mikael Mir[4]
Shika M Jain[5]
Aishwarya R Korsapati[6]
Swechchha Silwal[7]
Ibtisam Rauf[8]
Nitesh Jain[9]
and Syed Anjum Khan [9]
[1]Department of Internal Medicine, BronxCare Health System, Bronx, New York, USA
[2]Department of Internal Medicine, KFS University, KFS, Egypt
[3]Department of Internal Medicine, Abington Memorial Hospital, Abington, Pennsylvania, USA
[4]Department of Medicine, University of Minnesota Medical school, Minneapolis, Minnesota, USA
[5]Department of Medicine, MVJ medical college and research hospital, Bengaluru, India
[6]Department of Medicine, University of Buckingham medical school, UK
[7]Department of Internal Medicine Wayne state University, Detroit, Michigan, USA
[8]Department of Medicine, St. George's University Medical school, True Blue, Grenada
[9]Department of Critical Care, Mayo Clinic Health System, Mankato, Minnesota, USA

* Corresponding Author's Email: anwarkhedr8@gmail.com.

In: Histoplasmosis
Editors: Salim Surani, Syed Anjum Khan and Reena Shah
ISBN: 979-8-89113-129-3

Abstract

Histoplasma capsulatum is one of the most common causes of fungal endocarditis and has a high mortality rate. It is more common in endemic areas in the Americas but can also happen worldwide. This prevalence is due to the subtle and prolonged course of symptoms and mostly negative blood cultures, which leads to delays in providing effective treatment. Histoplasma capsulatum endocarditis is more common in prosthetic valves but can also occur in native valves, especially in immunosuppressed patients. It can take the histopathological forms of small intracellular yeast or septate branching hyphae. Symptoms and signs are diverse and non-specific, making the need for a high suspicion index a must for proceeding with further investigations. Transthoracic and transesophageal play a massive role in discovering vegetations. Positive serology can provide the first clue to the diagnosis, and cultures, especially from bone marrow, can confirm it. Mortality rates are higher without treatment, and better outcomes have been reported after receiving both antifungal and surgical interventions.

Keywords: histoplasmosis, infective endocarditis, echocardiography, prosthetic valve, antifungals

Introduction

Histoplasma capsulatum, a dimorphic fungus, is a highly uncommon cause of infectious endocarditis, and it typically affects people with prosthetic heart valves and HIV infection [1 - 4]. Histoplasmosis is a common mycosis in endemic locations, particularly in North and Central America. Although it typically has no symptoms, it can cause a severe sickness with a wide range of symptoms [3]. For endocarditis cases, a male predominance was found [5, 6]. In the United States, the age range of those affected is between 17 and 74 years, with a mean of 48 years. Most patients are residents of the Ohio-Mississippi Valley region and the eastern United States [5]. Some cases have also been reported worldwide, especially in Thailand [1, 7] and Mexico [8].

The mortality rate for fungal endocarditis is about 50%. Infections caused by Histoplasma capsulatum account for an even smaller subset of instances of fungal endocarditis, making it extremely rare [9]. Negative endocarditis cultures frequently cause delays in diagnosis and specific, life-saving treatments, making the requirement of a high level of suspicion an absolute necessity [10].

Discussion

Risk Factors

The most common risk factor for Histoplasma capsulatum endocarditis is the presence of a prosthetic heart valve. This has been reported in many cases [7, 11-15]. Other reported risk factors included immunosuppression due to HIV infection16 and rheumatoid arthritis [17].

A literature review that evaluated the cases of fungal endocarditis from 1995 to 2000 found other risk factors such as underlying IV drug use, central venous catheters, and underlying cardiac abnormalities such as rheumatic heart disease, atrial myxoma, bicuspid aortic valve, and luetic aortopathy [5, 14]. Additionally, one of these abnormalities was Lautenbacher Syndrome, which is a rare cardiac abnormality characterized by any combination of a congenital or iatrogenic atrial septal defect (ASD) and a congenital or acquired mitral stenosis (MS), that led to vegetative endocarditis of the mitral valve [18, 19].

Histoplasma Capsulatum endocarditis was also reported to occur following heart surgeries and procedures. One case of Histoplasma capsulatum endocarditis in a 57-year-old white male following an open mitral commissurotomy was previously described three months following the surgery. Another case reported the incidence of Histoplasma capsulatum endocarditis six months following cardiac catheterization [20].

Histopathology

The histopathological forms of Histoplasma capsulatum causing endocarditis are varied. Histoplasma capsulatum typically takes the shape of a small intracellular yeast. However, several cases of Histoplasma capsulatum Endocarditis with a thorough pathologic description were discovered to have hyphal forms [21]. Another case report described Histoplasma capsulatum endocarditis, simultaneously affecting mitral and aortic prosthetic valves, demonstrating various histological morphologies, including typical, intracellular, small yeast cells, septate, branching hyphae, and unusual hyphae with vesicular swellings [22].

Clinical Presentation

Histoplasma Capsulatum endocarditis usually presents with non-specific symptoms, including fever, chills, fatigue5, night sweats [23], hemoptysis [2], chest pain [24], dyspnea, near-syncope [9], vomiting [16], transient hemiparesis [2], altered mental status, failure to thrive, and weight loss [11].

Signs include elevated temperature [7], hypotension [9], peripheral edema [3], heart murmurs, embolic skin phenomena [11], oropharyngeal ulcers [5], systemic embolization [25], hepatomegaly, splenomegaly [5], and polyadenopathies [16].

Sixty-one cases of Histoplasma capsulatum endocarditis recorded between 1945 and 2020 were studied in a recent literature review in order to compare endocarditis affecting native and prosthetic valves. Weight loss, fatigue, and embolic complications were more common in patients with affected native valves. However, fever, chills, and night sweats were more common in diseased prosthetic valves [23].

Diagnosis

Before a diagnosis is made, symptoms can persist for weeks to months. Aortic grafts and prosthetic and native valves can all be impacted by Histoplasma capsulatum [26].

Anemia and leukopenia or leukocytosis will be present in most patients [5]. Histoplasma antigens detected in urine and/or serum can provide the first clue to diagnosing histoplasmosis for several patients [27]. A rise in complement fixation titers can also hint at the diagnosis [28]. Positive bone marrow, liver, oropharyngeal ulcers, or urine cultures were utilized to confirm the diagnosis in several cases [5, 28]. Blood cultures are rarely positive [5, 27] or take a very long time for incubation [29], so a high index of suspicion is necessary for the appropriate clinical context [5].

Transthoracic and transesophageal echocardiography is crucial for diagnosis as they show vegetations attached to the valve [3]. They can also monitor the progression of the valve lesions [30]. Excision of these vegetations and isolation of the organism from tissue culture can aid in confirming the diagnosis [7]. In one case report, applying the Histoplasma capsulatum AccuProbe directly to an excised valve that contained several yeast forms compatible with Histoplasma capsulatum was also used to confirm the diagnosis [31]. Sometimes, the diagnosis can only be made by microscopic examination and culture of the excised valve [32]. Due to the elusive presentation and course of the disease, the diagnosis was only made post-mortem in some cases [13].

Diagnosis can also occur only after the development of complications. Aspiration thrombectomy was used to diagnose Histoplasma capsulatum endocarditis complicated with anterior STEMI [10].

Treatment

Antifungal treatment of Histoplasma Capsulatum endocarditis includes amphotericin B, liposomal amphotericin, itraconazole, isavuconazole, ketoconazole, and/or voriconazole as a single agent or in combination [23]. The duration of treatment is typically six weeks [7]. Amphotericin B is the first line of treatment [27]. Isavuconazole is an ideal therapeutic choice in case of kidney disease [33]. Oral itraconazole therapy can be used for suppressive treatment for a duration that ranges from 11 months to lifelong administration [27]. Oral fluconazole was used before for long-term suppressive oral therapy [33].

The modalities of surgical intervention used are valve replacement and/or embolectomy [23]. One notable case described reoperative aortic root replacement with an allograft in a Jehovah's Witness patient with minimal blood loss and discussed different techniques for bloodless cardiac surgeries for such patient populations [34].

According to a review of the literature, the best course of treatment is probably a combination of high doses of amphotericin B and surgical replacement of the affected valve. However, if surgery is not a feasible treatment option, amphotericin B alone may be used to treat the condition successfully [35]. Similar to bacterial endocarditis, surgical valve replacement has comparable indications [25]. Anticoagulation is a must after valve replacement [36].

Complications and Outcomes

Complications may occur as a result of or in association with Histoplasma capsulatum Endocarditis. A case of fatal reactive hemophagocytic syndrome was reported in a patient with disseminated histoplasmosis and fungal endocarditis.37 Chronic meningitis has also been reported in association with a case of Histoplasma endocarditis [38].

Mortality rates were found to be similar between native and prosthetic valve cases. Patients who did not receive any pharmacologic or surgical treatment had a 100% mortality rate. Patients who received only antifungal therapy had a 50% mortality rate. Patients receiving antifungal therapy and surgical intervention had a 0% mortality rate. Generally, mortality rates have decreased from 88% between 1940 to 1970 to 21% from 1971 to 2020, indicating significant advancements in surgical intervention methods and the widespread use of antifungal treatment. In addition, the percentage of prosthetic valve infections has also risen due to the increased use and application of prosthetic valves [23].

Conclusion

Endocarditis is a rare manifestation of Histoplasma Capsulatum. Clinicians should have a high index of suspicion in order to diagnose in the appropriate clinical context, especially in cases with culture-negative endocarditis. Antifungal therapy should be started as soon as possible once the diagnostic confirmation has been made using either serology or cultures. More studies are vital to identify more effective and faster ways of confirming the diagnosis of Histoplasma Capsulatum infective endocarditis.

Better outcomes have been observed in patients who received antifungal therapy and surgical intervention, so this should be the first line of management. Additional research is needed to discover more antifungal therapies, as antimicrobial resistance may occur at any point.

References

[1] Amnuay K, Sirinawin C, Theerasuwipakorn N, Chattranukulchai P, Suankratay C. Native Valve Infective Endocarditis Caused by Histoplasma capsulatum in an Immunocompetent Host: The First Case in Asia and Literature Review in Asia and Australia. *Case Rep. Infect. Dis*. 2021;2021:9981286.

[2] Hartley R A, Remsberg J R, Sinaly N P. Histoplasma endocarditis. Case report and review of the literature. *Arch. Intern. Med.* 1967;119(5):527-31.

[3] Konik E A, Bremer M, Lin P T, Pislaru S V. Severe pulmonic valve regurgitation due to histoplasma endocarditis. *Echo. Res. Pract*. 2015;2(1):K21-4.

[4] Weaver D K, Batsakis J G, Nishiyama R H. Histoplasma endocarditis. *Arch. Surg.* 1968;96(1):158-62.

[5] Blair T, Raymond L. Histoplasma capsulatum endocarditis. *Chest.* 1981;79(6):620.

[6] Boland J M, Chung H H, Robberts F J, Wilson W R, Steckelberg J M, Baddour L M, Miller D V. Fungal prosthetic valve endocarditis: Mayo Clinic experience with a clinicopathological analysis. *Mycoses.* 2011;54(4):354-60.

[7] Lorchirachonkul N, Foongladda S, Ruangchira-Urai R, Chayakulkeeree M. Prosthetic valve endocarditis caused by Histoplasma capsulatum: the first case report in Thailand. *J. Med. Assoc. Thai.* 2013;96 Suppl 2:S262-5.

[8] Méndez-Tovar L J, Rangel-Delgado P M, Hernández-Hernández F, Flores-García A, Galicia-Castelán G, Manzano-Gayosso P, Córdova Martínez E. [First report of infectious endocarditis due to Histoplasma capsulatum in Mexico]. *Rev. Med. Inst. Mex Seguro Soc.* 2019;57(3):181-6.

[9] Manning E M, Zorach B, Kumar A. Rare case of Histoplasma capsulatum endocarditis in a patient with a prosthetic valve. *Eur. Heart J. Case Rep.* 2022;6(3):ytac086.

[10] Alzayer H, Winter J, Alshatti A, Nair V, Sheth T, Whitlock R P, Dyub A, Belley-Côté EP. Histoplasma Endocarditis Diagnosed by Thrombus Aspiration. *Can. J. Cardiol.* 2018;34(10):1370.e9-.e11.

[11] Adigun R O, Baddour L M, Geske J B. A case report of Histoplasma capsulatum prosthetic valve endocarditis: an extremely rare presentation with characteristic findings. *Eur. Heart J. Case Rep.* 2019;3(3):ytz127.

[12] Alexander W J, Mowry R W, Cobbs C G, Dismukes W E. Prosthetic valve endocarditis caused by Histoplasma capsulatum. *Jama.* 1979;242(13):1399-400.

[13] Lieu A, Parkes LO, Longtin Y, Weiss K, Zaharatos GJ. Progressive disseminated histoplasmosis in an apparently immunocompetent patient with a bioprosthetic aortic valve. *J. Assoc. Med. Microbiol. Infect. Dis. Can.* 2020;5(1):49-52.

[14] Pierrotti L C, Baddour L M. Fungal endocarditis, 1995-2000. *Chest.* 2002;122(1):302-10.

[15] Head S J, Dewey T M, Mack M J. Fungal endocarditis after transfemoral aortic valve implantation. *Catheter Cardiovasc. Interv.* 2011;78(7):1017-9.

[16] Scapellato P G, Desse J, Negroni R. Acute disseminated histoplasmosis and endocarditis. *Rev. Inst. Med. Trop. Sao Paulo.* 1998;40(1):19-22.

[17] Letranchant L, Debourgogne A, Doco-Lecompte T, Contet-Audonneau N, May T, Machouart M. Fatal Histoplasma capsulatum mitral endocarditis in a French patient treated for rheumatoid arthritis. *Mycopathologia.* 2012;173(2-3):183-6.

[18] Aminde L N, Dzudie A, Takah N F, Ngu K B, Sliwa K, Kengne A P. Current diagnostic and treatment strategies for Lutembacher syndrome: the pivotal role of echocardiography. *Cardiovasc. Diagn. Ther.* 2015;5(2):122-32.

[19] Korns M E. Coincidence of mycotic (Histoplasma capsulatum) vegetative endocarditis of the mitral valve and the Lutembacher syndrome. Report of a case. *Circulation.* 1965;32(4):589-92.

[20] Canlas M S, Dillon M L, Jr. Histoplasma capsulatum endocarditis: report of a case following heart surgery. *Angiology.* 1977;28(7):454-63.

[21] Hutton J P, Durham J B, Miller D P, Everett E D. Hyphal forms of Histoplasma capsulatum. A common manifestation of intravascular infections. *Arch. Pathol. Lab. Med.* 1985;109(4):330-2.

[22] Svirbely J R, Ayers L W, Buesching W J. Filamentous Histoplasma capsulatum endocarditis involving mitral and aortic valve porcine bioprostheses. *Arch. Pathol. Lab. Med.* 1985;109(3):273-6.

[23] Boyanton B L, Jr., Boamah H, Lauter C B. Native vs Prosthetic Valve Histoplasma capsulatum Infective Endocarditis: A Case Report and Systemic Literature Review Comparing Patient Presentation, Treatment Modalities, Clinical Outcomes, and Diagnostic Laboratory Testing. *Open Forum Infect. Dis.* 2021;8(8):ofab360.

[24] Choi J I, Chang A S, Cook R C, Fordyce C B. Histoplasma capsulatum culture-negative prosthetic valve endocarditis presenting as a cystic mass. *BMJ Case Rep.* 2022;15(2).

[25] Bhatti S, Vilenski L, Tight R, Smego R A, Jr. Histoplasma endocarditis: clinical and mycologic features and outcomes. *J. Infect.* 2005;51(1):2-9.

[26] Ledtke C, Rehm S J, Fraser T G, Shrestha N K, Tan C D, Rodriguez E R, Tomford JW, Jain A, Lytle B, Johnston D, Sabik J, Gordon SM, van Duin D. Endovascular infections caused by Histoplasma capsulatum: a case series and review of the literature. *Arch. Pathol. Lab. Med.* 2012;136(6):640-5.

[27] Riddell J 4th, Kauffman C A, Smith J A, Assi M, Blue S, Buitrago M I, Deresinski S, Wright P W, Drevets D A, Norris S A, Vikram H R, Carson P J, Vergidis P, Carpenter J, Seidenfeld SM, Wheat LJ. Histoplasma capsulatum endocarditis: multicenter case series with review of current diagnostic techniques and treatment. *Medicine* (Baltimore). 2014;93(5):186-93.

[28] Blair T P, Waugh R A, Pollack M, Ashworth H E, Young N A, Anderson S E, Bem T P. Histoplasma capsulatum endocarditis. *Am. Heart J.* 1980;99(6):783-8.

[29] Pasha A K, Lee J Z, Low S W, Desai H, Lee K S, Al Mohajer M. Fungal Endocarditis: Update on Diagnosis and Management. *Am. J. Med.* 2016;129(10):1037-43.

[30] Isotalo P A, Chan K L, Rubens F, Beanlands D S, Auclair F, Veinot JP. Prosthetic valve fungal endocarditis due to histoplasmosis. *Can. J. Cardiol.* 2001;17(3):297-303.

[31] Chemaly R F, Tomford J W, Hall G S, Sholtis M, Chua J D, Procop G W. Rapid diagnosis of Histoplasma capsulatum endocarditis using the AccuProbe on an excised valve. *J. Clin. Microbiol.* 2001;39(7):2640-1.

[32] Jinno S, Gripshover B M, Lemonovich T L, Anderson J M, Jacobs M R. Histoplasma capsulatum prosthetic valve endocarditis with negative fungal blood cultures and negative histoplasma antigen assay in an immunocompetent patient. *J. Clin. Microbiol.* 2010;48(12):4664-6.

[33] Penk A, Pittrow L. Role of Fluconazole in the long-term suppressive therapy of fungal infections in patients with artificial implants. *Mycoses.* 1999;42 Suppl 2:91-6.

[34] Hussain S T, Blackstone E H, Pettersson G B. Successful allograft root re-replacement for prosthetic valve endocarditis with improvement of renal function in a Jehovah's Witness patient. *J. Thorac. Cardiovasc. Surg.* 2014;148(4):e199-200.

[35] Kanawaty D S, Stalker M J, Munt P W. Nonsurgical treatment of Histoplasma endocarditis involving a bioprosthetic valve. *Chest.* 1991;99(1):253-6.

[36] Wiley Z, Woodworth M H, Jacob J T, Lockhart S R, Rouphael N G, Gullett J C, Guarner J, Workowski K. Diagnostic Importance of Hyphae on Heart Valve Tissue in Histoplasma Endocarditis and Treatment with Isavuconazole. *Open Forum Infect. Dis.* 2017;4(4):ofx241.

[37] Wang Z, Duarte A G, Schnadig V J. Fatal reactive hemophagocytosis related to disseminated histoplasmosis with endocarditis: an unusual case diagnosed at autopsy. *South Med. J.* 2007;100(2):208-11.

[38] Gerber H J, Schoonmaker F W, Vazquez M D. Chronic meningitis associated with Histoplasma endocarditis. *N. Engl. J. Med.* 1966;275(2):74-6.

Chapter 11

Occupational Histoplasmosis

Maryam Ahmed[1]
Lokesh Goyal[2]
Deborat Mallick[2]
Munish Sharma[3]
and Salim Surani[4,*]

[1]Department of Medicine, Punjab Medical College, Faisalabad, Pakistan
[2]Department of Medicine, Christus Spohn Hospital- Corpus Christi, Texas, USA
[3]Department of Medicine, Baylor Scott & White, Temple, Texas, USA
[4]Department of Medicine & Pharmacology, Texas A&M University, Texas, USA

Abstract

Occupational histoplasmosis is currently one of the most common systemic illnesses globally. The outbreaks typically result from actions that disturb the soil, particularly samples that contain bird or bat droppings. Over 50% of the world's population lives in endemic regions. There is a potential for any person who lives in Histoplasma endemic areas to be infected by the *H. capsulatum* during work or specific activities. Jobs that expose workers to soil contaminated with bird or bat droppings in places where Histoplasma is endemic may put them at risk for histoplasmosis. This category includes people who work in agriculture, forestry, and hunting and those who engage in construction and extraction. There is also laboratory-acquired histoplasmosis. The prevention of histoplasmosis exposures in the workplace involves the use of a 'Hierarchy of Controls' which involves elimination as the most effective way of prevention (removal of physical hazards), substitution

* Corresponding Author's Email: srsurani@hotmail.com.

In: Histoplasmosis
Editors: Salim Surani, Syed Anjum Khan and Reena Shah
ISBN: 979-8-89113-129-3

(replacement of the hazards), engineering control (isolation of people from the hazards), administrative controls (changing the way people are working), and PPE (protection of the workers through PPEs). In this chapter, we will discuss the details concerning occupational histoplasmosis.

Keywords: histoplasmosis, epidemiology, prevention, elimination, engineering control, occupational histoplasmosis

Introduction

Histoplasmosis is a fungal illness caused by breathing conidia, spore-like particles produced by the genus Histoplasma (1). Darling Samuel described the condition for the first time in 1906. *H. capsulatum duboisii* and *H. capsulatum capsulatum* can be distinguished by humans. *H. capsulatum*, which is found in the environment as saprobic filaments, belongs to the Ajellomycetaceae family and possesses septate hyphae [1]. Further investigation found that *H. capsulatum* produces two forms of asexual conidia, known as "microconidia" and "macroconidia," respectively. The microconidia are aerosolized and presumably inhaled when biological or abiotic disruption of the numerous *H. capsulatum* colonies happens during occupational activities [2].

Once microconidia are introduced into the body, and the temperature is optimal, they transform into the pathogenic polar budding yeast phase. *H. capsulatum*'s dimorphic switching, which allows the yeast to survive and reproduce within the cell (intracellular milieu of the phagolysosome), impairs the host immune system and leads to systemic infection [2]. *Although H. capsulatum* can be found worldwide, it is primarily indigenous to the Mississippi River basin and Ohio in the East and Central United States. Hemolytic uremic syndrome (HUS) is an infection induced by inhaling Histoplasma that is more prevalent in people whose employment requires them to work in areas containing bat and bird droppings.

General Epidemiology

According to current data, occupational histoplasmosis is one of the most prevalent systemic diseases worldwide [3]. Typically, the outbreaks are caused by operations that disrupt the soil, particularly the collection of samples containing bird or bat droppings [4]. Each continent has had an outbreak of histoplasmosis. According to a study4, more than 50% of the world's population resides in endemic zones. This endemic species is found in West Africa (Zimbabwe, Congo), Australia, South America, Southeast Asia (Malaysia, Taiwan, India, and Taiwan), South Africa, Europe, and Central and North America.4 However, indicates that the incidence of histoplasmosis varies significantly around the globe, ranging from 2 to 300 cases per 100,000 individuals. About 100,000 persons have disseminated histoplasmosis worldwide [5].

Any resident of a region where Histoplasma is endemic has the potential to contract H. capsulatum during work or specific activities [6]. It is observed that most people affected do not exhibit any symptoms. Consequently, only a tiny proportion of infections are manifested by individuals exhibiting diverse symptoms. And those with symptoms indicate shortness of breath, fever, and cough lasting between three- and seventeen-days during incubation. It is not always possible to distinguish these symptoms from those of other respiratory disorders, such as community-acquired pneumonia.

In most cases, these nonspecific symptoms lead to a delayed or incorrect diagnosis, resulting in inadequate treatment. As indicated in a review by Linder et al, it has also been observed in the Yangtze region of China. Some HIV-positive individuals in Thailand have also been diagnosed with the disease [7].

Histoplasmosis has expanded considerably in recent years, primarily due to the rise in immunocompromised individuals, particularly HIV patients. According to the Centers for Disease Control and Prevention, histoplasmosis is most prevalent among HIV/AIDS patients globally, particularly in places where HIV has been inadequately controlled by ART. According to the article, histoplasmosis is a big issue in Latin America, where an estimated 30% of HIV patients perish. Histoplasmosis and AIDS have been connected since the 1980s, when most disseminated histoplasmosis cases were observed in newly diagnosed HIV patients. Histoplasmosis among HIV-positive individuals has been observed in countries such as Thailand and Trinidad, which had never seen a case [8]. Histoplasmosis cases have been documented in Thailand, even in non-endemic regions, as the number of newly diagnosed HIV/AIDS patients has increased.

Understanding where the disease is most widespread can aid in its prevention and control. The high frequency of positive reactions to Histoplasma antigen in specific locations determined the approximate geographic distribution of the organism. Large-scale skin-testing studies undertaken in the 1940s and 1950s confirmed its validity. As indicated by P.H. surveillance, environmental data, and epidemic studies, histoplasmosis is likely more prevalent than previously believed due to underreporting and misinterpretation. Case frequencies and incidence estimates are also likely to be erroneous.

Settings, Jobs, and Activities Associated with Histoplasmosis

In locations where Histoplasma is endemic, occupations that expose workers to soil polluted with bird or bat droppings may put them at risk for histoplasmosis. This category comprises persons who work in agriculture, forestry, and hunting and those in the construction and extraction industries. Histoplasmosis is more prevalent among persons whose occupations or hobbies expose them to bird or bat droppings. According to a previous study, about one-third of all verified cases of histoplasmosis were linked to occupational settings. Histoplasmosis has historically affected numerous occupations, including bridge workers, construction workers, demolition workers, farmers, landscapers, tree removers, and microbiology lab workers [9].

Ecology or Histoplasma habitat disruption is a common trigger for histoplasmosis epidemics. The disturbance can be trivial, like treading on contaminated ground, or significant, like a construction site causing the windborne dispersal of Histoplasma conidia that infects hundreds of individuals throughout a city. Workers exposed to an epidemic virus at their place of employment but who had nothing to do with its spread, such as secretaries infected with staph after a building was renovated, were nonetheless affected. In almost 40% of observed outbreaks, disturbance of significant accumulations of bats and droppings is a frequent trait. Workers who clean chicken coops, remove bird poop from a bridge, or remove bat guano from attics are all at risk of contracting a disease that spreads rapidly through the population. There is a risk to employees beyond those directly responsible for cleaning up droppings, as more than 75% of all histoplasmosis outbreaks and 86% of work-related outbreaks are associated with the sheer presence of birds or bats. Further examples of environmental disruptions in histoplasmosis epidemics include work with the soil (such as digging and excavation in one-third of outbreaks) or plant materials (such as chopping trees or lumber, gardening, or landscaping [9]. About one-fourth of histoplasmosis outbreaks are preceded by demolition, construction, or remodeling. The activities associated with histoplasmosis is shown in Figure 1.

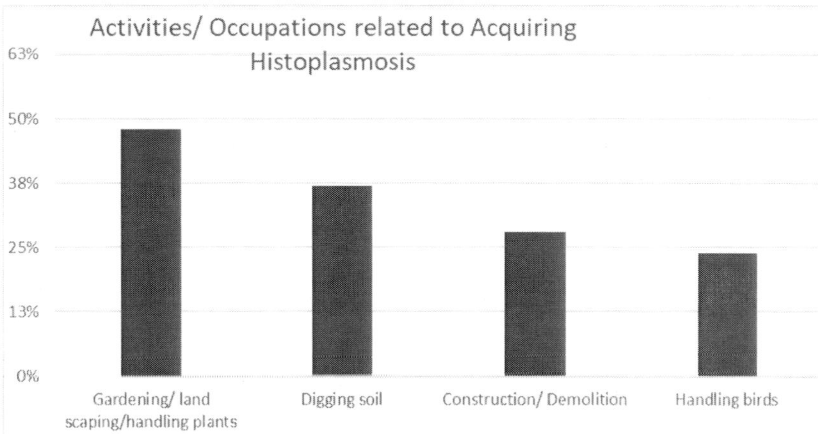

Figure 1. Activities / Occupations related to Acquiring Histoplasmosis.

However, these pursuits appear to be potential exposure routes for histoplasmosis cases that are not connected with an outbreak (i.e., cases that occur spontaneously). However, with regular P.H. surveillance, it is relatively uncommon for activities at work and play that may seldom be linked to infection to be overlooked. Nearly half of histoplasmosis patients interviewed in 2018-2019 in nine states (Arkansas, Indiana, Kentucky, Louisiana, Michigan, Minnesota, Nebraska, and Wisconsin) reported having contact with landscaping, trees, or plants in the wild. Nearly a third (37%) were continuously excavating, while 28% were engaged in construction, remodeling, and demolition activities, 48% were gardening, and 24% were bird handlers [9]. Two-thirds of those polled also said they had to deal with bird or bat poop. Therefore, specific exposures appear less common or prominent in occasional instances than in outbreaks. It may be challenging to ascertain if such exposures are work-related, mainly if people engage in recreational activities that also present a risk for Histoplasma exposure.

Immunocompromised people, who are more likely to experience severe histoplasmosis symptoms, may want to avoid the activities mentioned above in areas where Histoplasma is common. This was reported in a study of a histoplasmosis epidemic among Dominican Republic tunnel workers [10]. Using no respiratory protection, the study discovered that a crew of 36 men removed tones of bat guano from tunnels in a median of 24 days per worker (range, 1–25 days). They ranged in age from 18 to 62, and everyone was in good health (median 32). Thirty (83% of the workforce) were unwell enough to meet the case definition; among them, 9 (30%) needed intensive care, 6 (20%) required to be intubated, and 3 (10%) died while hospitalized. Antifungal treatment initiation interval (mean, six days) (range, 1–11 days). Out of the total of 34 employees, 22 (or 65%) were found to be infected by laboratory tests. Exposure to large numbers of *H. capsulatum* spores in an enclosed space, the lack of respiratory protection, and the delay in identification and treatment have all been linked to severe illness and mortality [10]. Histoplasmosis education for doctors, increased laboratory capacity for identifying fungal infections, and occupational health recommendations to protect workers from endemic fungus should all be implemented in the Dominican Republic.

According to research on histoplasmosis outbreaks [11], the majority of outbreaks occurred in structures (19 outbreaks), poultry coops (17 outbreaks), farms (12 outbreaks), and unidentifiable outdoor places (11 outbreaks). Those locations often involve fewer cases despite the frequency of outbreaks in particular regions. These instances were believed to have been caused by environmental disturbances near a stream bank (2 outbreaks), a golf course (1 outbreak), and either an obsolete amusement park or tennis complex (1 outbreak) (1 outbreak). Most outbreaks (28/29) associated with farms and poultry coops occurred between 1943 and 1969, the most recent being in 1985. Current (i.e., between 1987 and 2013) outbreaks were associated with several circumstances. The nine outbreaks associated with caverns occurred in some of the most southern states, including Florida, Texas, and Puerto Rico; four outbreaks in Puerto Rico were tied to caves.

In 42 (40%) cases, the outbreak was related to the disruption of bird or bat feces accumulations, in 34 (32%), in 21 (20%) to the disturbance of plant detritus, and in 26 (25%) to demolition or construction activities [11]. Inadequate data prohibited the identification of a single etiology for nine distinct epidemics. None of the papers specifically mentioned these acts. In 24 (23%) of the outbreaks, bats or bat guano were reported, whereas, in 59 (56%), it was birds, 81 (77%), it was bats, and in 2 (2%), both birds and bats were responsible. Blackbirds, mainly starlings, grackles, and unidentified blackbirds, accounted for 19 (32%) of the 59 bird-related infections reported, pigeons for 9 (15%), and gulls for 1 (2%) of the outbreaks. The bird species is implicated in 8 cases (14%). Thirty-five outbreaks, or 33% of all outbreaks, were attributable to workplace circumstances; 26 only affected employees, whereas nine outbreaks affected employees and non-employees. Sixteen (17%) workplace outbreaks occurred outside buildings, including four on bridges and two on water towers. The majority of workplace outbreaks occurred in the construction and maintenance industries. Thirty (86%) of the workplace outbreaks were associated with the presence of bats, birds, or their droppings. In eight non-work-related outbreaks, most patients were exposed in the workplace but were not involved in the actions that led to the outbreak. In 43 outbreaks (41%), occupational exposure was indicated as a contributing cause in the disease's spread. In at least four of these situations, a public health investigator or laboratory worker developed histoplasmosis while working to contain an epidemic.

Laboratory Acquired Histoplasmosis

Histoplasmosis contracted at a research facility was first reported in 1952. Seven people with influenza-like illness with a positive histoplasmin skin test and X-ray findings associated with histoplasmosis were diagnosed with pulmonary histoplasmosis in this study of 56 workers at the U.S. A PH Field Station in Kansas City, Kansas. Positive histoplasmin tests indicated that these workers' infection rate was 2.5 times higher than that of Kansas schoolchildren. The report's authors conclude that the laboratory setting favors human infection. After this study, between 1953 and 1966, a further 35 instances of L.A. histoplasmosis were documented [2]. Histoplasmosis is increasingly recognized as a spontaneously acquired disease, but laboratory acquired. *Histoplasma capsulatum* infections are rarely reported. In 1951, Sulkin and Pike compiled data on 1,342 illnesses in the U.S. that were thought to have been contracted in a laboratory setting. About a third of these diseases are documented in published works, while the rest were uncovered by sending out a questionnaire to almost 5,000 laboratories.

Clinicians and researchers working with clinical samples or cultures containing live *H. capsulatum* must be aware of the risk of laboratory-acquired histoplasmosis. Laboratory-acquired histoplasmosis has been reported in the scientific literature in the United States since the 1950s. The yeast and filamentous forms of *H. capsulatum* can be encountered in the laboratory. Inhalation of infectious *H. capsulatum* aerosols during laboratory procedures, unintentional inoculation, and transfer to skin and mucosal membranes have all been reported as potential routes of occupational exposure for the laboratorian.

Avoiding contact with *H. capsulatum* in the lab is essential, and one should follow the steps outlined in the laboratory protocols. Workers' exposure to *H. capsulatum* can be mitigated through aseptic microbiological methods, medical surveillance, and understanding the facility's laboratory safety manual. Elimination and substitution are impractical in a clinical and research laboratory. Exposure to *H. capsulatum* can be reduced by using a biosafety level (BSL)-3 laboratory, if available, and a laminar flow Biological Safety Cabinet (BSC), together with the proper personal protective equipment (PPE). Shrink-wrapping or taping closed culture plates, skipping slide cultures, and conducting molecular and proteomic studies early in the culture of Histoplasma are all other methods used to prevent exposure in the laboratory. Since histoplasmosis infections may be asymptomatic, have varying incubation periods, and occur even in non-endemic areas, determining exposure in the laboratory may be difficult [2]. Accidents and accidental exposures at work that cause histoplasmosis symptoms should be reported following the facility's policies and procedures, and an occupational physician should be consulted as soon as possible.

Prevention of *H. Capsulatum* at the Workplace

Working to limit the danger of histoplasmosis exposure in the workplace is attainable with this concept. The most efficient strategies for decreasing occupational hazards are elimination (totally doing away with the hazard) and substitution (effectively replacing the hazard with something else) (effectively replacing the hazard with something else). However, these strategies can be tough to adopt when dealing with infectious species like Histoplasma. Large quantities of bird and bat feces may demand the assistance of a licensed company to deal with such waste [9].

Engineering controls are adjustments to a work process that physically eliminates or isolates the hazard from personnel. Changes in the procedure are the outcome of administrative controls [12]. The last defense against an occupational hazard is a person's PPE. PPE is the least effective method of control since it calls for a structured program with a high level of worker participation and dedication to be applied efficiently. It is vital to limit risks in the workplace by adopting a site safety policy with the involvement of representatives of the employees, management, and health and safety professionals. The critical components of the strategy are the ability to recognize probable dangers and outline the activities that will be taken to minimize, remove, or otherwise deal with those threats. Engineering and administrative controls and personal protective equipment should be employed [12].

Elimination

It is the most effective method of histoplasmosis prevention. It can be accomplished in four ways: excluding birds and bats from buildings, controlling dust production and aerosolization, ensuring proper waste disposal, and disinfecting potentially contaminated materials [9].

Exclusion of the Birds Along with the Bats from Buildings

According to the hierarchy of controls, the most effective strategy to reduce the risk of exposure to Histoplasma at work is to eliminate the potential for bird and bat feces to accumulate in the first place. Best practices for bat and bird exclusion procedures have been established. Step one is to prevent anyone from entering or leaving the building. Put up lights in their daytime roosts and construct bat houses close to abandoned roosts to help eradicate bats. Unfortunately, ultrasonic devices and chemical repellents are ineffective at driving bats away from their roosting site [13]. In addition to using audible and visual deterrents, installing a mechanical anti-roosted system consisting of angled and spiky stainless-steel wires may be necessary to prevent birds from roosting.

Control of Generation and Aerosolization of Dust

Finding a roosting site in a building or other structure requires developing exclusion strategies and assessing the contamination level [9]. Occasionally, the next step is not to clean up a bat or bird droppings. When deciding whether or not to remove accumulations, numerous factors must be considered, including the material's volume and location, the building's structural integrity, weather, and the proximity of people. Eliminating or drastically reducing dust production through safe work practices and dust control methods would reduce the risk of infection during removal. Water can be used as an alternative to shoveling or sweeping to minimize the amount of aerosolized debris. Adding a wetting or surfactant agent to the water is another way to reduce aerosolization. Instead of manually collecting dust and debris, a powerful industrial vacuum with a filter could be utilized [9].

A truck-mounted or trailer-mounted vacuum system is required to remove large quantities of bat or bird feces. Histoplasma conidia can always be aerosolized during cleaning, building excavation, and demolition, even without a significant accumulation of bat and bird droppings. Once released into the air, Conidia can be carried great distances by wind currents and spread throughout an indoor space via an air handler or natural ventilation, potentially infecting people not even near the work site. Using dust suppression techniques and water sprays, the proportion of dust aerosolized during building excavation or demolition can be reduced in areas where Histoplasma is prevalent. Earth-moving operations should cease when strong winds or standard dust control measures are ineffective [14]. For the safety of the operators, it is best to equip all bulldozers and other earthmovers with fully enclosed cabs that include air conditioning and HEPA filtration. To prevent the spread of dirt and debris from a construction site, all trucks must pass through a cleaning station and have their beds covered.

Proper Waste Disposal

Material suspected of being contaminated with Histoplasma should not be moved to a location where it poses a health risk before being properly discarded. It is essential to comply with state and local regulations when removing, transporting, and disposing of potentially contaminated material. If municipal or state landfill guidelines classify Histoplasma-contaminated material as infectious waste, it may need to be burned or disposed of in another manner [15].

Disinfection of Probably Contaminated Materials

Environmental Protection Agency's list of "environmentally preferable" products does not include Histoplasma-effective soil disinfectants or other chemicals [16]. During previous histoplasmosis outbreaks, Histoplasma-contaminated materials were sterilized with formaldehyde. In contrast, the negative health effects of formaldehyde make this a bad idea. An additional method of preventing occupational histoplasmosis is administrative control. It can be accomplished in two ways: through communication and training about hazards and by posting health risk warnings. Bird and bat roosts, attics, and entire structures with bat and bird droppings accumulations should all be marked with signs warning of the potential health risk of [16]. Before beginning work that may disturb materials that Histoplasma can contaminate, employees must be aware of the dangers and how to protect themselves. Employers are required by OSHA's Hazard Communication Standard to provide their employees with information about potential workplace hazards and the necessary precautions. Risk factors, S & S, treatment, and exposure prevention are all recommended components of a documented histoplasmosis hazard communication program.

PPEs

Employers may benefit from implementing changes to working practices or an Occupational Safety and Health Administration-compliant respiratory protection program if they are aware of the risk factors for transmission and have conducted a comprehensive risk assessment [16]. It would be easier to detect histoplasmosis outbreaks in the workplace if surveillance included the systematic collection of occupational data. For sporadic and outbreak-associated histoplasmosis cases, recording information on the affected individuals' industry and occupation could assist public health officials in assessing the risks posed by various aspects of the workforce. Not all states with an endemic level of histoplasmosis collect data on industries and occupations, and those that do so utilize multiple methods. Examples include "check boxes" for industries or professions of interest and "free-text fields" for occupations.

The National Institute for Occupational Safety and Health Surveillance Program at the Centers for Disease Control and Prevention recommends standardizing occupational questions, collecting information on industry and occupation, and analyzing data with standard coding to better monitor disease trends in specific industries or occupations and protect worker health. For histoplasmosis surveillance, the company name, workplace address, nature of the work, and inquiries regarding specific exposures and preventative measures are also helpful.

To aid in identifying histoplasmosis infections, employers should also provide public health organizations with personnel rosters. Project owners and employers should also report histoplasmosis cases among employees to government health departments. Hospitalizations of employees due to illness must be reported to OSHA programs. Public health authorities must arrange with occupational safety and health organizations to share data for surveillance purposes. Healthcare providers in both endemic and non-endemic regions can benefit from efforts to raise awareness of occupational histoplasmosis through outreach [15].

Conclusion

Occupational histoplasmosis results from activities and occupations that disturb the soil. Especially the soils that contain birds or bats droppings. About 50% of the world lives in histoplasmosis-endemic areas. The disease has been found in every continent but is most endemic in West Africa, South Asia, and Central and North America. 60% to 90% of those living in the Mississippi River and Ohio have been exposed to these fungi at least once. Jobs that expose workers to soil contaminated with bird or bat droppings in areas where Histoplasma is endemic may put them at risk for histoplasmosis. This category includes people who work in agriculture, forestry, and hunting and those who engage in construction and extraction. When handling specimens, those working in the laboratory can also be infected with histoplasmosis. The prevention of histoplasmosis exposures in the workplace involves the use of a 'Hierarchy of Controls' which involves elimination as the most effective way of prevention (removal of physical hazards), substitution (replacement of the hazards), engineering control (isolation of people from the hazards), administrative controls (changing the way people are working), and PPE (protection of the workers through PPEs).

References

[1] Akram S M, Koirala J. Histoplasmosis. In Treasure Island (FL); 2022.

[2] Gugnani H C, Randhawa H S. Laboratory-Acquired Fungal Infections: A Review. *Arch. Microbiol. Immunol.* 2020;04(02):51–6.

[3] Rodrigues A M, Beale M A, Hagen F, Fisher M C, Terra P P D, de Hoog S, Brilhante RSN, de Aguiar Cordeiro R, de Souza Collares Maia Castelo-Branco D, Rocha M F G, Sidrim J J C, de Camargo ZP. The global epidemiology of emerging Histoplasma species in recent years. *Stud. Mycol.* [Internet]. 2020;97:100095. Available from: https://doi.org/10.1016/j.simyco.2020.02.001.

[4] Sami M. Akram J K. Histoplasmosis. *Stat. Pearls*. 2022. https://pubmed.ncbi.nlm.nih.gov/28846361/.

[5] Bongomin F. S G. Global and multi-national prevalence of fungal diseases—estimate precision. *J. Fungi.* [Internet]. 2017;49(3):408–9. Available from: https://www.sciencedirect.com/science/article/pii/S016606162030004X#bib1.

[6] Rahim M A, Zaman S, Amin M R, Uddin K N, Chowdhury M A J. Histoplasmosis: An emerging or neglected disease in Bangladesh? A systematic review. *Oman Med. J. [Internet].* 2020;35(1):1–17. Available from: https://www.ncbi.nlm.nih.gov/pmc/articles/PMC5773084/pdf/pntd.0006046.pdf.

[7] Linder K A, Kauffman C A. *Histoplasmosis : Epidemiology, Diagnosis, and Clinical Manifestations*. 2019;120–8. Available from: https://link.springer.com/content/pdf/10.1007/s12281-019-00341-x.pdf.

[8] Hatakeyama S, Okamoto K, Ogura K, Sugita C, Nagi M. Histoplasmosis among HIV-Infected Patients in Japan: a Case Report and Literature Review. *Jpn. J. Infect. Dis.* 2019 Sep;72(5):330–3.

[9] de Perio M A, Benedict K, Williams S L, Niemeier-Walsh C, Green B J, Coffey C, Di Giuseppe M, Toda M, Park J H, Bailey R L, Nett R J. Occupational Histoplasmosis: Epidemiology and Prevention Measures. *J. fungi.* (Basel, Switzerland). 2021 Jun;7(7).

[10] Armstrong P A, Beard J D, Bonilla L, Arboleda N, Lindsley M D, Chae S R, Castillo D, Nuñez R, Chiller T, de Perio M A, Pimentel R, Vallabhaneni S. Outbreak of Severe Histoplasmosis Among Tunnel Workers—Dominican Republic, 2015. *Clin. Infect. Dis. [Internet].* 2018 May 2;66(10):1550–7. Available from: https://doi.org/10.1093/cid/cix1067.

[11] Benedict K, Mody R K. Epidemiology of Histoplasmosis Outbreaks, United States, 1938-2013. *Emerg. Infect. Dis.* 2017 Mar;22(3):370–8.

[12] CDC. Who gets histoplasmosis? [Internet]. Center. 2021. Available from: https://www.cdc.gov/fungal/diseases/histoplasmosis/risk-prevention.html. Accessed on 12/20/22.

[13] Diaz J H. Environmental and Wilderness-Related Risk Factors for Histoplasmosis: More Than Bats in Caves. Wilderness Environ Med. 2018 Dec;29(4):531–40.

[14] CDC. Histoplasmosis in the Workplace [Internet]. Center for Disease and Prevention. 2022. Available from: https://www.cdc.gov/niosh/newsroom/feature/histoplasmosis.html. Accessed on 12/20/2022.

[15] Azar MM, Hage CA. Clinical Perspectives in the Diagnosis and Management of Histoplasmosis. Clin Chest Med. 2017 Sep;38(3):403–15.

[16] Mazi P B, Arnold S R, Baddley J W, Bahr N C, Beekmann S E, McCarty T P, Polgreen P M, Rauseo A M, Spec A. Management of Histoplasmosis by Infectious Disease Physicians. *Open Forum Infect. Dis. [Internet].* 2022 Jul 1;9(7):ofac313. Available from: https://doi.org/10.1093/ofid/ofac313.

Chapter 12

Neuro-Histoplasmosis

Simmy Lahori[1]
Tanya Amal[2]
Gaurang Bhatt[3]
Ruman Khurshid[4]
Rahul Kashyap[5]
and Salim Surani[6]

[1]Department of Anesthesiology, Research Scholar, Mayo Clinic, Department of Radiology, Rochester, Minnesota, United States of America
[2]Department of Medicine, Maulana Azad Medical College, New Delhi, India
[3]Department of Medicine, Junior Resident, Department of Burns and Plastic Surgery, All India Institute of Medical Sciences, Rishikesh, India
[4]Department of Medicine, Sher-i -Kashmir Institute of Medical Sciences, Srinagar, Jammu and Kashmir, India
[5]Department of Research, WellSpan Health, York, Pennsylvania, USA; Department of Anesthesiology and Critical Care Medicine, Rochester, Minnesota, United States of America; Harvard Medical School, Boston, Massachusetts, United States of America
[6]Adjunct Clinical Professor, Department of Medicine & Pharmacology, Texas A&M University, Research Collaborator, Mayo Clinic, Rochester, Minnesota, USA

Abstract

Histoplasmosis is a dimorphic fungus that can cause disseminated infection in 5-10% of patients. The most common reported presentations are central nervous system (CNS) inflammatory syndromes like encephalitis or chronic meningitis, focal lesions involving the brain and spinal cord. The major risk factors for developing CNS infections are Solid Organ transplantation, Tumor necrotic factor-Alpha (TNF-Alpha)

In: Histoplasmosis
Editors: Salim Surani, Syed Anjum Khan and Reena Shah
ISBN: 979-8-89113-129-3

inhibitors, and HIV with CD4 count < 150 cells/microL. Diagnosis can be made based on history and physical examination, Laboratory findings, cerebrospinal fluid (CSF) analysis, and radiological findings. The diagnosis can be confirmed with antigen and antibody testing, cytology, histopathology, and culture. Malignancy, bacterial, and other fungal infections should be ruled out before making the diagnosis. Treatment of CNS Histoplasmosis can be challenging, and hence aggressive management is suggested. Induction therapy with Liposomal Amphotericin B (5 mg/kg daily for 4-6 weeks is suggested. Itraconazole twice or thrice daily is used for maintenance therapy for 12 months. The treatment is continued till the antigen becomes undetected from the CSF. Hence, monitoring for Histoplasma antigen concentrations is necessary. Drug interactions with other medications should be kept in mind while treating for Neuro-Histoplasmosis.

Keywords: histoplasmosis, central nervous system, hiv, inflammation, disseminated histoplasmosis, histoplasma capsulatum, histoplasma duboisii

Introduction

Histoplasma Capsulatum is a dimorphic fungus that is prevalent in Central America [1]. It occurs in 2 forms H. Capsulatum var. Capsulatum and H. Capsulatum var Duboisii. The exact reason for this particular geographic distribution is unknown, but it could be because of a certain characteristic of soil, climate, and moisture [1]. Although it most commonly causes pulmonary infections, it can affect the central nervous system, causing chronic meningitis, arachnoiditis, hydrocephalus, focal parenchymal lesions, etc., [1]. The involvement of the central nervous system or any extra-pulmonary system can be considered a disseminated disease. CNS Histoplasmosis is a common complication of H. Capsulatum occurring in 2-20% of disseminated cases. The major risk factor for disseminated infection is the state of immunosuppression. The infection developing in immunocompetent individuals is self-limited or can be asymptomatic. The diagnosis of neuro histoplasmosis can be made by culture and microbiological stains, histopathology, cytopathology, antigen detection, serology, or molecular methods. The gold standard for the diagnosis is the detection of septate hyphae with spherical, thick-walled tuberculate conidia on a microscope in the culture. Antigen detection is a rapid, non-invasive, and highly sensitive method of detection as well as a useful way for treatment response [2]. Delay in diagnosis leads to a rise in morbidity and mortality [3]. The initial treatment is started with Amphotericin B and then, switched to the Azole group of drugs. The length of treatment depends on the immune status of the patient as well the severity of the infection [4]. The resolution of symptoms and improvement in fatigue can be noticed after a period of about 1 and a half months. In contrast, weight gain is noticed after a period of 2 weeks. Monitoring for the antigens and antibodies from the urine and serum is quite important. Preventing exposure in immunocompromised hosts can help in the prevention of disease [5].

Etiopathogenesis

H. Capsulatum occurs in 2 forms, mold or mycelial form and yeast form [6]. It belongs to the family of Ascomycetes [7]. The mycelial form exists in the environment in nitrogen-enriched soil where it is contaminated with bird or bat droppings. The hyphae measure from 1.25 to 2 micrometers in diameter. These hyphal forms can cause human infections such as endocarditis, etc., [8]. The two forms of conidia exist depending upon their sizes. Macroconidia range from 8 to 15 micrometers in diameter, and microconidia range from 2 to 5 micrometers in diameter. The yeast form is ovoid and measures from 2 to 5 micrometers in diameter. Temperature changes largely influence the mycelial to yeast transition in H. Capsulatum. At 370, the yeast phase predominates in host tissues [9]. The smaller conidia can be easily aerosolized and inhaled into the lungs, where alveolar macrophages phagocytize them. There they convert to yeast form and are disseminated widely through the lymphatics and bloodstream [4]. In immunocompetent individuals, even though the dissemination occurs, it is rarely symptomatic. This is because the T-lymphocytes become sensitized to the H. Capsulatum antigens and release cytokines that cause the macrophages to kill the intracellular organism. Thus, the infection is contained [10]. However, in immunocompromised hosts, the cell-mediated immunity does not function, and the organism remains viable in the macrophages causing disseminated infections.

Epidemiology

Histoplasmosis is one of the dimorphic fungi that can produce human disease. Histoplasmosis was once described as "Darling's disease" as it was first discovered in 1905 by pathologist Samuel Darling. He described it to be a protozoan. However, da Rocha-Lima in 1912, described its resemblance to yeast, which later was revealed as a dimorphic organism. 5-10% of patients with disseminated histoplasmosis develop CNS infections [3]. Over 1/3rd of cases reported have occurred in immunocompetent individuals [11]. Histoplasmosis occurred in 5-17% of patients with advanced HIV in endemic areas of the United States early in the HIV epidemic [3]. Although found in the temperate zones, specific endemic areas are the Mississippi and Ohio river valleys, the Caribbean, Southern Mexico, and certain parts of Central and South America, Africa, and Asia [12]. It is commonly found in contaminated soil by bird and bat guano. Certain activities like farming, spelunking, and demolition increase the risk of exposure. The source of infections is transmission via inhaling the conidia of the fungus from the soil [13]. In endemic areas, the incidence rate of HIV approaches 5%/year [14]. Histoplasmosis of the CNS is a common complication of H. Capsulatum, as it occurs in 2-20% of disseminated cases. The diagnosis of CNS Histoplasmosis is frequently missed due to misdiagnosis or failure to include histoplasmosis as a differential diagnosis in non-endemic regions [15]. Around 50-90% of immunocompetent individuals who are infected by it remain asymptomatic [16]. There are a series of case reports with disseminated histoplasmosis that are misdiagnosed as primary hematological malignancies [17]. The annual incidence rate approaches 5% in the endemic areas among individuals with HIV. Of which CD4 count of < 150 cells/mm3 is associated with increased symptomatic illness [3, 18].The diagnosis of Chronic histoplasmosis is delayed by over a month in 60% of the cases as the diagnosis is overlooked. Infection of the CNS with histoplasmosis may occur with or without dissemination in up to 10% of the cases [19]. Infection of CNS Histoplasmosis was first recognized in an infant in 1934 [20]. However, for the clinician, diagnosing the CNS infection can be a challenge as the symptoms can be subtle and poor sensitivity of the fungal culture of CSF [19]. CNS Histoplasmosis can mimic CNS metastasis [21].

The five-year transplant-associated surveillance network (TRANSNET) study reported 48 cases of histoplasmosis among solid organ transplant recipients, and the incidence rate was 0.1% [22]. The occurrence was bimodal, with 40% of cases occurring within the first six months but can occur at 18-20 years post-transplantation. Kidney and liver transplant patients account for half a quarter of histoplasmosis cases [23]. In such patients, the illness was severe and occurred early after transplantation, especially during the time of maximal immunosuppression [24, 25]. In some patients, H. Capsulatum was found in the donor organ during the time of or post-transplantation. The recipients were treated pre-emptively and successfully with the antifungal agents even before they developed the symptoms of histoplasmosis [22, 25].

Agents

H. Capsulatum is an endemic thermally dimorphic fungi occurring in 2 forms. The forms infecting the human are H. Capsulatum var. Capsulatum and H. Capsulatum var. Duboisii. H. Capsulatum var. Capsulatum, which is the most common variety, is found worldwide. H. Capsulatum var. Duboisii exists only in Africa [5]. H. Capsulatum occurs as hyaline, septate hyphae with spherical, thick-walled tuberculate conidia and smaller microconidia microscopically. The budding yeasts are found both inside and outside of the macrophages. Gomori methenamine silver (GMS) and periodic-acid Schiff (PAS) are the most common stains that can be used to stain these broad-spectrum fungi. It helps to distinguish fungi based on morphologic features such as size, type of budding, presence of hyphae, and branching. They are identified as 2-4 micrometers in size with round to oval uninucleate yeast cells having narrow-based budding. [26].

Risk Factors for Disseminated Histoplasmosis

The following are considered the risk factors for disseminated histoplasmosis include extremes of age, AIDS, hematological malignancies, solid organ transplants, hematopoietic stem cell transplant, immunosuppressive agents, congenital T-cell deficiencies [27].

Clinical Features

Histoplasma primarily affects the lungs and mediastinum; however, in some patients, the disease might get disseminated and involve the CNS too. CNS is involved in about one out of ten patients with disseminated histoplasmosis. However, it accounts for only half the cases of the disease. Although immunocompromised individuals are more prone to develop CNS histoplasmosis, about one-third of the cases are reported in unsuspecting immunocompetent individuals. CNS histoplasmosis must be considered a differential in individuals residing in the endemic regions with an otherwise unexplained acute, subacute or chronic neurological illness like meningitis, stroke syndromes, mass lesions, or hydrocephalus [15].

Most reported presentations include CNS inflammatory syndromes like encephalitis or chronic meningitis, focal lesions involving the brain and spinal cord, hydrocephalus, and stroke syndromes [15]. Patients present with headache, altered sensorium, cranial nerve deficits, focal deficits, and seizures depending on the location of the lesion [1]. Patients with disseminated histoplasmosis might also present with fever, malaise, anorexia, hepatosplenomegaly, and lymphadenopathy due to the involvement of the reticuloendothelial system. Less commonly, abscesses or ulcers are seen involving the skin or the gastrointestinal system. Other organ systems involved include bone marrow, adrenal glands, etc, [28].

Immunocompromised patients with HIV represent a significant at-risk population due to poor cellular defense mechanisms. Apart from constitutional symptoms like weight loss, fever, and abdominal pain, these patients with CNS histoplasmosis may present with headache, ataxia, spatiotemporal disorientation, dysarthria, meningeal syndromes, and ideomotor slowdown [29]. There have been reports of Immune reconstitution inflammatory syndrome in patients with HIV and histoplasmosis and Post Infectious Inflammatory Response Syndrome in patients with HCV who contracted CNS histoplasmosis [30].

Due to its relatively rare occurrence, most diagnostic recommendations are based on evidence gathered from case reports and case series. This has also led to comparatively poor characterization of the clinical features associated with the disease, resulting in delayed diagnosis due to poor clinical suspicion [15].

Diagnosis

Neuro histoplasmosis, which is a disseminated form of the disease, should be suspected in patients with risk factors such as immunosuppression, and extremes of age, in combination with the clinical features of the disseminated form of the disease, making the diagnosis highly likely.

Suspicion about disseminated histoplasmosis can be in the presence of the above-mentioned risk factors and the clinical symptoms. Table 1 describes the

Physical Exam findings, Laboratory, and radiographic abnormalities in patients with disseminated histoplasmosis that can help in the diagnosis [31].

Table 1. Histoplasmosis findings on physical examination, laboratory, Cerebrospinal Fluid (CSF) and radiology

Physical Examination	Labs	CSF	Radiology
1. Peripheral Lymphadenopathy 2. Hepatosplenomegaly 3. Skin and Mucosal Lesions 4. Altered Mental Status and other neurological abnormalities.	1. Pancytopenia 2. Elevated Serum Aminotransferases, Alkaline Phosphatase, and/or Bilirubin 3. Markedly elevated Serum Lactate Dehydrogenase and Ferritin	1. Lymphocytic Pleocytosis with elevated protein and low glucose concentration.	1. Chest X-ray shows interstitial or reticulonodular infiltrates. Rarely, Mediastinal Adenopathy or Cavitation can occur [32] 2. Abdominal CT scan can show enlargement of the spleen, adrenal glands, or lymph nodes. 3. CT scan or MRI displays Single or Multiple enhancing lesions [3].

The following confirmation tests can help in the diagnosis of the Disseminated Histoplasmosis diagnosis.

1. Antigen testing: Antigen testing in cerebrospinal fluid, urine, and serum is extremely helpful in diagnosis. Antigens are detected in CSF of patients with CNS involvement. In cases where antigen detection is negative in urine, they may be positive in the serum [33, 34]. Antigen testing is usually done by enzyme immunoassay (EIA), which detects antigens in 75% of non-immunocompromised and 95% of immunocompromised patients [35]. A few conditions can have false-positive results in the urine and serum antigen assay. Infections such as Blastomycosis, Para Coccidiomycosis, Penicilliosis, and African histoplasmosis can have a false positive urine antigen assay. Serum antigen assay is seen positive with Rheumatoid factor as well as treatment with rabbit antithymocyte globulin [27].
2. Cytology and histopathology: a cytological and histopathological examination of various tissue and fluid samples [36] using fungal stains such as methenamine silver or periodic acid-Schiff. CSF fluid

analysis shows findings of lymphocytic pleocytosis, elevated protein, and low glucose concentration. Biopsy results of bone marrow and other involved organs can yield positive results

3. Fungal culture: Fungal cultures are usually considered the gold standard for diagnosis, but culture results usually take up to a month, and they are negative in less severe cases [36]. Fungal cultures are usually positive for blood, [37, 38]. BAL, and bone marrow aspirate.
4. Antibody testing: H. Lasmosis infection with central nervous system involvement is often diagnosed when assays for IgG/IgM antibody and antigen are performed [3, 15, 16, 39].
5. Radiological imaging: Computed tomography scan or Magnetic resonance imaging shows single or multiple enhancing brain lesions [40].
6. Further diagnostic evaluation: Tests of lymphocyte proliferative response to H. Capsulatum antigens and Interferon Gamma release assay in response to H. Capsulatum antigens are being developed in the future [41].

Differential Diagnosis

The common symptoms of Disseminated Histoplasmosis are fever, fatigue, and weight loss. The differential diagnosis includes malignancy, infections such as Tuberculosis, and other Fungal Diseases. Inflammatory bowel diseases and sarcoidosis [42] are a few other inflammatory conditions that can mimic Neuro-Histoplasmosis. Certain therapeutics, such as glucocorticoids, cytotoxic agents, or TNF-Alpha Inhibitors, must be ruled out before making the disseminated Histoplasmosis diagnosis.

Imaging

A case of NeuroHistoplasmosis in an Immunocompetent adult demonstrates significant MRI findings. It was a unique finding as the brain MRI demonstrated two of them had multiple ring-enhancing lesions, restricted diffusion, and thickened wall with hemosiderin deposits [43]. Projections from the wall of the abscess into the cavity with a low apparent diffusion coefficient and no enhancement is a typical finding of fungal etiology [44]. Certain patients with CNS histoplasmosis are misdiagnosed as CNS gliosarcoma [45]. Some cases are associated with isolated CNS Neuro Histoplasmosis, or some are in the form of dissemination [27, 46].

Impact of COVID-19 on Neuro Histoplasmosis

Cases of Pulmonary Histoplasmosis have been found. However, CNS Neuro Histoplasmosis has not been noted during or after post-COVID-19 [47]. Although Neuro Histoplasmosis can occur because of its dissemination and hence a differential should be kept in mind while treating the patients of COVID-19.

Treatment

Primary Prevention

1. Decreasing exposure: Patients with HIV with CD 4+ counts < 150 should avoid exposure to activities that create dust containing Histoplasma Capsulatum. These include going to areas with possible contamination with bird or bat droppings: caves, demolishing old buildings, and areas undergoing remodeling and cleaning. They should also avoid activities like cleaning chicken coops, and gardening [48].
2. Antimicrobial prophylaxis: Prophylactic treatment with Itraconazole (200 mg daily) is recommended in patients with HIV having CD 4+ counts < 150, particularly in those who are at increased risk of exposure due to the nature of their occupation or being in a hyperendemic area (> 10 cases/100 patient-years).

Secondary Prevention

Medical management is the mainstay for treating neuro histoplasmosis. The major barriers faced in treatment are limited penetration of drugs into the central nervous system [3]. and underlying conditions like HIV, organ transplant, and pregnancy. Surgical treatment is not routinely recommended but has proven beneficial in selected cases [49].

Antimicrobial Therapy

Treatment of CNS Histoplasmosis can be challenging because of poor penetration of antifungal agents through the blood-brain barrier. Hence, aggressive treatment is recommended for successful results.

Antimicrobial treatment is given in two phases:

1. Induction therapy: Induction is done with liposomal Amphotericin B (5 mg/kg daily) for 4-6 weeks (target dose being 175 mg/kg over the course of treatment [50]. Significant side effects, including acute kidney injury, can be managed with dose reduction or early transition to itraconazole.
   Lipid formulations are preferred in pregnant females. However, in the pediatric population, amphotericin B deoxycholate (1 mg/kg) is better tolerated.
2. Maintenance therapy: Itraconazole (200 mg), twice or thrice daily, is given for 12 months as maintenance therapy in adults. The pediatric dose is 5-10 mg/kg (the upper limit is 400 mg). The treatment is also continued until CSF abnormalities resolve and Histoplasma antigen becomes undetectable in the same.

Treatment courses of > 12 months may be needed for immunosuppressed patients or those with primary immunodeficiency syndromes. Lifelong therapy with itraconazole may be considered in situations with a high risk of relapse [50]. Treatment is also guided by monitoring antigen levels in the serum and urine. Persistence of the antigen in body fluids necessitates prolongation of therapy [33].

Itraconazole may not be tolerated in some patients, while others may not be able to achieve therapeutic levels. Fluconazole (400 mg daily) is a less effective but possible alternative in these cohorts or Voriconazole [51].

Surgical Management

Occasional reports of resection of brain and spinal cord abscesses exist in literature. However, surgical techniques are not routinely applied in the management of Histoplasmosis.

Monitoring

For the first few months, Histoplasma antigen concentrations should be checked monthly in the urine and serum as they fall after effective antifungal therapy. Later on, they can be checked every 3 months [33]. Absence of such a fall even after 3 months of therapy suggests ineffective treatment [31]. A few reasons for treatment failure or relapse can be as follows:

- Low Itraconazole concentration.
- Poor adherence to medications.
- Resistance to antifungal agents.

Only 60-80% of patients responded to treatment with amphotericin B, and up to half of the responders relapsed during the subsequent years [3]. Further consultation with infectious diseases is needed in case of treatment failure or relapse.

Drug Interactions

ll Azole antifungal agents' drug interactions involve oxidative drug metabolism via the cytochrome P450 enzyme system. They are metabolized and affect the hepatic cytochrome P450 (CYP) enzymes to varying degrees [52].

The common clinical side effects [48]. of azoles are as follows:

- Long QT syndrome and Sudden cardiac death due to torsade de pointes with concomitant use of drugs that prolong QT interval, such as Amiodarone, Cisapride, Haloperidol, etc.
- Concomitant use of Triazolam and Midazolam can cause excessive sedation. Lorazepam which is not metabolized by CYP3A4 is preferred.
- Use of concomitant statins like Simvastatin, Lovastatin, and Atorvastatin can cause rhabdomyolysis as they are metabolized by CYP3A4. Pravastatin, Fluvastatin or Rosuvastatin are not metabolized by CYP3A4 and are preferred.

Latest Clinical Trials

The largest clinical study of CNS Histoplasmosis was conducted to understand the clinical presentation, diagnosis, and outcomes. A retrospective multicentric study was conducted of cases occurring between 1997 and 2010 by taking a survey from physicians about the cases of CNS Histoplasmosis. The disease was classified as mild, moderate, and severe based on the severity of the infection and how it was managed. Mild for patients who were managed without hospitalization, moderate if the patient was hospitalized, and severe if the patient required critical care unit admission. Functional impairment was also classified as none, mild, moderate, and severe. The proven diagnosis was done by isolation of Histoplasma from fungal culture or visualization of fungi in the brain, CSF, or spinal cord tissue. Probable diagnosis required a positive antigen or antibody test from CSF. Possible diagnoses required laboratory confirmation of pulmonary or disseminated histoplasmosis without another cause of CNS infections depending upon the clinical findings, symptoms, and examination in the absence of any proven or probable CNS Histoplasmosis. The study showed that CNS disease was the first manifestation in 84% of patients, and relapse of dissemination occurred in 16% of them. Relapse presentation occurs more often in AIDS patients. The risk of death increased with the advancement of age, ICU management, and duration of Amphotericin B treatment. However, the findings were not statistically significant [53].

Future Clinical Trials

No clinical trials were found on clinicaltrials.gov while searching for Neuro histoplasmosis at the time of writing this article.

Conclusion

Neurohistoplasmosis is a disseminated form of Histoplasmosis infection caused by H. Capsulatum var. Capsulatum and H. Capsulatum var Duboisii. Prevention of exposure in immunocompromised patients can help in prevention of the disease. Monitoring the antigens in urine and serum is very important. Diagnosis can be done with physical examination, Laboratory findings, CSF analysis and imaging findings. CT scan and MRI demonstrates single or multiple ring-enhancing lesions. Confirmation is done by Antigen testing, Cytology and histopathology tests, fungal culture, and antibody testing. Medical management is the mainstay therapy for patients with Neuro histoplasmosis. Induction is done with liposomal Amphotericin B (5 mg/kg daily) for 4-6 weeks. Itraconazole (200 mg), twice or thrice daily, is given for 12 months as maintenance therapy in adults. Only one clinical trial was done on CNS Histoplasmosis. Further clinical trials must be conducted in order to learn more about the disease.

References

[1] Saccente M. Central nervous system histoplasmosis. *Curr. Treat. Options Neurol.* 2008;10(3):161-167.

[2] Azar M M, Hage C A. Laboratory Diagnostics for Histoplasmosis. *J. Clin. Microbiol.* 2017;55(6):1612-1620.

[3] Wheat L J, Batteiger B E, Sathapatayavongs B. Histoplasma capsulatum infections of the central nervous system. A clinical review. *Med. Baltim.* 1990;69(4):244-260.

[4] Kauffman C A. Management of histoplasmosis. *Expert Opin. Pharmacother.* 2002;3(8):1067-1072.

[5] Myint T. HIV-Associated Histoplasmosis: Current Perspectives. *HIV AIDS Auckl.* 2020;12:113-125.

[6] Nosanchuk J D, Gacser A. Histoplasma capsulatum at the host-pathogen interface. *Microbes Infect.* 2008;10(9):973-977.

[7] Kwon-Chung K J, Weeks R J, Larsh H W. Studies on Emmonsiella capsulata (Histoplasma capsulatum). II. Distribution of the two mating types in 13 endemic states of the United States. *Am. J. Epidemiol.* 1974;99(1):44-49.

[8] Hutton J P. Hyphal forms of Histoplasma capsulatum. A common manifestation of intravascular infections. *Arch. Pathol. Lab. Med.* 1985;109(4):330-332.

[9] Mittal J. Histoplasma Capsulatum: Mechanisms for Pathogenesis. *Curr. Top. Microbiol. Immunol.* 2019;422:157-191.

[10] Newman SL. Cell-mediated immunity to Histoplasma capsulatum. *Semin. Respir. Infect.* 2001;16(2):102-108.

[11] Schestatsky P. Isolated central nervous system histoplasmosis in immunocompetent hosts: a series of 11 cases. *Scand. J. Infect. Dis.* 2006;38(1):43-48.

[12] Bahr N C. Histoplasmosis infections worldwide: thinking outside of the Ohio River valley. *Curr. Trop. Med. Rep.* 2015;2(2):70-80.

[13] Wheat L J. Disseminated histoplasmosis in the acquired immune deficiency syndrome: clinical findings, diagnosis and treatment, and review of the literature. *Med. Baltim.* 1990;69(6):361-374.

[14] Masur H. Prevention and treatment of opportunistic infections in HIV-infected adults and adolescents: Updated Guidelines from the Centers for Disease Control

and Prevention, National Institutes of Health, and HIV Medicine Association of the Infectious Diseases Society of America. *Clin. Infect. Dis.* 2014;58(9):1308-1311.

[15] Wheat J. Central nervous system histoplasmosis: Multicenter retrospective study on clinical features, diagnostic approach and outcome of treatment. *Med. Baltim.* 2018;97(13):0245.

[16] Wheat L J, Musial C E, Jenny-Avital E. Diagnosis and management of central nervous system histoplasmosis. *Clin. Infect. Dis.* 2005;40(6):844-852.

[17] Hariri O R. Histoplasmosis with Deep CNS Involvement: Case Presentation with Discussion and Literature Review. *J. Neurol. Surg. Rep.* 2015;76(1):167-172.

[18] McKinsey D S. Prospective study of histoplasmosis in patients infected with human immunodeficiency virus: incidence, risk factors, and pathophysiology. *Clin. Infect. Dis.* 1997;24(6):1195-1203.

[19] Riddell J, Wheat L J. Central Nervous System Infection with Histoplasma capsulatum. *.J Fungi.* 2019;5(3):70.

[20] Dodd K, Tompkins E H. A Case of Histoplasmosis of Darling in an Infant. *Am. J. Trop. Med.* 1934;14(2).

[21] Liu B. Histoplasmosis mimicking metastatic spinal tumour. *J. Int. Med. Res.* 2017;45(4):1440-1446.

[22] Kauffman C A. Endemic fungal infections in solid organ and hematopoietic cell transplant recipients enrolled in the Transplant-Associated Infection Surveillance Network (TRANSNET. *Transpl. Infect. Dis.* 2014;16(2):213-224.

[23] Kauffman C A, Miceli M H. Histoplasmosis and Blastomycosis in Solid Organ Transplant Recipients. *J. Fungi. Basel.* 2015;1(2):94-106.

[24] Assi M. Histoplasmosis after solid organ transplant. *Clin. Infect. Dis.* 2013;57(11):1542-1549.

[25] Cuellar-Rodriguez J. Histoplasmosis in solid organ transplant recipients: 10 years of experience at a large transplant center in an endemic area. *Clin. Infect. Dis.* 2009;49(5):710-716.

[26] Rajeshwari M. Acid-Fastness of Histoplasma in Surgical Pathology Practice. *J. Pathol. Transl. Med.* 2017;51(5):482-487.

[27] Kauffman C A. Histoplasmosis: a clinical and laboratory update. *Clin. Microbiol. Rev.* 2007;20(1):115-132.

[28] Wheat L J. Histoplasmosis. *Infect. Clin. North Am.* 2016;30(1):207-227.

[29] Epelboin L. Histoplasmosis of the Central Nervous System: A Case Series between 1990 and 2019 in French Guiana. *Am. J. Trop. Med. Hyg.* 2021;105:125-129.

[30] Jabr R. Histoplasmosis-Associated Hemophagocytic Lymphohistiocytosis: A Review of the Literature. The Canadian journal of infectious diseases &amp. *Med Microbiol J. Can. Mal. Infect. Microbiol. Medicale.* Published online 2019: 7107326. doi:10.1155/2019/7107326.

[31] Wheat LJ. Improvements in diagnosis of histoplasmosis. *Expert Opin. Biol. Ther.* 2006;6(11):1207-1221.

[32] Sathapatayavongs B. Clinical and laboratory features of disseminated histoplasmosis during two large urban outbreaks. *Med. Baltim.* 1983;62(5):263-270.

[33] Hage C A. Histoplasma antigen clearance during treatment of histoplasmosis in patients with AIDS determined by a quantitative antigen enzyme immunoassay. *Clin. Vaccine Immunol.* 2011;18(4):661-666.

[34] Hage CA. Recognition, diagnosis, and treatment of histoplasmosis complicating tumor necrosis factor blocker therapy. *Clin. Infect. Dis.* 2010;50(1):85-92.

[35] Hage C A. A multicenter evaluation of tests for diagnosis of histoplasmosis. *Clin Infect. Dis.* 2011;53(5):448-454.

[36] Assi MA. Systemic histoplasmosis: a 15-year retrospective institutional review of 111 patients. *Med Baltim.* 2007;86(3):162-169.

[37] Fuller D D. Comparison of BACTEC Plus 26 and 27 media with and without fastidious organism supplement with conventional methods for culture of sterile body fluids. *J. Clin. Microbiol.* 1994;32(6):1488-1491.

[38] Lyon R, Woods G. Comparison of the BacT/Alert and Isolator blood culture systems for recovery of fungi. *Am. J. Clin. Pathol.* 1995;103(5):660-662.

[39] Bloch K C. Improvement in Diagnosis of Histoplasma Meningitis by Combined Testing for Histoplasma Antigen and Immunoglobulin G and Immunoglobulin M Anti-Histoplasma Antibody in Cerebrospinal Fluid. *Clin. Infect. Dis.* 2018;66(1):89-94.

[40] Gonzalez H H. Disseminated Central Nervous System Histoplasmosis: A Case Report. *Cureus.* 2019;11(3):4238.

[41] Rubio-Carrasquilla M. An interferon gamma release assay specific for Histoplasma capsulatum to detect asymptomatic infected individuals: A proof of concept study. *Med. Mycol.* 2019;57(6):724-732.

[42] Wheat L J, French M L, Wass J L. Sarcoid like manifestations of histoplasmosis. *Arch. Intern. Med.* 1989;149(11):2421-2426.

[43] Ines Andrade A, Donato M, Previgliano C, Hardjasudarma M. Histoplasmosis Brain Abscesses in an Immunocompetent Adult. *Neuroradiol. J.* 27(3):334-338. doi:10.15274/NRJ-2014-10038.

[44] Luthra G, Parihar A, Nath K, Jaiswal S, Prasad K N, Husain N, Husain M, Singh S, Behari S, Gupta RK. Comparative evaluation of fungal, tubercular, and pyogenic brain abscesses with conventional and diffusion MR imaging and proton MR spectroscopy. *AJNR Am. J. Neuroradiol.* 2007;28(7):1332-1338. doi:10.3174/ajnr.A0548.

[45] Khalaf S A, Patel P, Caruso C R, Parrett T, Bran A. CNS Histoplasmosis as a Gliosarcoma mimicker: The diagnostic dilemma of solitary brain lesions. *IDCases.* 2021;27:e01364. doi:10.1016/j.idcr.2021.e01364.

[46] Levi G C, Pozzi C M, Hirschheimer S M D S, Chahade W H, Gomes H R, Granato C. [Central nervous system involvement by histoplasmosis as the unique manifestation of this disease in immunocompetent patients: presentation of two cases]. *Arq. Neuropsiquiatr.* 2003;61(3B):859-863. doi:10.1590/s0004-282x2003000500029.

[47] de Macedo P M, Freitas A D, Bártholo T P, Bernardes-Engemann A R, Almeida M A, Almeida-Silva F, Zancopé-Oliveira R M, Almeida-Paes R. Acute Pulmonary Histoplasmosis Following COVID-19: Novel Laboratorial Methods Aiding Diagnosis. *J. Fungi. Basel Switz.* 2021;7(5):346. doi:10.3390/jof7050346.

[48] Dodds Ashley E. Pharmacology of azoles. https://www.uptodate.com/contents/pharmacology-of-azoles?sectionName=DRUG%20INTERACTIONS&search=histoplasmosis%20CNS%20treatment&topicRef=2461&anchor=H31&source=see_link#H31.

[49] Srinivasan J, Ooi W W. Successful treatment of histoplasmosis brain abscess with voriconazole. *Arch. Neurol.* 2008;65(5):666-667.

[50] Wheat L J. Clinical practice guidelines for the management of patients with histoplasmosis: 2007 update by the Infectious Diseases Society of America. *Clin. Infect. Dis*. 2007;45(7):807-825.

[51] McKinsey D S. Fluconazole therapy for histoplasmosis. The National Institute of Allergy and Infectious Diseases Mycoses Study Group. *Clin. Infect. Dis*. 1996;23(5):996-1001.

[52] Venkatakrishnan K, Moltke L L, Greenblatt D J. Effects of the antifungal agents on oxidative drug metabolism: clinical relevance. *Clin. Pharmacokinet*. 2000;38(2):111-180.

[53] Wheat J. Central nervous system histoplasmosis: Multicenter retrospective study on clinical features, diagnostic approach and outcome of treatment. *Medicine (Baltimore)*. 2018;97(13):0245.

Chapter 13

Disseminated Histoplasmosis

Akshat Banga[1]
Riecha Joshi[2]
Rahul Kashyap[3]
Reena Shah[4]
and Salim Surani[4,5,*]

[1]Department of Medicine, Sawai Man Singh Medical College, Jaipur, India
[2]Department of Medicine, Government Medical College, Kota, India
[3]Department of Research, WellSpan Health, York, Pennsylvania, USA
[4]Department of Medicine, Aga Khan University Hospital, Nairobi, Kenya
[5]Department of Medicine & Pharmacology, Texas A&M University, College Station, Texas, USA

Abstract

Histoplasmosis is a systemic mycosis caused by the dimorphic fungus Histoplasma capsulatum, a facultative intracellular parasite of the system. It is predominantly found in North America, primarily Midwestern and Southeastern United States. Transmitted by inhalation of airborne fungal conidia, H. capsulatum can cause mild to severe respiratory illness. Dissemination of histoplasmosis occurs in immunocompromised patients following initial infection, reinfection, or reactivation of the latent foci. Histoplasma initially disseminates to organs rich in reticuloendothelial cells, but it can infect any organ/organ system, including central nervous system (CNS), gastrointestinal tract (GIT), skin, and adrenal glands, etc. Disseminated histoplasmosis is considered one of the acquired immunodeficiency syndrome (AIDS)-

* Corresponding Author's Email: srsurani@hotmail.com.

In: Histoplasmosis
Editors: Salim Surani, Syed Anjum Khan and Reena Shah
ISBN: 979-8-89113-129-3

defining infections, and it usually occurs in HIV-infected individuals with a CD4 count<200/mm^3.

Keywords: histoplasmosis, disseminated histoplasmosis, AIDS, immunocompromised, TNF-alpha, CNS histoplasmosis, GI histoplasmosis

Introduction

Histoplasmosis is an airborne mycotic disease caused by the fungus Histoplasma capsulatum. First described by Dr. Samuel Darling in 1906. H. capsulatum is an encapsulated dimorphic fungus found in a moist environment contaminated by bird and bat droppings [1].

Histoplasma capsulatum inhabits the temperate zone regions. It is commonly found in North America, Central America, and South America. It is the most common endemic mycosis in the United States of America (USA), prevalent in the Midwestern and Southeastern United States around the Ohio River valley and lower Mississippi River [2]. Although the significant burden of the disease is concentrated in the Americas, cases of histoplasmosis have also been reported in some Asian (India, China, Myanmar, Taiwan), African (Congo, Zimbabwe, South Africa), and European (Italy) countries [3]. It is transmitted by inhalation of fungal spores, and the lungs are the primary site of infection. Immunocompetent hosts generally remain asymptomatic or present with self-limiting flu-like illness. However, it can also lead to systemic mycoses, manifesting in different, less common clinical forms, including acute pulmonary histoplasmosis, chronic pulmonary histoplasmosis, cutaneous histoplasmosis, and rarely, central nervous system histoplasmosis. In some cases, it can also lead to a severe disseminated infection [4].

Pathogenesis

Histoplasma capsulatum belongs to the family ascomycetes. It is a thermally dimorphic fungus found as mold in nature (20 degree centigrade) and as yeast in warmer conditions, such as inside the host (human) body (37 degree centigrade) [5]. Moist, fertile soil contaminated by birds (e.g., Starlings) and bat droppings is a rich source of H. capsulatum [5]. The mold gets transmitted into the environment through the air. Histoplasma Infection occurs via inhalation of its asexual reproductive spores, called microconidia, into the lungs, where the fungus converts into its yeast form at body temperature e(37C), which is the tissue-invasive form [6]. The typical incubation period is 7-21 days. Although the lungs are the primary site of infection, the extra-pulmonary dissemination of Histoplasma can occur throughout the body, especially in immunocompromised patients [7].

Neutrophils, macrophages, lymphocytes, and Natural Killer (NK) cells respond to Histoplasma infection [8]. T-cell-mediated immunity plays a crucial role in preventing and controlling severe histoplasmosis. Cytokines Interferon - Gamma (IFN-γ), Tumor Necrosis Factor - Alpha (TNF-α), and interleukin 12 (IL-12) are responsible for triggering the macrophages to kill the yeast [9-12]. The host defense mechanism usually sustains Histoplasma invasion in an immunocompetent host, leading to either an asymptomatic course or a self-limited acute disease [9].

Failure of the cellular immunity to attain enough response to eradicate the fungus from the body completely leads to disseminated histoplasmosis infection [13]. This can be corroborated by the occurrence of severe disseminated infections in immunocompromised individuals, including those undergoing TNF-α inhibitor therapy and those with HIV infection [14, 15]. Individuals with IL-12 receptor deficiency and IFN-γ receptor deficiency are also more susceptible to disseminated infection due to the inability of such individuals to generate a cellular immune response [16, 17]. However, dissemination of Histoplasma infection can also develop in immunocompetent subjects, as in the case of children, due to poor immunological development, and in the geriatric age group, probably due to constitutive immunosenescence [1, 4].

Reinfection and reactivation of the infection in patients with a history of histoplasmosis are also possible, especially when there is immunosuppression. An overwhelming infectious load in immunocompromised patients hampers the host defense's ability to control the infection and leads to reinfection [18, 19].

Reactivation of latent histoplasmosis occurs when viable organisms persist in the tissues following recovery from the initial histoplasmosis infection. In immunocompromised individuals, the protective immunity from previous exposure wanes off quickly and promotes reactivation of the latent infection. However, the incidence of reactivation is 1-2 per 10,000 population, which is much less than expected, the reason for which hasn't been established other than the effectiveness of cellular immunity to protect against the infection [14, 19-21].

Pathophysiology

The pathophysiology of disseminated histoplasmosis typically resembles the pathophysiology of Tuberculosis (TB) [22]. The dissemination process begins with the engulfment of the yeast by macrophages, similar to TB. In contrast to a localized acute Histoplasma infection, neutrophil, lymphocyte, and plasma cell infiltration are not observed in disseminated infection. Failure of activation of the full fungicidal capacity of macrophages, as in immunocompromised patients, prevents the clearance of the yeast from the body. This promotes intracellular proliferation of the engorged fungus inside the macrophages, leading to uncontrolled growth of the organism in multiple organ systems [2].

As the inhaled fungus gets phagocytosed by alveolar macrophages, the ingested yeast multiplies inside the macrophages [2]. These macrophages further aid in the lymphatic spread of the organism through the lymphatics to the lymph nodes, primarily the perihilar and mediastinal lymph nodes. The infection spreads throughout the body via the hematogenous route, especially to the reticuloendothelial system (liver, spleen, and bone marrow) rich in reticuloendothelial cells, producing inflammatory foci in the infected organs [13, 23].

Pathology

Histiocytosis is the phenomenon in which the infection of macrophages causes the recruitment of more macrophages in the tissues [24]. The Tissue responses that have been demonstrated in disseminated histoplasmosis are shown in Table 1:

Risk Factors

Disseminated Histoplasmosis usually affects people with suppressed immunity, such as transplant recipients on immunosuppressants, HIV infected, on TNF-Alpha inhibitors.

(a) Transplant Recipients

Solid organ transplant recipients are susceptible to disseminated histoplasmosis. The infection may be a result of reinfection, relapse, or transmission from the donor [25]. In order to differentiate between reinfection and relapse, molecular typing of Histoplasma capsulatum can be done [26]. Concurrent infections can be seen with disseminated infections such as infections with the Herpes virus, especially Cytomegalovirus (CMV), bloodstream infections by Gram-positive cocci, and Gram-negative bacilli [25].

(b) TNF- Alpha Inhibitors

TNF-alpha is the cytokine that is responsible for the activation of macrophages to act against the fungal species [11]. When it is inhibited, the macrophages cannot prevent infection dissemination. TNF- alpha inhibitors Include adalimumab, infliximab, and etanercept. These are used for the treatment of rheumatoid arthritis, Crohn's disease, Ulcerative colitis, and ankylosing spondylitis. Since TNF-alpha plays a crucial role in limiting the infection by Histoplasma capsulatum, its inhibitor causes the patient to be susceptible to infection [14, 19].

Table 1. Tissue responses seen in disseminated histoplasmosis

Types of Tissue reaction	Diffuse histiocytosis	Focal Histiocytosis	Tuberculoid Granuloma
Location and pathology	The infected histiocytes are present diffusely throughout the monocyte phagocyte system (such as in lymph nodes, spleen, liver, and bone marrow).	In focal histiocytosis, the histiocytes are only limited to a single area.	These are usually formed by a cellular necrotic central region being surrounded by a tight aggregation of parasitized macrophages, multinuclear giant cells, and lymphocytes. The pathology is similar to the one seen in Tuberculosis.
Incidence	More common	This type of histiocytosis is less common in disseminated histoplasmosis.	These are present only rarely in disseminated histoplasmosis.

(c) HIV Infection

HIV-infected individuals have low cellular immunity, thus, are more likely to be infected by Histoplasma capsulatum. In AIDS patients, histoplasmosis is a severe, often fatal disease that occurs when the level of CD4 is below 200 cells/mm^3. Although disseminated histoplasmosis is prevalent in HIV patients in Latin America, In the US, due to the early use of antiretroviral agents, the infection has declined [15, 27, 28].

(d) Others

The infection is more likely to be seen in patients with low cellular immunity, such as those on corticosteroids or those with congenital immunodeficiencies. Pregnancy is also suspected to be a risk factor for disseminated histoplasmosis [29].

Clinical Manifestations

I. Natural History of the Disease

Clinical presentation of disseminated histoplasmosis and the acuteness of the disease manifestation depends upon the host's immune response and the degree of fungus exposure [1, 4]. Disseminated histoplasmosis can present acutely within a few weeks of exposure, or it can manifest years after exposure [1]. Sometimes patients may experience prolonged asymptomatic periods followed by symptomatic relapses. Disseminated histoplasmosis occurs in two classical forms:

(a) Acute Infection

- Acute infection mainly occurs in infants and immunocompromised patients (e.g., HIV infection, transplant recipients, etc.).
- Patients presents with non-specific symptoms such as fever, malaise, nausea, vomiting, anorexia, and weight loss. Diarrhea and dyspnea are less commonly seen. Hepatosplenomegaly and lymphadenopathy can be observed on physical examination [4].

- Some HIV patients may present with Histoplasmosis-associated Immune Reconstitution Inflammatory Syndrome (IRIS) upon starting Antiretroviral therapy (ART) [30].
- Disseminated histoplasmosis can have grievous complications in severely immunocompromised individuals. Patients are at risk of developing shock, coagulopathy, hepatic failure, renal failure, respiratory failure, and obtundation [21].

(b) Chronic Infection

Chronic progressive disseminated histoplasmosis primarily occurs in immunocompetent older patients [2, 4].

Symptoms include pancytopenia, hepatosplenomegaly, oropharyngeal lesions, and adrenal insufficiency. They may also have skin, mucosal, and gastrointestinal involvement [2].

II. Systemic Manifestations

Evidence of H. capsulatum, even at a single extrapulmonary site (e.g., extrathorasic lymphadenopathy, hepatomegaly, isolated Central nervous system (CNS) involvement), is sufficient to classify the infection as disseminated histoplasmosis. Findings in such cases are usually related to the predominantly affected organ, as seen below.

(a) Lung Involvement

Lungs are usually the primary foci of infection which then leads to dissemination. Thus, involvement of the lungs is very common, affecting about 25% of patients [1]. Pulmonary involvement can present as acute mild histoplasmosis (resembles community-acquired pneumonia), acute severe (diffuse) histoplasmosis, chronic (progressive) pulmonary pneumonia, broncholithiasis (granulomatous calcification in lungs and lymph nodes), mediastinal granuloma, mediastinal lymphadenitis, and fibrosing mediastinitis [1-4, 6, 7, 22-24, 31-37].

(b) Skin Infestation

- Skin involvement is commonly seen in disseminated histoplasmosis. Skin lesions are reported more frequently in patients suffering from advanced/severe HIV infection [38].

- Characteristic lesions of disseminated histoplasmosis include papules, pustules, plaques, nodules, vesicles, ulcers, and abscesses. Generalized dermatitis is a common manifestation of the disease [4, 22, 24].
- Cellulitis, panniculitis, petechiae, purpura, ecchymoses, exfoliative erythroderma, and necrotizing vasculitis are uncommon manifestations of disseminated histoplasmosis [39-41].
- Infiltrates composed of H. capsulatum-infected macrophages are characteristically seen on histopathological examination. Histiocytes are present in the center of the lesion, and only a small number of parasitized macrophages are seen in the margins. This finding may resemble leukocytoclastic vasculitis, which makes the diagnosis of skin infestation difficult [40, 41].

(c) Adrenal Disease

- Clinically apparent adrenal insufficiency is not common (<10% cases), but adrenal involvement has been a frequent finding on autopsies [4, 42].
- Adrenal involvement may be unilateral or bilateral.
- Macrophages infected with H. capsulatum can be either diffusely distributed throughout the adrenal sinusoids or limited to focal collections within the medulla, corticomedullary junction, or the cortical zona reticularis [43].
- Adrenal insufficiency could occur due to perivasculitis, leading to thrombosis and infarction of adrenal glands [1].
- Thus, adrenal insufficiency should be considered in patients with disseminated histoplasmosis, especially those who present with electrolyte disturbances, hypoglycemia, or orthostatic hypotension [42, 43].

(d) Central Nervous System (CNS) Involvement

- CNS involvement has been reported in around 5-20 percent of cases of disseminated histoplasmosis. CNS disease is more common in immunocompromised patients.

- CNS involvement most commonly manifests as meningitis. Other clinical features include focal cerebritis, encephalitis, cerebral vasculitis, and localized spinal cord compression [1, 44, 45].

(e) Gastrointestinal (GIT) Disease

- Gastrointestinal tract involvement is seen in approximately 70% of disseminated histoplasmosis cases. Gastrointestinal disease most commonly affects the ileum, especially the ileocecal area; however, it can involve the entire gastrointestinal tract [1].
- In most cases, gastrointestinal tract disease remains subclinical. But when symptomatic, it presents with nausea, vomiting, abdominal pain, and, less commonly, diarrhea. Rarely gastrointestinal histoplasmosis can also cause dysphagia, esophagitis, gastrointestinal (GI) bleeding, and colonic perforation [4, 46, 47].
- Endoscopic examination findings involve intestinal ulcerations (resembling Inflammatory bowel disease) and polypoid mass (resembling malignancy) [48].
- Patients from endemic regions who present with non-specific symptoms such as fever, nausea, vomiting, and abdominal pain and have intestinal lesions on colonoscopy should be evaluated for histoplasmosis [1].

(f) Others

- Pancreatitis, cholecystitis, hypercalcemia, thrombotic microangiopathy, hemophagocytic lymphohistiocytosis, Chorioretinitis, osteomyelitis, and prostatitis [49-55].
- Other uncommon manifestations include Pleuritis, pericarditis, endocarditis, and peritonitis [56-60].
- Hypercalcemia occurs due to the excessive production of calcitriol by the activated macrophages. Hypercalcemia in disseminated histoplasmosis can get aggravated by vitamin D. Thus, disseminated histoplasmosis diagnosis can be misdiagnosed as sarcoidosis [50, 61].
- H. capsulatum-associated endocarditis can affect both native and prosthetic valves, as well as aortic grafts. The aortic valve is the most commonly affected valve in Histoplasma endocarditis [62].

Disseminated Histoplasmosis in Patients with Underlying HIV Infection

- HIV-infected individuals have low cellular immunity, thus, are more likely to be infected by H. capsulatum. Disseminated histoplasmosis is symptomatic in a majority of AIDS patients and is usually fatal in the absence of appropriate treatment. The extrapulmonary form of histoplasmosis is considered an AIDS-defining illness [27, 63].
- A CD4 count of <200 cells/microL is a major risk factor for the development of disseminated Histoplasmosis, along with the activities or occupations that involve the handling of soil contaminated with bird or bat droppings [64].
- In HIV patients with >200 cells/microL, histoplasmosis usually occurs as a self-limiting illness; however, patients with <200 cells/microL and disseminated histoplasmosis report a rapidly progressive disease with high-grade fever, severe anorexia, and weight loss, miliary or interstitial pattern of pulmonary involvement, along with extrapulmonary sites such as gastrointestinal tract, liver, skin, and adrenals getting affected [65].
- Physical signs include hepatosplenomegaly, generalized lymphadenopathy, bone marrow lesions manifesting as pancytopenia, and mucosal and skin lesions. Cutaneous symptoms are more common in Latin America than in the United States [65].
- Immune Reconstitution Inflammatory Syndrome (IRIS) associated with Histoplasmosis is very rare, but uncommon symptoms such as splenic infarction and skin lesions have been reported in patients who have started on ART [66].

Diagnosis

Disseminated histoplasmosis is considered in individuals with risk factors for the disease, along with clinical signs and symptoms suggestive of the same [6]. Usual findings on physical examination and laboratory evaluations of patients with disseminated histoplasmosis include:

- Fever, weight loss, nausea, vomiting, cough, dyspnea, abdominal pain, and altered mental status.

- Peripheral lymphadenopathy, hepatosplenomegaly, splenomegaly, mucosal and skin lesions
- Anemia, Leukopenia, Thrombocytopenia, and pancytopenia
- Deranged Liver function tests (LFT), including elevations in serum aminotransferases (ALT and AST), alkaline phosphatase (ALP), bilirubin, serum ferritin, and lactate dehydrogenase enzyme (LDH).

Establishing the diagnosis of histoplasmosis is necessary to prompt rapid treatment initiation. Microscopic detection of Histoplasma or its isolation from an extrapulmonary site indicates dissemination of the disease from the primary pulmonary foci. Various diagnostic modalities [4, 19, 21, 311, 37, 46, 67] used to diagnose disseminated histoplasmosis are as follows:

1. Cultures
2. Cytology and histopathology
3. Antibody testing
4. Antigen testing
5. Imaging
6. Bronchoalveolar Lavage (BAL)

1. Cultures

Blood cultures, bone marrow cultures, and cultures from infected organs (e.g., respiratory samples) remain the gold standard for the diagnosis of disseminated histoplasmosis. However, the culture of H. capsulatum takes up to 4-6 weeks to grow [1, 4, 19, 21, 31, 37, 46, 67, 68-70].

- Blood cultures are recommended in all suspected cases. Blood cultures have a sensitivity of 65%; however, it usually varies depending on the disease burden and specimen type. The lysis centrifugation technique gives a higher yield than standard blood cultures [68, 69].
- As the lungs are the primary site of infection, H. capsulatum can be cultured from the respiratory secretions, and lung tissue in most patients with diffuse pulmonary infiltrates.
- A culture of bone marrow aspirate is taken in patients who have anemia, leukopenia, and/or thrombocytopenia.

- Depending on the infection sites, culture can yield H. capsulatum from tissue biopsies of involved organs, adrenal glands, gastrointestinal tract, liver, lymph nodes, oral mucosa, skin, etc.

2. Cytology and Histopathology

Tissue biopsy specimens visualized under the microscope can reveal the typical yeast structure of the fungus [1, 4, 19, 21, 31, 37, 46, 67, 69, 70].

- Methamine silver stain and periodic Acid-Schiff stains are used for H. capsulatum visualization in tissue specimens. Giemsa stain is used for bone marrow aspirates. Hematoxylin and eosin stain can be used as an alternative; however, it is not preferred due to poorer visualization of the organism.
- Granulomas with yeasts resembling H. capsulatum in extrapulmonary tissues are consistent with the disseminated disease.
- In rare cases, H. capsulatum can cause endocarditis which affects the vascular structures. Histopathological examination of these vascular structures may reveal the presence of both yeast-like structures and hyphae. This is an unusual finding as hyphae are not a typical finding of disseminated histoplasmosis [71].

3. Antibody Testing

Antibodies against H. capsulatum antigens may appear as early as two weeks after the infection; however, acutely presenting histoplasmosis usually fails to produce a positive result on antibody assays. That is why Histoplasma antibody assays are more useful in diagnosing chronic disseminated infection [1, 4, 19, 21, 31, 37, 46, 67, 69-71].

- The presence of antibodies in the blood can be tested using an immunodiffusion test and complement fixation test in patients with suspected disseminated histoplasmosis.
- The sensitivity and specificity of the complement fixation test for histoplasmosis is between 60-70%. A fourfold increase in the antibody titer is used to diagnose acute H. capsulatum infection [72].

- Serodiagnosis of histoplasmosis is based on Histoplasmin, a product of H. capsulatum. It predominantly consists of three antigens: C, H, and M antigens. C antigen is composed of the carbohydrate Galactomannan, which is responsible for the cross-reaction with other fungal organisms. H antigen is a beta-glucosidase, and M antigen is a catalase enzyme. These are the antigens that are detected in the complement antibody fixation testing [73].
- Latex agglutination has a higher sensitivity and specificity than the complement fixation and immunodiffusion test; however, it fails to differentiate Histoplasma from Blastomyces and, thus, is not commonly used in Histoplasma diagnosis.
- Antibody titers may be negative in immunocompromised patients (e.g., HIV infection, transplant recipients, immunosuppressive medications, etc.). This occurs due to the suppressive action of the underlying disease or medication on the immune system, leading to antibody production inhibition and attenuation of immune response generation. This results in the low sensitivity of antibody assays in such individuals [74].
- Recent developments have led to the introduction of newer enzyme immunoassays which are more sensitive and specific than immunodiffusion tests and complement fixation test, especially in acute pulmonary histoplasmosis, but their efficacy in the diagnosis disseminated disease is still under investigation [75, 76].

4. Antigen Testing

Antigen testing of serum and urine should be performed in all suspected cases of disseminated histoplasmosis. It is the most sensitive test for disseminated histoplasmosis detection. A positive antigen test strongly supports histoplasmosis diagnosis [4, 74, 77, 78].

- H. capsulatum antigen can also be detected in the bronchoalveolar lavage (BAL) fluid in patients with pulmonary involvement, while cerebrospinal fluid (CSF) can be assessed for antigen in case of central nervous system (CNS) infestation [78, 79].
- Antigen detection is done using Enzyme immunoassay (EIA). A negative urine antigen EIA does not rule out a positive serum assay.

Likewise, a negative serum or urine antigen assay does not rule out disseminated histoplasmosis diagnosis. This occurs due to a difference in sensitivity of the various enzymes in immunoassay being used [80, 81].

- Another disadvantage of EIA for H. capsulatum is its high false-positive rate. False positive results have been reported in patients with Blastomycosis, coccidioidomycosis, paracoccidioidomycosis, and talaromycosis. False-positive results are also observed on bronchoalveolar lavage (BAL) fluid antigen assay in Aspergillosis [82].
- Combining antigen and antibody detection by using EIA increases the sensitivity up to 96%, thus is a new, improved method for the diagnosis of Histoplasmosis.[74].

5. Imaging

Different imaging modalities are used in the diagnosis of disseminated histoplasmosis depending upon the involved organ [4, 70].

- Chest radiographs are abnormal in the majority of patients with disseminated histoplasmosis. Pulmonary infestation leads to diffuse infiltration of the lungs, which presents as interstitial and reticulonodular infiltrates on chest X-ray. The presence of diffuse reticulonodular infiltrates suggestive of disseminated disease, especially in immunocompromised individuals [4, 83].
- Computed tomography (CT) scan is the imaging modality preferred in case of gastrointestinal involvement. An abdominal CT scan is used to visualize the liver, spleen, adrenal glands, and abdominal lymph nodes, which appear enlarged when infected [4, 47, 48].
- In comparison to a non-invasive abdominal CT scan, the assessment of lesions inside the stomach, small intestine, and large intestine (colon) is done with invasive gastrointestinal endoscopy [47, 48].
- Both computed tomography (CT) scan and magnetic resonance imaging (MRI) can be used in case of central nervous system (CNS) involvement. CNS histoplasmosis presents as single or multiple enhancing brain lesions on imaging [4, 42, 79].

6. Polymerase Chain Reaction (PCR)

Although PCR has not been widely used in the diagnosis of histoplasmosis yet, a new, nested, real-time PCR assay with a higher sensitivity (>75%) than previous assays has been developed and is under evaluation [4, 84-87].

Diagnosing Disseminated Histoplasmosis with Meningitis

Patients with suspected Histoplasma meningitis need to undergo cerebrospinal fluid (CSF), serum, and urine testing [44, 45, 80].

- In the case of isolated meningitis, diagnosis is made by antigen detection and/or antibody assay of the cerebrospinal fluid (CSF). A diagnostic approach involving both antigen detection and IgG/IgM antibody test provides a better result than a single test [88].
- Positive culture of the organism can be obtained from CSF, blood, or other tissues (e.g., bone marrow), but the fungal stain of CSF is mostly negative during the histopathological examination. CSF cultures yield the best diagnostic results when a large volume of CSF (10-20 mL) is used on at least two occasions. However, a negative culture (even with a large volume CSF sample) does not rule out Histoplasma infection [44, 45].
- In rare cases, when all these tests, antigen detection, antibody titers, and cultures are negative, a brain parenchymal or meningeal biopsy is performed to establish the diagnosis [44].
- The 1,3-beta-D-glucan test of CSF is a new test based on 1,3-beta-D-glucan, which is a cell wall component of many fungi. Although it is a valuable tool in the investigation of this condition, a positive 1,3-beta-D-glucan test alone is neither sensitive nor specific enough to identify a specific causative organism. A positive test only helps in raising suspicion of Histoplasma infection and prompting further testing with antigen detection, antibody complement fixation, Enzyme immunoassay, culture, etc. [89-91].

Differential Diagnosis

The differential diagnosis for disseminated histoplasmosis includes entities with similar symptoms and signs (e.g., Fever, weight loss, night sweats, hepatosplenomegaly, lymphadenopathy.)

(i) Tuberculosis

Tuberculosis is the most common infection considered in the differential of disseminated histoplasmosis. Tuberculosis and disseminated histoplasmosis can present as co-infections as well. It is very difficult to differentiate the two based on just clinical manifestations and laboratory evidence, thus, almost always requiring culture and histopathology for the diagnosis [92].

(ii) Disseminated Cryptococcosis

Disseminated Cryptococcosis presents clinical signs such as hepatomegaly, lymphadenopathy, and skin lesions. Serum Cryptococcal antigen testing is required for diagnosis.

(iii) Other Endemic Fungi

Other endemic fungi such as Blastomycosis, Coccidioidomycosis, Paracoccidioidomycosis, and Talaromycosis also may present as disseminated infections. Fungal infections are difficult to differentiate from each other [82].

(iv) Sarcoidosis

Sarcoidosis presents with similar clinical manifestations as disseminated histoplasmosis (e.g., Fever, weight loss, night sweats, hepatosplenomegaly, lymphadenopathy, skin lesion). Thus, infectious causes need to be excluded first before making the diagnosis of Sarcoidosis [50, 61].

(v) Malignancy

Hematological malignancies (e.g., Lymphomas) have manifestations similar to histoplasmosis, such as fever, night sweats, weight loss, lymphadenopathy, and pancytopenias and may also present with pulmonary and GI symptoms.

(vi) Multicentric Castleman Disease (MCD)

MCD presents with symptoms such as fever, weight loss, and cytopenias. MCD can be diagnosed by histopathology. Hypogammaglobinemia is common with MCD but not seen in histoplasmosis [93].

Treatment

The treatment of disseminated histoplasmosis follows the guidelines published by the Infectious Diseases Society of America (IDSA, 2007) and the World Health Organization (WHO, 2020) [94, 95]. Drug and drug-regimen selection in patients infected with Disseminated Histoplasmosis depends on the severity of the infection, the involvement of the central nervous system, and the presence of underlying HIV infection. Untreated acute disseminated histoplasmosis spreads progressively, becoming fatal within a course of 2-to-12 weeks [6, 37, 46, 67, 94].

Indications for the initiating treatment of Disseminated Histoplasmosis:

- Treatment is indicated for all patients with disseminated histoplasmosis.
- If the symptoms persist for less than four weeks, treatment with antifungal drugs is not necessary.

Treatment of Disseminated Histoplasmosis follows a 2-phase treatment and commonly involves the use of the antifungal agent's Amphotericin B and azoles, including Itraconazole, Fluconazole, and newer agents like voriconazole, Posaconazole, and Isavuconazole [95-97].

Amphotericin B

Amphotericin B is considered the first-line therapy for severe disseminated histoplasmosis, disseminated histoplasmosis with CNS involvement, and in AIDS patients suffering from disseminated histoplasmosis. Its fungicidal properties, ability to clear fungemia faster than other antifungal agents, greater efficacy, better overall survival, and lower toxicity compared to other antifungal options make it the preferred choice [94, 98].

Amphotericin B is used in two different formulations - Liposomal formulation (e.g., AmBisome or Abelcet) and Deoxycholate formulation. The liposomal formulation is found to produce better outcomes than the deoxycholate formulation. Liposomal formulation AmBisome is the preferred formulation for CNS histoplasmosis as it is found to achieve a higher concentration in CNS compared to other lipid formulations and Amphotericin B deoxycholate. However, administration of Amphotericin B requires a central venous catheter, long line catheter, or peripheral venous catheter, and needs regular monitoring as it can lead to infusion-related toxicity and nephrotoxicity [99, 100].

Adverse effects of Amphotericin B include infusion-related phlebitis and other reactions, including nausea, vomiting, chills, and rigor. In order to lessen the effect of phlebitis, the addition of hydrocortisone or heparin may be added [101].

Azoles

Itraconazole is the preferred oral azole for histoplasmosis [97, 102]. It is found to have better *in-vitro* activity against H. capsulatum than other azoles [103]. Along with it, the absence of any reports suggestive of Itraconazole resistance makes it suitable for histoplasmosis treatment [104]. Itraconazole is commonly given in a capsule formulation; however, its liquid formulation has better absorption and 30% higher bioavailability. SUBA-Itraconazole, a new formulation with even higher bioavailability, was approved in the USA in 2018 [105, 106].

Itraconazole requires several days of loading dose to achieve a steady state concentration in the blood; that's why Amphotericin B is preferred for the treatment induction, while Itraconazole is started later for maintenance therapy [102]. The serum concentration of Itraconazole should be maintained at 1-2 mcg/mL, and regular monitoring is suggested once the drug reaches this steady-state concentration [94].

Fluconazole is usually reserved for patients who cannot tolerate Itraconazole [107]. Inferior *in-vitro* activity against H. capsulatum, higher rate of relapse amongst recipients, and increasing drug resistance cases limit Fluconazole's usability in Histoplasmosis [103, 108-110]. Despite achieving significantly higher concentration in CSF compared to Itraconazole, its inefficacy in treating the infection limits its application in histoplasmosis [111, 112].

Voriconazole, Posaconazole, and Andisavuconazole are new drugs used for Histoplasmosis management. They are considered in patients unable to tolerate both Itraconazole and Fluconazole. There are no clinical trials conducted to report the efficacy of these agents [113-119].

Adverse effects of Azoles include GI symptoms such as nausea, vomiting, abdominal pain, and diarrhea. Hepatic abnormalities such as hepatitis, cholestasis, and fulminant hepatic failures are associated with azoles [120].

The approach to the management of Disseminated Histoplasmosis will be discussed under the following headings:

1. Disseminated Histoplasmosis without HIV infection and CNS involvement
2. Disseminated Histoplasmosis with underlying HIV infection
3. Disseminated Histoplasmosis with CNS involvement

1. Disseminated Histoplasmosis without HIV Infection and CNS Involvement

Treatment of Disseminated Histoplasmosis typically involves Amphotericin B (preferably liposomal formulation) and an azole drug, preferably Itraconazole. Dosing recommendations depend on the disease severity.

A. Mild-Moderate Disease

Itraconazole (200 mg BD x 12 months) is the treatment of choice for patients with mild-to-moderate symptoms [102, 121].

B. Moderately Severe-Severe Disease

Patients with severe disease require hospitalization and initial therapy with IV Amphotericin B (Lipid formulation: 3 mg/kg daily or deoxycholate formulation: 0.7-1 mg/kg daily). Following its quick response to fungemia, treatment is transitioned to oral Itraconazole (loading dose 200 mg TDS x 3 days followed by 200mg BID) over 1-2 weeks. This transition is initiated only when a patient becomes afebrile and does not require vitals monitoring, intravenous fluid management, or mechanical ventilation support [94-97, 99].

The treatment, in both conditions, should be continued for a period of at least 12 months to reduce the risk of relapse [94, 95]. Lifelong suppressive antifungal therapy with Itraconazole 200mg OD/BID can be considered in high-risk patients, such as transplant patients on lifelong immunosuppressants [14, 19, 122, 123].

Special Consideration: Management of disseminated histoplasmosis in pregnant women is challenging due to the risk of teratogenicity posed by azoles which are contraindicated in the first trimester.

2. Disseminated Histoplasmosis with Underlying HIV Infection

Disseminated histoplasmosis in patients with Human Immunodeficiency Virus (HIV) is fatal without therapeutic intervention. Patients with HIV are indicated to undergo rapid initiation of acute-phase induction therapy followed by long-term maintenance therapy due to the high mortality of the disseminated disease. Concurrent management of HIV infection with anti-retroviral therapy (ART) is highly recommended [94, 95].

The treatment strategy for AIDS patients is based on their immune status and the severity of Histoplasma infection.

A. Mild-Moderate disease

Disseminated histoplasmosis presenting with mild clinical symptoms and a single disease focus, not including the central nervous system, is considered to have mild-to-moderate disease. Itraconazole is the preferred treatment choice for induction therapy in AIDS patients with mild-to-moderate severity histoplasmosis and non-meningeal involvement [102, 121].

Itraconazole is also the drug of choice for maintenance therapy and treatment of mild-to-moderate disseminated histoplasmosis without meningeal involvement. The duration of the maintenance therapy should be at least 12 months. Treatment should be continued until clinical symptoms have resolved [94, 95].

Lower *in-vitro* activity, higher rates of relapse from treatment, and reports of known cases of drug resistance against Fluconazole limit its utility to only cases where Itraconazole is not tolerated [109, 110].

B. Moderately Severe-Severe Disease

Severe immunosuppression (CD4 count ≤150 cells/microL), a disseminated disease involving ≥2 foci, sepsis, high-grade fever, clinical instability, organ dysfunction, respiratory failure, or pancytopenia are considered as features of moderately severe to severe histoplasmosis.

Multiple guidelines recommend Liposomal Amphotericin B (3mg/kg/daily) as the drug of choice for initial treatment. It should be given for two weeks or until clinical improvement is noticed [94, 95, 124]. Transition to Itraconazole (200mg TDS for 3 days followed by 200mg BD) occurs after the induction therapy. The consolidation therapy continues for at least 12 months [125, 126].

Itraconazole is not recommended for induction therapy for patients with severe disseminated histoplasmosis. A slow fungemia clearance rate (blood culture sterilization rate) of this fungistatic drug compared to Amphotericin B and a longer time period (days) to achieve steady-state serum concentration for Itraconazole makes Amphotericin B the preferred drug for treatment initiation [96, 99].

Itraconazole suppressive therapy in patients with HIV is indicated in either highly immunosuppressed individuals or in patients who do not achieve an immune recovery on Anti-Retroviral Therapy (ART) to reduce the risk of relapse [95, 124, 127]. A relapse rate of >50% is observed amongst AIDS patients with histoplasmosis when prolonged suppressive therapy is discontinued [128]. Lifelong prophylaxis should also be considered in patients who experience a relapse after the completion of an initial course of therapy. Itraconazole suppressive therapy could be discontinued if [127, 129, 130]:

- The patient completes at least 12 months of maintenance therapy.
- Histoplasma antigen levels come negative or remain at the lower level of detection.
- Negative blood cultures.
- Positive response to ART with the rise in CD4 cell counts to >150 cells/microL for ≥6 months, and the patient continues ART with a suppressed HIV viral load.

3. Disseminated Histoplasmosis with CNS Involvement

Patients with CNS involvement require aggressive therapy due to poor penetration of antifungal agents into the CSF [44, 45, 80, 112].

Table 2. Pharmacological approach to the management of disseminated histoplasmosis

Manifestation	Treatment Approach	Response Monitoring
1. Progressive disseminated histoplasmosis		
A. Mild to Moderate	Itraconazole (200 mg BD x 12 months)	(I) Fall in urine concentration of Histoplasma antigen. Initially, checked monthly and later every three months till therapy continued. (II) Treatment is ineffective if urine antigen concentration doesn't decrease after three months of therapy. (III) In responders, urine antigen concentration monitoring should continue for 1-2 years after completion of the treatment. (IV) A rising antigen level may raise concern for relapse. (V) Probable cause of treatment failure or infection relapse: A. Low serum Itraconazole concentration B. Poor Adherence to treatment C. Drug resistance D. Major side effects
B. Moderately severe to severe	**Induction Therapy** - Amphotericin B ((Lipid formulation: 3 mg/kg daily or deoxycholate formulation: 0.7-1 mg/kg daily) x 1-2 weeks) **Maintenance Therapy** - Itraconazole (loading dose 200 mg TDS x 3 days followed by 200mg BD/TDS x 12 months) or Fluconazole (400 mg/day x 12 months)	
2. Disseminated Histoplasmosis with underlying HIV infection		
Mild to Moderate	Itraconazole (200 mg BD x 12 months)	
Moderately severe to severe	**Induction Therapy** - Liposomal Amphotericin B (3 mg/kg daily x 1-2 weeks) **Maintenance Therapy** - Itraconazole (loading dose 200 mg TDS x 3 days followed by 200mg BD/TDS x 12 months) or Fluconazole (400 mg/day x 12 months)	

Manifestation	Treatment Approach	Response Monitoring
3. Disseminated Histoplasmosis with CNS involvement		
Without underlying HIV infection	**Induction Therapy** - Liposomal Amphotericin B (5 mg/kg daily x 4-6 weeks) **Maintenance Therapy** - Itraconazole (loading dose 200 mg BD/TDS x 12 months) or Fluconazole (800 mg/day x 12 months)	Close monitoring and regular follow-up of CNS histoplasmosis patients who respond to initial therapy for signs of relapse. The patient's response to treatment is evaluated by repeat lumbar puncture to analyze CSF protein, glucose, white blood cell count, culture, and Histoplasma antigen. Concurrent testing of urine and serum for Histoplasma antigen is carried out. A rise in serum or urine antigen level or reversion from a negative test result to positive are indicative of relapse and require to follow-up CSF analysis for evaluation.
With underlying HIV infection	**Induction Therapy** - Liposomal Amphotericin B (5 mg/kg daily x 4-6 weeks) **Maintenance Therapy** - Itraconazole (200 mg TDS x 12 months)	Serum and urine Antigen levels should be assayed every three months during therapy to assess treatment response. Antigen levels should also be measured for 6-12 months post treatment completion to determine any early signs of relapse Antigen monitoring should be considered if relapse is suspected based on clinical symptoms or if CD4 cell counts decline to <100 cells/microL. Regular monitoring of itraconazole serum levels is recommended to determine the adequacy of drug treatment, particularly in light of potential drug interactions.

A. Without Underlying HIV

Patients not infected with HIV who develop CNS infection are started with Liposomal Amphotericin B (AmBisome 5mg/kg IV daily) for 4-6 weeks. Patients with renal impairment require dose reduction or transition to Itraconazole early in the treatment due to nephrotoxicity caused by Amphotericin B.

Induction therapy is followed by a switch to Itraconazole (200 mg oral BID/TDS) which should be given for at least 12 months to prevent relapse. Thrice-a-day administration is preferred for Itraconazole due to its poor penetration into the CNS. Some clinicians prefer lifelong prophylaxis with an azole drug (Itraconazole) due to the risk of relapse [80].

Patients who are unable to tolerate Itraconazole are treated with alternative azole drugs like high-dose Fluconazole (800 mg daily) or voriconazole, both of which achieve excellent drug concentrations in the Cerebrospinal fluid (CSF) but have poor activity and efficacy against the fungus.

B. With Underlying HIV

The Infectious Diseases Society of America (IDSA) and the Centers for Disease Control and Prevention (CDC) recommend liposomal amphotericin B (5 mg/kg daily) given over four to six weeks (for a total of 175 mg/kg) followed by Itraconazole (200 mg oral TDS) for at least 12 months or until the resolution of cerebrospinal fluid (CSF) abnormalities (including CNS Histoplasma antigen) [94, 95].

The initial course of histoplasmosis treatment therapy is highly recommended to be a minimum of one year. But treatment continuation should be considered until the resolution of the clinical symptoms, even if it is more than 12 months. Concurrent management of HIV infection with Anti-Retroviral treatment (ART) is highly recommended [124]. The therapeutic details are summarized in Table 2

Conclusion

- Histoplasmosis is the most prevalent endemic mycosis in the United States. A dimorphic fungus, Histoplasma capsulatum, causes it. Infection occurs via inhalation of fungal spores, and lungs are the primary site of infection. Most of the infections are asymptomatic, but in some cases, it leads to acute pulmonary histoplasmosis or severe disseminated histoplasmosis.

- Immunosuppression and extremes of age are risk factors for the dissemination of infection. Diagnosis of disseminated histoplasmosis should be suspected in patients with risk factors who present with signs and symptoms consistent with disseminated histoplasmosis.
- Histopathological examination using fungal stains, the culture of the organism from the extrapulmonary site, antigen detection, and Histoplasma-specific antibody tests are used to diagnose the disease. Imaging modalities, including chest radiographs, computed tomography (CT) scans, and magnetic resonance imaging (MRI), aid in the diagnosis.
- Treatment is indicated in all disseminated histoplasmosis patients. Treatment typically consists of Amphotericin B during the initial induction phase, followed by azole, particularly Itraconazole, for the maintenance phase. The total duration of treatment should be at least one year.

References

[1] Goodwin, R. A., Jr. Shapiro, J. L., Thurman, G. H., Thurman, S. S., and Des Prez, R. M. (1980). Disseminated histoplasmosis: clinical and pathologic correlations. *Medicine (Baltimore).*, 59(1), 1-33.

[2] Knox., K. S., and Hage, C. A. (2010). Histoplasmosis. *Proc Am Thorac Soc.*, 7(3), 169-172. doi:10.1513/pats.200907-069AL.

[3] Bahr, N. C., Antinori, S., Wheat, L. J., and Sarosi, G. A. (2015). Histoplasmosis infections worldwide: thinking outside of the Ohio River valley. *Curr Trop Med Rep.*, 2(2), 70-80. doi:10.1007/s40475-015-0044-0.

[4] Kauffman, C. A. (2007). Histoplasmosis: a clinical and laboratory update. *Clin Microbiol Rev.*, 20(1), 115-132. doi:10.1128/CMR.00027-06.

[5] Mittal, J., Ponce, M. G., Gendlina, I., and Nosanchuk, J. D. (2019). Histoplasma Capsulatum: Mechanisms for Pathogenesis. *Curr Top Microbiol Immunol.*, 422, 157-191. doi:10.1007/82_2018_114.

[6] Joseph Wheat. (1994). "Histoplasmosis: Recognition and Treatment." *Clinical Infectious Diseases*, vol. 19, pp. S19–27. *JSTOR*, http://www.jstor.org/stable/4458030. Accessed 30 Jan. 2023.

[7] Deepe, Jr., and George, S. (2005). "Histoplasma capsulatum." *Mandell, Douglas, and Bennett's principles and practice of infectious diseases*, 3012-3026.

[8] Newman, S. L. (2001). Cell-mediated immunity to *Histoplasma capsulatum. Semin Respir Infect*, 16, 102–108.

[9] Valdez, A. F., Miranda, D. Z., Guimarães, A. J., Nimrichter, L., and Nosanchuk, J. D. (2022). Pathogenicity & virulence of *Histoplasma capsulatum* - A multifaceted organism adapted to intracellular environments. *Virulence.*, 13(1), 1900-1919. doi:10.1080/21505594.2022.2137987.

[10] Scheckelhoff, M., and Deepe, G. S. Jr. (2005). A deficiency in gamma interferon or interleukin-10 modulates T-cell-dependent responses to heat shock protein 60 from *Histoplasma capsulatum. Infect Immun*, 73, 2129–2134.

[11] Deepe, G. S. Jr. (2005). Modulation of infection with histoplasma capsulatum by inhibition of tumor necrosis factor-alpha activity. *Clin Infect Dis*, 41, S204–S207.

[12] Cain, J. A., and Deepe, G. S Jr. (2000). Interleukin-12 neutralization alters lung inflammation and leukocyte expression of cd80, cd86, and major histocompatibility complex class II in mice infected with *Histoplasma capsulatum. Infect Immun*, 68, 2069–2076.

[13] Zhou, P., Sieve, M. C., Tewari, R. P., and Seder, R. A. (1997). Interleukin-12 modulates the protective immune response in SCID mice infected with Histoplasma capsulatum. *Infect Immun.*, 65(3), 936-942. doi:10.1128/IAI.65.3.936-942.1997.

[14] Vergidis, P., Avery, R. K., Wheat, L. J., Dotson, J. L., Assi, M. A., Antoun, S. A., Hamoud, K. A., Burdette, S. D., Freifeld, A. G., McKinsey, D. S., Money, M. E., Myint, T., Andes, D. R., Hoey, C. A., Kaul, D. A., Dickter, J. K., Liebers, D. E., Miller, R. A., Muth, W. E., Prakash, V., Steiner, F. T., Walker, R. C., and Hage, C. A. (2015). Histoplasmosis complicating tumor necrosis factor-α blocker therapy: a retrospective analysis of 98 cases. *Clin Infect Dis.*, 61(3), 409-417. doi:10.1093/cid/civ299.

[15] Wheat, L. J., Chetchotisakd, P., Williams, B., Connolly, P., Shutt, K., and Hajjeh, R. (2000). Factors associated with severe manifestations of histoplasmosis in AIDS. *Clin Infect Dis.*, 30(6), 877-881. doi:10.1086/313824.

[16] Zerbe, C. S., and Holland, S. M. (2005). Disseminated histoplasmosis in persons with interferon-gamma receptor 1 deficiency. *Clin Infect Dis.*, 41(4), e38-e41. doi:10.1086/432120.

[17] de Beaucoudrey, L., Samarina, A., Bustamante, J., Cobat, A., Boisson-Dupuis, S., Feinberg, J., Al-Muhsen, S., Jannière, L., Rose, Y., de Suremain, M., Kong, X. F., Filipe-Santos, O., Chapgier, A., Picard, C., Fischer, A., Dogu, F., Ikinciogullari, A., Tanir, G., Al-Hajjar, S., Al-Jumaah, S., Frayha, H. H., AlSum, Z., Al-Ajaji, S., Alangari, A., Al-Ghonaium, A., Adimi, P., Mansouri, D., Ben-Mustapha, I., Yancoski, J., Garty, B. Z., Rodriguez-Gallego, C., Caragol, I., Kutukculer, N., Kumararatne, D. S., Patel, S., Doffinger, R., Exley, A., Jeppsson, O., Reichenbach, J., Nadal, D., Boyko, Y., Pietrucha, B., Anderson, S., Levin, M., Schandené, L., Schepers, K., Efira, A., Mascart, F., Matsuoka, M., Sakai, T., Siegrist, CA., Frecerova, K., Blüetters-Sawatzki, R., Bernhöft, J., Freihorst, J., Baumann, U., Richter, D., Haerynck, F., De Baets, F., Novelli, V., Lammas, D., Vermylen, C., Tuerlinckx, D., Nieuwhof, C., Pac, M., Haas, W. H., Müller-Fleckenstein, I., Fleckenstein, B., Levy, J., Raj, R., Cohen, A. C., Lewis, D. B., Holland, S. M., Yang, K. D., Wang, X., Wang, X., Jiang, L., Yang, X., Zhu, C., Xie, Y., Lee, P. P. W., Chan, K. W., Chen, T. X., Castro, G., Natera, I., Codoceo, A., King, A., Bezrodnik, L., Di, Giovani, D., Gaillard, M. I., de Moraes-Vasconcelos, D., Grumach, A. S., da

Silva Duarte, A. J., Aldana, R., Espinosa-Rosales, F. J., Bejaoui, M., Bousfiha, A. A., Baghdadi, J. E., Özbek, N., Aksu, G., Keser, M., Somer, A., Hatipoglu, N., Aydogmus, Ç., Asilsoy, S., Camcioglu, Y., Gülle, S., Ozgur, T. T., Ozen, M., Oleastro, M., Bernasconi, A., Mamishi, S., Parvaneh, N., Rosenzweig, S., Barbouche, R., Pedraza, S., Lau, Y. L., Ehlayel, M. S., Fieschi, C., Abel, L., Sanal, O., and Casanova, J. L. (2010). "Revisiting Human IL-12Rβ1 Deficiency: A Survey of 141 Patients From 30 Countries." *Medicine*, vol. 89, no. 6, p. 381, https://doi.org/10.1097/MD.0b013e3181fdd832. Accessed 30 Jan. 2023.

[18] Goodwin, R. A., Loyd, J. E., and Des Prez, R. M. (1981). Histoplasmosis in normal hosts. *Medicine (Baltimore).*, 60(4), 231-266. doi:10.1097/00005792-198107000-00001.

[19] Hage, C. A., Bowyer, S., Tarvin, S. E., Helper, D., Kleiman, M. B., and Wheat, L. J. (2010). Recognition, diagnosis, and treatment of histoplasmosis complicating tumor necrosis factor blocker therapy. *Clin Infect Dis.*, 50(1), 85-92. doi:10.1086/648724.

[20] Keath, E. J., Kobayashi, G. S., and Medoff, G. (1992). Typing of Histoplasma capsulatum by restriction fragment length polymorphisms in a nuclear gene. *J Clin Microbiol.*, 30(8), 2104-2107. doi:10.1128/jcm.30.8.2104-2107.1992.

[21] Wheat, L. J., Connolly-Stringfield, P. A., Baker, R. L., Curfman, M. F., Eads, M. E., Israel, K. S., Norris, S. A., Webb, D. H., and Zeckel, M. L. (1990). Disseminated histoplasmosis in the acquired immune deficiency syndrome: clinical findings, diagnosis and treatment, and review of the literature. *Medicine (Baltimore).*, 69(6), 361-374. doi:10.1097/00005792-199011000-00004.

[22] Wheat, L. J., Azar, M. M., Bahr, N. C., Spec, A., Relich, R. F., and Hage, C. (2016). Histoplasmosis. *Infect Dis Clin North Am.*, 30(1), 207-227. doi:10.1016/j.idc.2015.10.009.

[23] Lapitz, A., Goldman, M., and Sarosi, G. A. (2008). "Histoplsmosis," in *Clinical Infectious Disease*, D. Sclossberg, Ed., pp. 1211–1214, Cambridge University Press, New York, NY, USA.

[24] Goodwin, R. A, Jr. Shapiro, J. L., Thurman, G. H., Thurman, S. S., and Des Prez, R. M. (1980). Disseminated histoplasmosis: clinical and pathologic correlations. *Medicine (Baltimore).*, 59(1), 1-33.

[25] Kauffman, C. A., Freifeld, A. G., Andes, D. R., Baddley, J. W., Herwaldt, L., Walker, R. C., Alexander, B. D., Anaissie, E. J., Benedict, K., Ito, J. I., Knapp, K. M., Lyon, G. M., Marr, K. A., Morrison, V. A., Park, B. J., Patterson, T. F., Schuster, M. G., Chiller, T. M., and Pappas, P. G. (2014). Endemic fungal infections in solid organ and hematopoietic cell transplant recipients enrolled in the Transplant-Associated Infection Surveillance Network (TRANSNET). *Transpl Infect Dis.*, 16(2), 213-224. doi:10.1111/tid.12186.

[26] Limaye, A. P., Connolly, P. A., Sagar, M., Fritsche, T. R., Cookson, B. T., Wheat, L. J., and Stamm, W. E. (2000). Transmission of Histoplasma capsulatum by organ transplantation. *N Engl J Med.*, 343(16), 1163-1166. doi:10.1056/NEJM200010193431605.

[27] Hajjeh, R. A., Pappas, P. G., Henderson, H., Lancaster, D., Bamberger, D. M., Skahan, K. J., Phelan, M. A., Cloud, G., Holloway, M., Kauffman, C. A., Wheat, L.

J., National Institute of Allergy and Infectious Diseases Mycoses Study Group. (2001). Multicenter case-control study of risk factors for histoplasmosis in human immunodeficiency virus-infected persons. *Clin Infect Dis.*, 32(8), 1215-1220. doi:10.1086/319756.

[28] Wheat, L. J., Chetchotisakd, P., Williams, B., Connolly, P., Shutt, K., and Hajjeh, R. (2000). Factors associated with severe manifestations of histoplasmosis in AIDS. *Clin Infect Dis.*, 30(6), 877-881. doi:10.1086/313824.

[29] Whitt, S. P., Koch, G. A., Fender, B., Ratnasamy, N., and Everett, E. D. (2004). Histoplasmosis in pregnancy: case series and report of transplacental transmission. *Arch Intern Med.*, 164(4), 454-458. doi:10.1001/archinte.164.4.454.

[30] Walker, N. F., Scriven, J., Meintjes, G., and Wilkinson, R. J. (2014). "Immune Reconstitution Inflammatory Syndrome in HIV-Infected Patients." *HIV/AIDS (Auckland, N.Z.)*, vol. 7, pp. 49-64, https://doi.org/10.2147/HIV.S42328. Accessed 30 Jan. 2023.

[31] Wheat, L. J., Conces, D., Allen, S. D., Blue-Hnidy, D., and Loyd, J. (2004). Pulmonary histoplasmosis syndromes: recognition, diagnosis, and management. *Semin Respir Crit Care Med.*, 25(2), 129-144. doi:10.1055/s-2004-824898

[32] Kataria, Y. P., Campbell, P. B., and Burlingham, B. T. (1981). Acute pulmonary histoplasmosis presenting as adult respiratory distress syndrome: effect of therapy on clinical and laboratory features. *South Med J.*, 74(5), 534-542. doi:10.1097/00007611-198105000-00007

[33] Goodwin, R. A., Jr., Owens, F. T., Snell, J. D., Hubbard, W. W., Buchanan, R. D., Terry, R. T., and Des Prez, R. M. (1976). Chronic pulmonary histoplasmosis. *Medicine (Baltimore).*, 55(6), 413-452. doi:10.1097/00005792-197611000-00001.

[34] Conces, D. J., Jr. Tarver, R. D., and Vix, V. A. (1991). Broncholithiasis: CT features in 15 patients. *AJR Am J Roentgenol.*, 157(2), 249-253. doi:10.2214/ajr.157.2.1853800.

[35] Landay, M. J., and Rollins, N. K. (1989). Mediastinal histoplasmosis granuloma: evaluation with CT. *Radiology.*, 172(3), 657-659. doi:10.1148/radiology.172.3.2772173.

[36] Staszak, J. K., Zmijewski, P., Arnold, S., Bagga, B., and Williams, R. F. (2019). Mediastinal Lymphadenopathy in Children With Histoplasmosis. *J Surg Res.*, 244, 558-565. doi:10.1016/j.jss.2019.06.062.

[37] Azar, M. M., Loyd, J. L., Relich, R. F., Wheat, L. J., and Hage, C. A. (2020). Current Concepts in the Epidemiology, Diagnosis, and Management of Histoplasmosis Syndromes. *Semin Respir Crit Care Med.*, 41(1), 13-30. doi:10.1055/s-0039-1698429.

[38] Cohen, P. R., Bank, D. E., Silvers, D. N., and Grossman, M. E. (1990). Cutaneous lesions of disseminated histoplasmosis in human immunodeficiency virus-infected patients. *J Am Acad Dermatol.*, 23(3 Pt 1), 422-428. doi:10.1016/0190-9622(90)70235-a.

[39] Karimi, K., Wheat, L. J., Connolly, P., Cloud, G., Hajjeh, R., Wheat, E., Alves, K., Lacaz Cd Cda, S., and Keath, E. (2002). Differences in histoplasmosis in patients

with acquired immunodeficiency syndrome in the United States and Brazil. *J Infect Dis.*, 186(11), 1655-1660. doi:10.1086/345724.

[40] Morote, S., Nacher, M., Blaizot, R., Ntab, B., Blanchet, D., Drak Alsibai, K., Demar, M., Djossou, F., Couppié, P., and Adenis, A. (2020). Comparison of disseminated histoplasmosis with and without cutaneo-mucous lesions in persons living with HIV in French Guiana. *J Fungi (Basel)*, 6, 133.

[41] Eidbo, J., Sanchez, R. L., Tschen, J. A., and Ellner, K. M. (1993). Cutaneous manifestations of histoplasmosis in the acquired immune deficiency syndrome. *Am J Surg Pathol.*, 17(2), 110-116. doi:10.1097/00000478-199302000-00002.

[42] Wheat, L. J., and Kauffman, C. A. (2003). Histoplasmosis. *Infect Dis Clin North Am.*, 17(1), 1-vii. doi:10.1016/s0891-5520(02)00039-9.

[43] Robinson, L. J., Lu, M., Elsayed, S., and Joy, T. R. (2019). "Bilateral Adrenal Histoplasmosis Manifesting as Primary Adrenal Insufficiency." *CMAJ : Canadian Medical Association Journal*, vol. 191, no. 44, p. E1217, https://doi.org/10.1503/cmaj.190710. Accessed 31 Jan. 2023.

[44] Wheat, L. J., Batteiger, B. E., and Sathapatayavongs, B. (1990). Histoplasma capsulatum infections of the central nervous system. A clinical review. *Medicine (Baltimore).*, 69(4), 244-260. doi:10.1097/00005792-199007000-00006.

[45] Wheat, J., Myint, T., Guo, Y., Kemmer, P., Hage, C., Terry, C., Azar, M. M., Riddell, J., Ender, P., Chen, S., Shehab, K., Cleveland, K., Esguerra, E., Johnson, J., Wright, P., Douglas, V., Vergidis, P., Ooi, W., Baddley, J., Bamberger, D., Khairy, R., Vikram, H. R., Jenny-Avital, E., Sivasubramanian, G., Bowlware, K., Pahud, B., Sarria, J., Tsai, T., Assi, M., Mocherla, S., Prakash, V., Allen, D., Passaretti, C., Huprikar, S., and Anderson, A. (2018). Central nervous system histoplasmosis: Multicenter retrospective study on clinical features, diagnostic approach and outcome of treatment [published correction appears in Medicine (Baltimore). 2018 Apr, 97(16), e0537]. *Medicine (Baltimore).*, 97(13), e0245. doi:10.1097/MD.0000000000010245.

[46] McKinsey, D. S., McKinsey, J. P., and Brune, P. R. (2008). Diagnosis and management of histoplasmosis. *Curr Fungal Infect Rep*, 2, 94–102, https://doi.org/10.1007/s12281-008-0015-1.

[47] Lamps, L. W., Molina, C. P., West, A. B., Haggitt, R. C., and Scott, M. A. (2000). The pathologic spectrum of gastrointestinal and hepatic histoplasmosis. *Am J Clin Pathol.*, 113(1), 64-72. doi:10.1309/X0Y2-P3GY-TWE8-DM02.

[48] Suh, K. N., Anekthananon, T., and Mariuz, P. R. (2001). Gastrointestinal histoplasmosis in patients with AIDS: case report and review. *Clin Infect Dis.*, 32(3), 483-491. doi:10.1086/318485.

[49] Patrick, C. C., Flynn, P. M., Henwick, S., and Pui, C. H. (1992). Disseminated histoplasmosis presenting as a cystic duct obstruction. *Pediatr Infect Dis J.*, 11(7), 593-594. doi:10.1097/00006454-199207000-00017.

[50] Murray, J. J., and Heim, C. R. (1985). Hypercalcemia in disseminated histoplasmosis. Aggravation by vitamin D. *Am J Med.*, 78(5), 881-884. doi:10.1016/0002-9343(85)90300-6.

[51] Dwyre, D. M., Bell, A. M., Siechen, K., Sethi, S., and Raife, T. J. (2006). Disseminated histoplasmosis presenting as thrombotic microangiopathy. *Transfusion.*, 46(7), 1221-1225. doi:10.1111/j.1537-2995.2006.00873.x.

[52] Townsend, J. L., Shanbhag, S., Hancock, J., Bowman, K., and Nijhawan, A. E. (2015). Histoplasmosis-Induced Hemophagocytic Syndrome: A Case Series and Review of the Literature. *Open Forum Infect Dis.*, 2(2), ofv055. Published 2015 Apr 15. doi:10.1093/ofid/ofv055.

[53] Darouiche, R. O., Cadle, R. M., Zenon, G. J., Weinert, M. F., Hamill, R. J., and Lidsky, M. D. (1992). Articular histoplasmosis. *J Rheumatol.*, 19(12), 1991-1993.

[54] Macher, A., Rodrigues, M. M., Kaplan, W., Pistole, M. C., McKittrick, A., Lawrinson, W. E., and Reichert, C. M. (1985). Disseminated bilateral chorioretinitis due to Histoplasma capsulatum in a patient with the acquired immunodeficiency syndrome. *Ophthalmology.*, 92(8), 1159-1164. doi:10.1016/s0161-6420(85)33921-0.

[55] Zighelboim, J., Goldfarb, R. A., Mody, D., Williams, T. W., Bradshaw, M. W., and Harris, R. L. (1992). Prostatic abscess due to Histoplasma capsulatum in a patient with the acquired immunodeficiency syndrome. *J Urol.*, 147(1), 166-168. doi:10.1016/s0022-5347(17)37175-6.

[56] Kilburn, C. D., and McKinsey, D. S. (1991). Recurrent massive pleural effusion due to pleural, pericardial, and epicardial fibrosis in histoplasmosis. *Chest.*, 100(6), 1715-1717. doi:10.1378/chest.100.6.1715.

[57] Quinter, S., Cheng, C. L., Prakash, N., Currie, G., and Fleming, M. Disseminated histoplasmosis presenting as panniculitis in two immunosuppressed patients. *Dermatol Online J.* 2012, 18(11), 3. Published 2012 Nov 15.

[58] REDDY, P. A., Brasher, C. A., CHRISTIANSON, C., and Gorelick, D. F. (1970). Peritonitis due to histoplasmosis. *Annals of Internal Medicine.*, Jan 1, 72(1), 79-81

[59] Young, E. J., Vainrub, B., and Musher, D. M. (1978). Pericarditis due to histoplasmosis. *JAMA.*, 240(16), 1750-1751.

[60] Bhatti, S., Vilenski, L., Tight, R., and Smego, R. A. Jr. (2005). Histoplasma endocarditis: clinical and mycologic features and outcomes. *J Infect.*, 51(1), 2-9. doi:10.1016/j.jinf.2004.10.002.

[61] Bansal, A., and Drewek, R. (2015). Sarcoidosis and Histoplasmosis: Is One a Consequence of the Other? A Case Report and Review of the Literature. *Case Rep Rheumatol.*, 2015, 108459. doi:10.1155/2015/108459.

[62] Ledtke, C., Rehm, S. J., Fraser, T. G., Shrestha, N. K., Tan, C. D., Rodriguez, E. R., Tomford, J. W., Jain, A., Lytle, B., Johnston, D., Sabik, J., Gordon, S. M., and van Duin, D. (2012). Endovascular infections caused by Histoplasma capsulatum: a case series and review of the literature. *Arch Pathol Lab Med.*, 136(6), 640-645. doi:10.5858/arpa.2011-0050-OA.

[63] Arora, S., Ashta, K. K., Hashmi, S. A., Arun, N., and Dudani, S. (2022). Disseminated Histoplasmosis in HIV patients- Case series from a single tertiary care centre in India. *APIK J Int Med*, 10, 98-102.

[64] Myint, T., Leedy, N., Villacorta, Cari, E., and Wheat, L. J. (2020). HIV-Associated Histoplasmosis: Current Perspectives. *HIV AIDS (Auckl).*, 12, 113-125. Published 2020 Mar 19. doi:10.2147/HIV.S185631.

[65] Sarosi, G. A., and Johnson, P. C. (1992). Disseminated histoplasmosis in patients infected with human immunodeficiency virus. *Clin Infect Dis.*, 14 Suppl 1, S60-S67. doi:10.1093/clinids/14.supplement_1.s60.

[66] Melzani, A., de Reynal de Saint Michel, R., Ntab, B., Djossou, F., Epelboin, L., Nacher, M., Blanchet, D., Demar, M., Couppie, P., and Adenis, A. (2020). Incidence and Trends in Immune Reconstitution Inflammatory Syndrome Associated With Histoplasma capsulatum Among People Living With Human Immunodeficiency Virus: A 20-Year Case Series and Literature Review. *Clin Infect Dis.*, 70(4), 643-652. doi:10.1093/cid/ciz247.

[67] Wheat, L. J. (1989). Diagnosis and management of Histoplasmosis. *Eur. J. Clin. Microbiol. Infect. Dis.*, 8, 480–490. https://doi.org/10.1007/BF01964063.

[68] Lyon, R., and Woods, G. (1995). Comparison of the BacT/Alert and Isolator blood culture systems for recovery of fungi. *Am J Clin Pathol.*, 103(5), 660-662. doi:10.1093/ajcp/103.5.660.

[69] Assi, M. A., Sandid, M. S., Baddour, L. M., Roberts, G. D., and Walker, R. C. (2007). Systemic histoplasmosis: a 15-year retrospective institutional review of 111 patients. *Medicine (Baltimore).*, 86(3), 162-169. doi:10.1097/md.0b013e3180679130.

[70] Wheat, L. J. (2006). Improvements in diagnosis of histoplasmosis. *Expert Opin Biol Ther.*, 6(11), 1207-1221. doi:10.1517/14712598.6.11.1207.

[71] Riddell, J., 4th. Kauffman, C. A., Smith, J. A., Assi, M., Blue, S., Buitrago, M. I., Deresinski, S., Wright, P. W., Drevets, D. A., Norris, S. A., Vikram, H. R., Carson, P. J., Vergidis, P., Carpenter, J., Seidenfeld, S. M., and Wheat, L. J. (2014). Histoplasma capsulatum endocarditis: multicenter case series with review of current diagnostic techniques and treatment. *Medicine (Baltimore).*, 93(5), 186-193. doi:10.1097/MD.0000000000000034.

[72] Akram, S. M., Koirala, J. Histoplasmosis. [Updated 2022 Aug 8]. In: *StatPearls* [Internet]. Treasure Island (FL) : StatPearls Publishing, 2022 Jan-. Available from: https://www.ncbi.nlm.nih.gov/books/NBK448185/.

[73] Guimarães, A. J., Nosanchuk, J. D., and Zancopé-Oliveira, R. M. (2006). DIAGNOSIS OF HISTOPLASMOSIS. *Braz J Microbiol.*, 37(1), 1-13. doi:10.1590/S1517-83822006000100001.

[74] Hage, C. A., Ribes, J. A., Wengenack, N. L., Baddour, L. M., Assi, M., McKinsey, D. S., Hammoud, K., Alapat, D., Babady, N. E., Parker, M., Fuller, D., Noor, A., Davis, T. E., Rodgers, M., Connolly, P. A., El Haddad, B., and Wheat, L. J. (2011). A multicenter evaluation of tests for diagnosis of histoplasmosis [published correction appears in *Clin Infect Dis*. 2012 Feb 1, 54(3), 454]. *Clin Infect Dis*. 2011, 53(5), 448-454. doi:10.1093/cid/cir435.

[75] Richer, S. M., Smedema, M. L., Durkin, M. M., Herman, K. M., Hage, C. A., Fuller, D., and Wheat, L. J. (2016). Improved Diagnosis of Acute Pulmonary Histoplasmosis by Combining Antigen and Antibody Detection. *Clin Infect Dis.*, 62(7), 896-902. doi:10.1093/cid/ciw007.

[76] Zhang, C., Lei, G. S., Lee, C. H., and Hage, C. A. (2015). Evaluation of two new enzyme immunoassay reagents for diagnosis of histoplasmosis in a cohort of

clinically characterized patients. *Med Mycol.*, 53(8), 868-873. doi:10.1093/mmy/myv062.

[77] Connolly, P. A., Durkin, M. M., Lemonte, A. M., Hackett, E. J., and Wheat, L. J. (2007). Detection of histoplasma antigen by a quantitative enzyme immunoassay. *Clin Vaccine Immunol.*, 14(12), 1587-1591. doi:10.1128/CVI.00071-07.

[78] Wheat, L. J., Kohler, R. B., and Tewari, R. P. (1986). Diagnosis of disseminated histoplasmosis by detection of Histoplasma capsulatum antigen in serum and urine specimens. *N Engl J Med.*, 314(2), 83-88. doi:10.1056/NEJM198601093140205.

[79] Hage, C. A., Davis, T. E., Fuller, D., Egan, L., Witt, J. R., 3rd. Wheat, L. J., and Knox, K. S. (2010). Diagnosis of histoplasmosis by antigen detection in BAL fluid. *Chest.*, 137(3), 623-628. doi:10.1378/chest.09-1702.

[80] Wheat, L. J., Musial, C. E., and Jenny-Avital, E. (2005). Diagnosis and management of central nervous system histoplasmosis. *Clin Infect Dis.*, 40(6), 844-852. doi:10.1086/427880.

[81] Scheel, C. M., Samayoa, B., Herrera, A., Lindsley, M. D., Benjamin, L., Reed, Y., Hart, J., Lima, S., Rivera, B. E., Raxcaco, G., Chiller, T., Arathoon, E., and Gómez, B. L. (2009). Development and evaluation of an enzyme-linked immunosorbent assay to detect Histoplasma capsulatum antigenuria in immunocompromised patients. *Clin Vaccine Immunol.*, 16(6), 852-858. doi:10.1128/CVI.00066-09.

[82] Theel, E. S., Jespersen, D. J., Harring, J., Mandrekar, J., and Binnicker, M. J. (2013). Evaluation of an enzyme immunoassay for detection of Histoplasma capsulatum antigen from urine specimens. *J Clin Microbiol.*, 51(11), 3555-3559. doi:10.1128/JCM.01868-13.

[83] Wheat, J., Wheat, H., Connolly, P., Kleiman, M., Supparatpinyo, K., Nelson, K., Bradsher, R., and Restrepo, A. (1997). Cross-reactivity in Histoplasma capsulatum variety capsulatum antigen assays of urine samples from patients with endemic mycoses. *Clin Infect Dis.*, 24(6), 1169-1171. doi:10.1086/513647.

[84] Conces, D. J., Jr. Stockberger, S. M., Tarver, R. D., and Wheat, L. J. (1993). Disseminated histoplasmosis in AIDS: findings on chest radiographs. *AJR Am J Roentgenol.*, 160(1), 15-19. doi:10.2214/ajr.160.1.8416614.

[85] Babady, N. E., Buckwalter, S. P., Hall, L., Le Febre, K. M., Binnicker, M. J., and Wengenack, N. L. (2011). Detection of Blastomyces dermatitidis and Histoplasma capsulatum from culture isolates and clinical specimens by use of real-time PCR. *J Clin Microbiol.*, 49(9), 3204-3208. doi:10.1128/JCM.00673-11.

[86] Muraosa, Y., Toyotome, T., Yahiro, M., Watanabe, A., Shikanai-Yasuda, M. A., and Kamei, K. (2016). Detection of Histoplasma capsulatum from clinical specimens by cycling probe-based real-time PCR and nested real-time PCR. *Med Mycol.*, 54(4), 433-438. doi:10.1093/mmy/myv106.

[87] Alexandre Alanio, Maud Gits-Muselli, Fanny Lanternier, Aude Sturny-Leclère, Marion Benazra, Samia Hamane, Anderson Messias Rodrigues, Dea Garcia-Hermoso, Olivier Lortholary, Françoise Dromer, Stéphane Bretagne and the French Mycoses study group. (2021). Evaluation of a New Histoplasma spp. Quantitative RT-PCR Assay. *J Mol Diagn.*, 23(6), 698-709. doi:10.1016/j.jmoldx.2021.02.007

[88] Bloch, K. C., Myint, T., Raymond-Guillen, L., Hage, C. A., Davis, T. E., Wright, P. W., Chow, F. C., Woc-Colburn, L., Khairy, R. N., Street, A. C., Yamamoto, T.,

Albers, A., and Wheat, L. J. (2018). Improvement in Diagnosis of Histoplasma Meningitis by Combined Testing for Histoplasma Antigen and Immunoglobulin G and Immunoglobulin M Anti-Histoplasma Antibody in Cerebrospinal Fluid. *Clin Infect Dis*., 66(1), 89-94. doi:10.1093/cid/cix706.

[89] Myint, T., Chow, F. C., Bloch, K. C., Raymond-Guillen, L., Davis, T. E., Wright, P. W., Woc-Colburn, L., Khairy, R. N., Street, A. C., Yamamoto, T., Albers, A., Wheat, L. J., and Hage, C. A. (2018). Detection of (1,3)-β-d-Glucan in Cerebrospinal Fluid in Histoplasma Meningitis. *J Clin Microbiol*., 56(10), e00663-18. Published 2018 Sep 25. doi:10.1128/JCM.00663-18.

[90] Tran, T., and Beal, S. G. (2016). Application of the 1,3-β-D-Glucan (Fungitell) Assay in the Diagnosis of Invasive Fungal Infections. *Arch Pathol Lab Med*., 140(2), 181-185. doi:10.5858/arpa.2014-0230-RS.

[91] Lyons, J. L., Thakur, K. T., Lee, R., Watkins, T., Pardo, C. A., Carson, K. A., Markley, B., Finkelman, M. A., Marr, K. A., Roos, K. L., and Zhang, S. X. (2015). Utility of measuring (1,3)-β-d-glucan in cerebrospinal fluid for diagnosis of fungal central nervous system infection. *J Clin Microbiol*., 53(1), 319-322. doi:10.1128/JCM.02301-14.

[92] Agudelo, C. A., Restrepo, C. A., Molina, D. A., Tobón, A. M., Kauffman, C. A., Murillo, C., and Restrepo, A. (2012). Tuberculosis and histoplasmosis co-infection in AIDS patients. *Am J Trop Med Hyg*., 87(6), 1094-1098. doi:10.4269/ajtmh.2012.12-0292.

[93] Bower, M., Powles, T., Williams, S., Davis, T. N., Atkins, M., Montoto, S., Orkin, C., Webb, A., Fisher, M., Nelson, M., Gazzard, B., Stebbing, J., and Kelleher, P. (2007). Brief communication: rituximab in HIV-associated multicentric Castleman disease. *Ann Intern Med*., 147(12), 836-839. doi:10.7326/0003-4819-147-12-200712180-00003.

[94] Wheat, L. J., Freifeld, A. G., Kleiman, M. B., Baddley, J. W., McKinsey, D. S., Loyd, J. E., and Kauffman, C. A. (2007). Infectious Diseases Society of America. Clinical practice guidelines for the management of patients with histoplasmosis: 2007 update by the Infectious Diseases Society of America. *Clin Infect Dis*., 45(7), 807-825. doi:10.1086/521259.

[95] Pan American Health Organization and World Health Organization. Guidelines for Diagnosing and Managing Disseminated Histoplasmosis among People Living with HIV. https://iris.paho.org/handle/10665.2/52304 (Accessed on July 14, 2020).

[96] Wheat, L. J., Cloud, G., Johnson, P. C., Connolly, P., Goldman, M., Le Monte, A., Fuller, D. E., Davis, T. E., and Hafner, R. (2001). AIDS Clinical Trials Group: Mycoses Study Group of NIAID. Clearance of fungal burden during treatment of disseminated histoplasmosis with liposomal amphotericin B versus Itraconazole. *Antimicrob Agents Chemother*., 45(8), 2354-2357. doi:10.1128/AAC.45.8.2354-2357.2001.

[97] Kauffman, C. A. (2017). Treatment of the Midwestern Endemic Mycoses, Blastomycosis and Histoplasmosis. *Curr Fungal Infect Rep*, 11, 67–74 https://doi.org/10.1007/s12281-017-0281-x.

[98] Lanternier, F., and Lortholary, O. (2008). Liposomal amphotericin B: what is its role in 2008?. *Clin Microbiol Infect.*, 14 Suppl 4, 71-83. doi:10.1111/j.1469-0691.2008.01984.x.

[99] Johnson, P. C., Wheat, L. J., Cloud, G. A., Goldman, M., Lancaster, D., Bamberger, D. M., Powderly, W. G., Hafner, R., Kauffman, C. A., and Dismukes, W. E. (2002). U.S. National Institute of Allergy and Infectious Diseases Mycoses Study Group. Safety and efficacy of liposomal amphotericin B compared with conventional amphotericin B for induction therapy of histoplasmosis in patients with AIDS. *Ann Intern Med.*, 137(2), 105-109. doi:10.7326/0003-4819-137-2-200207160-00008.

[100] Hamill, R. J. (2013). Amphotericin B formulations: a comparative review of efficacy and toxicity. *Drugs.*, 73(9), 919-934. doi:10.1007/s40265-013-0069-4.

[101] Gallis, H. A., Drew, R. H., and Pickard, W. W. (1990). Amphotericin B: 30 years of clinical experience. *Rev Infect Dis.*, 12(2), 308-329. doi:10.1093/clinids/12.2.308.

[102] Wheat, J., Hafner, R., Korzun, A. H., Limjoco, M. T., Spencer, P., Larsen, R. A., Hecht, F. M., and Powderly, W. (1995). Itraconazole treatment of disseminated histoplasmosis in patients with the acquired immunodeficiency syndrome. AIDS Clinical Trial Group. *Am J Med.*, 98(4), 336-342. doi:10.1016/s0002-9343(99)80311-8.

[103] Wheat, L. J., Connolly, P., Haddad, N., Le Monte, A., Brizendine, E., and Hafner, R. (2002). Antigen clearance during treatment of disseminated histoplasmosis with Itraconazole versus fluconazole in patients with AIDS. *Antimicrob Agents Chemother.*, 46(1), 248-250. doi:10.1128/AAC.46.1.248-250.2002.

[104] Brooks, J. T., and Wheat, L. J. (1998). Histoplasmosis: update 1998. *AIDS Clin Care.*, 10(1), 4-5.

[105] Whitmore, T. J., Yaw, M., Lavender, M., Musk, M., Boan, P., and Wrobel, J. (2021). A novel highly bio-available itraconazole formulation (SUBA®-Itraconazole) for anti-fungal prophylaxis in lung transplant recipients. *Transpl Infect Dis.*, 23(4), e13587. doi:10.1111/tid.13587.

[106] Nield, B., Larsen, S. R., and van Hal, S. J. (2019). Clinical experience with new formulation SUBA®-itraconazole for prophylaxis in patients undergoing stem cell transplantation or treatment for haematological malignancies. *J Antimicrob Chemother.*, 74(10), 3049-3055. doi:10.1093/jac/dkz303.

[107] McKinsey, D. S., Kauffman, C. A., Pappas, P. G., Cloud, G. A., Girard, W. M., Sharkey, P. K., Hamill, R. J., Thomas, C. J., and Dismukes, W. E. (1996). Fluconazole therapy for histoplasmosis. The National Institute of Allergy and Infectious Diseases Mycoses Study Group. *Clin Infect Dis.*, 23(5), 996-1001. doi:10.1093/clinids/23.5.996.

[108] Wheat, L. J., Connolly, P., Haddad, N., Le Monte, A., Brizendine, E., and Hafner, R. (2002). Antigen clearance during treatment of disseminated histoplasmosis with Itraconazole versus fluconazole in patients with AIDS. *Antimicrob Agents Chemother.*, 46(1), 248-250. doi:10.1128/AAC.46.1.248-250.2002.

[109] Wheat, J., MaWhinney, S., Hafner, R., McKinsey, D., Chen, D., Korzun, A., Shakan, K. J., Johnson, P., Hamill, R., Bamberger, D., Pappas, P., Stansell, J., Koletar, S., Squires, K., Larsen, R. A., Cheung, T., Hyslop, N., Lai, K. K., Schneider, D., Kauffman, C., Saag, M., Dismukes, W., and Powderly, W. (1997).

Treatment of histoplasmosis with fluconazole in patients with acquired immunodeficiency syndrome. National Institute of Allergy and Infectious Diseases Acquired Immunodeficiency Syndrome Clinical Trials Group and Mycoses Study Group. *Am J Med.*, 103(3), 223-232. doi:10.1016/s0002-9343(97)00151-4.

[110] Wheat, L. J., Connolly, P., Smedema, M., Brizendine, E., and Hafner, R. (2001). AIDS Clinical Trials Group and the Mycoses Study Group of the National Institute of Allergy and Infectious Diseases. Emergence of resistance to fluconazole as a cause of failure during treatment of histoplasmosis in patients with acquired immunodeficiency disease syndrome. *Clin Infect Dis.*, 33(11), 1910-1913. doi:10.1086/323781.

[111] Tucker, R. M., Williams, P. L., Arathoon, E. G., Levine, B. E., Hartstein, A. I., Hanson, L. H., and Stevens, D. A. (1988). Pharmacokinetics of fluconazole in cerebrospinal fluid and serum in human coccidioidal meningitis. *Antimicrob Agents Chemother.*, 32(3), 369-373. doi:10.1128/AAC.32.3.369.

[112] Haynes, R. R., Connolly, P. A., Durkin, M. M., LeMonte, A. M., Smedema, ML., Brizendine, E., and Wheat, L. J. (2002). Antifungal therapy for central nervous system histoplasmosis, using a newly developed intracranial model of infection. *J Infect Dis.*, 185(12), 1830-1832. doi:10.1086/340825.

[113] Wheat, L. J., Connolly, P., Smedema, M., Durkin, M., Brizendine, E., Mann, P., Patel, R., McNicholas, P. M., and Goldman, M. (2006). Activity of newer triazoles against Histoplasma capsulatum from patients with AIDS who failed fluconazole. *J Antimicrob Chemother.*, 57(6), 1235-1239. doi:10.1093/jac/dkl133.

[114] Freifeld, A., Proia, L., Andes, D., Baddour, L. M., Blair, J., Spellberg, B., Arnold, S., Lentnek, A., and Wheat, L. J. (2009). Voriconazole use for endemic fungal infections. *Antimicrob Agents Chemother.*, 53(4), 1648-1651. doi:10.1128/AAC.01148-07.

[115] Dhawan, J., Verma, P., Sharma, A., Ramam, M., Kabra, S. K., and Gupta, S. (2010). Disseminated cutaneous histoplasmosis in an immunocompetent child, relapsed with Itraconazole, successfully treated with voriconazole. *Pediatr Dermatol.*, 27(5), 549-551. doi:10.1111/j.1525-1470.2010.01273.x.

[116] Clark, B., Foster, R., Tunbridge, A., and Green, S. (2005). A case of disseminated histoplasmosis successfully treated with the investigational drug posaconazole. *J Infect.*, 51(3), e177-e180. doi:10.1016/j.jinf.2005.01.001.

[117] Restrepo, A., Tobón, A., Clark, B., Graham, D. R., Corcoran, G., Bradsher, R. W., Goldman, M., Pankey, G., Moore, T., Negroni, R., and Graybill, J. R. (2007). Salvage treatment of histoplasmosis with posaconazole. *J Infect.*, 54(4), 319-327. doi:10.1016/j.jinf.2006.05.006.

[118] Schwartz, S., Cornely, O. A., Hamed, K., Marty, F. M., Maertens, J., Rahav, G., Herbrecht, R., and Heinz, W. J. (2020). Isavuconazole for the treatment of patients with invasive fungal diseases involving the central nervous system. *Med Mycol.*, 58(4), 417-424. doi:10.1093/mmy/myz103.

[119] Thompson, G. R., 3rd. Rendon, A., Ribeiro, Dos Santos, R., Queiroz-Telles, F., Ostrosky-Zeichner, L., Azie, N., Maher, R., Lee, M., Kovanda, L., Engelhardt, M., Vazquez, J. A., Cornely, O. A., and Perfect, J. R. (2016). Isavuconazole Treatment

of Cryptococcosis and Dimorphic Mycoses. *Clin Infect Dis.*, 63(3), 356-362. doi:10.1093/cid/ciw305.

[120] Zonios, D. I., and Bennett, J. E. (2008). Update on azole antifungals. *Semin Respir Crit Care Med.*, 29(2), 198-210. doi:10.1055/s-2008-1063858.

[121] Dismukes, W. E., Bradsher, R. W., Jr. Cloud, G. C., Kauffman, C. A., Chapman, S. W., George, R. B., Stevens, D. A., Girard, W. M., Saag, M. S., and Bowles-Patton, C. (1992). Itraconazole therapy for blastomycosis and histoplasmosis. NIAID Mycoses Study Group. *Am J Med.*, 93(5), 489-497. doi:10.1016/0002-9343(92)90575-v.

[122] Assi, M., Martin, S., Wheat, L. J., Hage, C., Freifeld, A., Avery, R., Baddley, J. W., Vergidis, P., Miller, R., Andes, D., Young, J. A., Hammoud, K., Huprikar, S., McKinsey, D., Myint, T., Garcia-Diaz, J., Esguerra, E., Kwak, E. J., Morris, M., Mullane, K. M., Prakash, V., Burdette, S. D., Sandid, M., Dickter, J., Ostrander, D., Antoun, S. A., and Kaul, D. R. (2013). Histoplasmosis after solid organ transplant. *Clin Infect Dis.*, 57(11), 1542-1549. doi:10.1093/cid/cit593.

[123] Freifeld, A. G., Iwen, P. C., Lesiak, B. L., Gilroy, R. K., Stevens, R. B., and Kalil, A. C. (2005). Histoplasmosis in solid organ transplant recipients at a large Midwestern university transplant center [published correction appears in Transpl Infect Dis. 2006 Mar, 8(1), 58] [published correction appears in Transpl Infect Dis. 2006 Sep, 8(3), 185. Dosage error in article text]. *Transpl Infect Dis.*, 7(3-4), 109-115. doi:10.1111/j.1467-8365.2005.00105.x.

[124] Panel on Opportunistic Infections in HIV-Infected Adults and Adolescents. Guidelines for the prevention and treatment of opportunistic infections in HIV-infected adults and adolescents: Recommendations from the Centers for Disease Control and Prevention, the National Institutes of Health, and the HIV Medicine Association of the Infectious Diseases Society of America. http://aidsinfo.nih.gov/contentfiles/lvguidelines/adult_oi.pdf (Accessed on June 14, 2017).

[125] Murray, M., and Hine, P. (2020). Treating progressive disseminated histoplasmosis in people living with HIV. *Cochrane Database Syst Rev.*, 4(4), CD013594. Published 2020 Apr 28. doi:10.1002/14651858.CD013594.

[126] Wheat, J. (1997). Histoplasmosis. Experience during outbreaks in Indianapolis and review of the literature. *Medicine (Baltimore).*, 76(5), 339-354. doi:10.1097/00005792-199709000-00002.

[127] Hecht, F. M., Wheat, J., Korzun, A. H., Hafner, R., Skahan, K. J., Larsen, R., Limjoco, M. T., Simpson, M., Schneider, D., Keefer, M. C., Clark, R., Lai, K. K., Jacobson, J. M., Squires, K., Bartlett, J. A., and Powderly, W. (1997). Itraconazole maintenance treatment for histoplasmosis in AIDS: a prospective, multicenter trial. *J Acquir Immune Defic Syndr Hum Retrovirol.*, 16(2), 100-107. doi:10.1097/00042560-199710010-00005.

[128] Drew, R. H. (1993). Pharmacotherapy of disseminated histoplasmosis in patients with AIDS. *Ann Pharmacother.*, 27(12), 1510-1518. doi:10.1177/106002809302701218.

[129] Goldman, M., Zackin, R., Fichtenbaum, C. J., Skiest, D. J., Koletar, S. L., Hafner, R., Wheat, L. J., Nyangweso, P. M., Yiannoutsos, C. T., Schnizlein-Bick, C. T.,

Owens, S., and Aberg, J. A. (2004). AIDS Clinical Trials Group A5038 Study Group. Safety of discontinuation of maintenance therapy for disseminated histoplasmosis after immunologic response to antiretroviral therapy. *Clin Infect Dis.*, 38(10), 1485-1489. doi:10.1086/420749.

[130] Myint, T., Anderson, A. M., Sanchez, A., Farabi, A., Hage, C., Baddley, J. W., Jhaveri, M., Greenberg, R. N., Bamberger, D. M., Rodgers, M., Crawford, T. N., and Wheat, L. J. (2014). Histoplasmosis in patients with human immunodeficiency virus/acquired immunodeficiency syndrome (HIV/AIDS): multicenter study of outcomes and factors associated with relapse. *Medicine (Baltimore).*, 93(1), 11-18. doi:10.1097/MD.0000000000000016.

Chapter 14

Pharmacological Management of Histoplasmosis

Ladan Panahi*
Niraj Patel
Augusta Udeani
Ricardo Ibarra
Kasey Torres
Meina Determan
Perfecto Rodriguez IV
Phoung Tran
Salim Surani
and Chinonso Paul
[1]Department of Pharmacy Practice,
Texas A&M Rangel School of Pharmacy and Reynolds Medical Building,
College Station, Kingsville, Texas, USA

Abstract

Histoplasma capsulatum is a fungus that causes Histoplasmosis in the human host. Most subclinical or mild histoplasmosis infections patients do not require treatment among immunocompetent patients. However, it is recommended to treat all immunocompromised patients, as well as those with chronic pulmonary disease or progressive disseminated

---

* Corresponding Author's Email: panahi@tamu.edu.

In: Histoplasmosis
Editors: Salim Surani, Syed Anjum Khan and Reena Shah
ISBN: 979-8-89113-129-3

disease. For severe or disseminated disease amphotericin B is the first line therapy, whereas itraconazole is suitable for milder cases and continuation therapy following response to amphotericin B. This chapter provides an overview of the evidence-based approaches to managing Histoplasmosis with antifungal medications, including safety concerns and treatment considerations for special populations like solid organ transplant and HIV patients.

Keywords: histoplasmosis, solid organ transplantation, infection, endemic mycoses, immunocompromised, antifungal, pharmacological management

Introduction

Histoplasmosis is an infection that occurs when H. capsulatum enters the lungs through inhalation and causes pneumonitis [1]. Histoplasmosis is a fungal infection caused by inhalation of the environmental fungus Histoplasma spp [2]. Histoplasma capsulatum var. capsulatum, commonly referred to as H. capsulatum, has a nearly worldwide distribution, while the var. duboisii is mainly restricted to western Africa [2].

Most exposures to H. capsulatum are through any activities involving the handling of bird or bat droppings, like farmers, or outdoor activities such as gardening, digging soil, handling plants, or construction [2]. Spontaneous cases still occur while exposure to bat or bird droppings make up more than three-quarters of histoplasmosis outbreaks [3]. Therefore, Histoplasmosis should never be completely ruled out as the cause of illness by clinicians if common exposures to bird or bat droppings or outdoor activities are absent [2].

Endemic mycoses, including Histoplasmosis, Coccidioidomycosis, Blastomycosis, Paracoccidioidomycosis, Talaromycosis, and Emergomycosis, are known to cause significant morbidity and mortality, especially in individuals with HIV/AIDS, other immunosuppressive medical conditions, or those taking immunosuppressive medications [4]. Histoplasmosis is a dimorphic fungus, existing in the mycelial phase in the environment as two types of conidia, macroconidia, and microconidia, with the latter being the infectious form. After inhalation, they are small enough to reach the terminal bronchioles and alveoli and convert to the yeast phase within macrophages, leading to acute infection, reactivation, or reinfection [5].

The main culprits of outbreaks are occupational exposures through a bird or bat feces from the soil [2]. Spores may remain active for several years, and exposure in endemic areas is virtually 100%, although few patients develop active disease [6].

Epidemiology and Diagnosis

The current distribution of Histoplasmosis is much broader than previously believed, with it being endemic in much of the world [4]. It is also likely that the disease is underdiagnosed due to a lack of available diagnostic tests and/or clinician awareness or misdiagnosis [4]. The selection and interpretation of the diagnostic test depend on the clinical syndrome, the host immune status, and the epidemiologic context [5]. Currently, the gold standard for laboratory-proven diagnosis of Histoplasmosis is the isolation of the mold in a clinical specimen culture [5].

Clinical Presentation

Clinical manifestations of Histoplasmosis vary depending on the extent of exposure, the presence of underlying lung disease, and the host immune response. Symptoms can range from a self-limiting flu-like syndrome to pneumonia, mediastinal fibrosis, or chronic cavitary disease in those with obstructive lung disease, and disseminated Histoplasmosis, which is more common in immunocompromised individuals and infants. After a 3 to 17-day incubation, infections can present as asymptomatic, acute or chronic pulmonary, or life-threatening disseminated infections, depending on the host's immune status and exposure intensity [2]. Common symptoms may include fever, shortness of breath, fatigue, cough, chest pain, chest tightness, headache, weight loss, diarrhea, diaphoresis, hoarseness (in patients with tonsillar abscess), and blurry vision (in those with central nervous system involvement). Radiologic studies, cultures, and/or histopathology typically show lung involvement, with positive culture results from different organs in some cases and radiographic evidence of involvement in other organs in others [7].

An unhindered immune system is vital to stop the dissemination of Histoplasma. Patients receiving immunosuppressive agents, particularly those receiving treatment for rheumatologic, gastrointestinal, or dermatologic diseases, are at increased risk of Histoplasmosis [1].

Table 1. Current Treatment Regimens for Pulmonary Histoplasmosis Infection [9-11]

	Mild-moderate infection	Acute or Severe Infection	Chronic cavitary
Treatment Regimen	Itraconazole 200 mg PO three times daily x 3 days Followed by Itraconazole 200 mg PO twice daily 6 to 12 weeks	Liposomal amphotericin B 3-5 mg/kg x 1-2 weeks Followed by Itraconazole 200 mg three times a day x 3 days Followed by Itraconazole 200 mg daily	Itraconazole 200 mg PO three times a day x 3 days Followed by Itraconazole 200 mg PO once or twice daily
Duration	1 to 3 months	> 3 months	≥ 1 year
Monitoring	Obtain blood levels of itraconazole after ≥2 weeks of treatment to assure absorption	Obtain blood levels of itraconazole after ≥2 weeks of treatment to assure absorption	
Alternative Regimens		Amphotericin B 0.7 mg/kg/d IV if patients are at low risk for nephrotoxicity	

Treatment

Since most acute primary Histoplasmosis resolves spontaneously on its own, hospitalization is unnecessary, and only outpatient care is needed for most cases of Histoplasmosis. However, immunocompromised patients exposed to a large inoculum of Histoplasma, or disseminated infection, typically require antifungal therapy. Histoplasmosis treatment involves two drug classes of antifungal agents: triazoles and polyenes. Furthermore, the foundation of histoplasmosis therapy has always been amphotericin B and/or itraconazole, with intravenous AmB being preferred for severe infections [8]. Echinocandin use is not supported because of insufficient data, but fluconazole has been used in place of ITZ in case of intolerance [8].

Triazole Drug Class

Triazoles inhibit the biosynthesis of an essential component of the fungal cell membrane, ergosterol [5]. Itraconazole (ITZ), voriconazole, and posaconazole are part of the triazole drug class and are the triazoles employed to treat Histoplasma infections. ITZ monotherapy, the preferred azole against H.

capsulatum, can be used in cases of mild or moderate disease, although treatment is usually unnecessary as the infection is typically self-limiting [8]. The parenteral formulation of itraconazole is no longer available in the US [9-11].

Posaconazole is highly active *in vitro,* and no resistance developing during exposure has been reported [9-11]. The experience of administering posaconazole for Histoplasmosis is limited. Random levels should be at least 0.5 μg/mL [9-11]. It is available in both oral and intravenous formulations [9-11]. Current treatment rgimens for pulmonary histoplasmosis infection is shown in Table 1.

Table 2. Treatment Regimen for Extrapulmonary/Mediastinal Histoplasmosis [9-11]

	Pericarditis and rheumatologic syndromes	Central Nervous System Involvement	Severe Disseminated Infection	Moderate Disseminated Infection
Treatment Regimen	NSAIDs	Liposomal amphotericin B 3-5 mg/kg/d IV x minimum of 4 to 6 weeks (or longer) Followed by Itraconazole 200 mg twice daily or three times a day	Liposomal amphotericin B 3 mg/kg q24 h x 1-2 weeks Followed by Itraconazole 200 mg PO three times a day x 3 day Followed by Itraconazole 200 mg PO twice daily	Itraconazole 200 mg PO three times a day x 3 day Followed by Itraconazole 200 mg PO twice daily
Duration		≥ 1 year and there is the resolution of all CSF abnormalities including clearance of Histoplasma antigen	≥ 1 year Possible lifetime for immunosuppressed	≥ 1 year Possible lifetime for immunosuppressed
Alternative Regimen	Prednisone 0.5-1 mg/kg/d with a taper over 1 to 2 weeks PLUS Itraconazole 200 mg PO three times a day x 3 days Followed by	Fluconazole 800 mg/day	Lipid complex amphotericin 5 mg/kg, if necessary	

	200 mg PO twice a day x 6 to 12 weeks if given steroids			

Fluconazole is less effective than itraconazole in treating H. capsulatum since fluconazole is believed only to inhibit the growth of the fungus [5]. Therefore, fluconazole is not considered a first-line option for managing Histoplasmosis [9-11]. However, fluconazole has more predictable absorption and fewer drug interactions and is often tolerated better by those who cannot tolerate itraconazole [9-11]. Generally, high doses of fluconazole (400 to 800 mg daily) are needed for treatment [9-11]. It is available in both oral and intravenous formulations [9-11]. Fluconazole can be used as an alternative for central nervous system (CNS) Histoplasmosis infections since fluconazole possesses the greatest penetration into the cerebrospinal fluid (CSF) [12].

Successful induction therapy usually consists of itraconazole (200 mg twice daily) for at least one year to treat disseminated infection [9]. In individuals with less severe disease, itraconazole is more effective than fluconazole; however, resistance to fluconazole has been reported in patients receiving fluconazole therapy [9-11]. Voriconazole, although active *in vitro,* is not typically recommended due to the development of resistance and likely inferiority to itraconazole [9-11]. Treatment regimen for extrapulmonary/mediastinal histoplasmosis is shown in Table 2.

Triazole Safety Concerns and Monitoring

Absorption issues with itraconazole use should be monitored. Itraconazole requires the solution to be taken on an empty stomach, and the capsules and tablets are taken with food or cola. For capsules, a low gastric pH is required, and with achlorhydria, the drug should be taken with an acidic soft drink (e.g., Coke, Pepsi, or orange juice) [9-11]. Oral posaconazole must be administered with a full meal, nutritional supplement, or acidic carbonated drink for adequate absorption. Oral voriconazole must be taken on an empty stomach one hour before or after meals.

Additionally, drug interactions should be monitored as itraconazole requires the P450 pathway; therefore, proton pump inhibitors, antacids, and H2 blockers should be avoided. Itraconazole toxicities include worsening of heart failure and liver function enzymes. Although hepatotoxicity and cardiac dysrhythmias have been observed with all azole antifungals, itraconazole also exhibits negative inotropic effects and has been associated with congestive heart failure. Due to its toxicities, itraconazole is not recommended in patients with a history of heart failure, elevated transaminases, liver disease, or a history of drug-induced hepatotoxicity.

If a provider is concerned about absorption, compliance, or drug interactions, itraconazole levels should be measured two hours after the dose is administered at the peak after at least two weeks of use; levels should be expected to be 1.0 μg/ml [9-11]. Successful treatment has been linked to Itraconazole levels of at least 1 mcg/ml. However, there is not a clear-cut serum concentration that increases the risk of toxicity, though concentrations greater than 5 mcg/ml have been linked to adverse effects [9-11].

The new SUBA-itraconazole formulation, marketed as Tolsura in the United States, has improved absorption capabilities compared to other itraconazole formulations. It is absorbed in the intestine, does not require an acidic environment for absorption, and has a bioavailability of around 95%. Studies are ongoing regarding its performance in Histoplasmosis [9-11].

Most systemic azole antifungals have been associated with QT prolongation and rare cases of arrhythmias, including torsade de pointes. Additionally, these agents inhibit the CYP3A4 isoenzyme which may increase the risk of QT prolongation in drugs metabolized by CYP3A4 and known to prolong the QT interval. The inhibitory potential of the azole agents on CYP3A4 varies. Posaconazole, ketoconazole, and itraconazole are more potent inhibitors than fluconazole and voriconazole. Triazole safety comparisons is shown in Table 3.

Table 3. Triazole Safety Comparisons [13-16]

Itraconazole	Fluconazole	Posaconazole	Voriconazole
CYP3A4 and P-glycoprotein inhibitor. There are many CYP3A4 substrates with which use is contraindicated or not recommended. May worsen heart failure; do not use in patients with a history of heart failure Check baseline liver function; avoid in patients with elevated transaminases, liver disease, or history of drug-induced hepatotoxicity May also interact with medications affecting P-glycoprotein efflux	Relatively low risk of liver enzyme elevation. Less risk of drug interactions compared to itraconazole	The IV formulation of should not be used in patients with a CrCl < 50 ml/min; the solvent used in these IV formulations (SBECD) may accumulate in patients with renal dysfunction May also interact with medications affecting P-glycoprotein efflux	The IV formulation of should not be used in patients with a CrCl < 50 ml/min; the solvent used in these IV formulations (SBECD) may accumulate in patients with renal dysfunction May cause visual disturbances

Possible neuropathy and hearing loss			

Polyenes Drug Class

Amphotericin B (AmB), like other polyenes, forms a complex with ergosterol in the fungal plasma membrane, disrupting the cell membrane and cell death [5]. Liposomal AmB is the favored formulation versus traditional deoxycholate because of reduced toxicity to the kidneys and the higher rate of survival when used in HIV patients and disseminated Histoplasmosis. Longer courses of AmB therapy are recommended in patients with central nervous system (CNS) disorders [8].

A randomized clinical trial concluded that IV liposomal amphotericin B (3 mg/kg daily) is more effective than standard IV amphotericin B deoxycholate (0.7 mg/kg daily) [17]. This liposomal formulation resulted in a quicker and more complete response, lower mortality rates, and decreased toxicity [17]. Therefore, it is recommended that patients with moderately severe to severe disseminated Histoplasmosis should be treated with IV liposomal amphotericin B (3 mg/kg daily) for at least two weeks or until they show signs of improvement. If cost is an issue or if the patient cannot tolerate liposomal amphotericin B, then amphotericin B lipid complex (5 mg/kg daily) should be used instead [17].

Polyenes Safety Concerns

Amphotericin B formulations are currently only available in IV formulation and associated with renal and electrolyte and infusion-related toxicities [9-11].

NSAID: Non-steroidal anti-inflammatory drug; CSF: cerebrospinal fluid.

Drugs in the Pipeline

Other antifungal or FDA-approved drugs with different indications exist as alternative medications and may help manage Histoplasma [8]. For instance, encochleated amphotericin B deoxycholate is a newly developing polyene formulation that uses a novel lipid nanocrystal for oral administration [8]. Tetrazoles are developing azoles that will help avoid drug interactions because of their greater selectivity for fungal Cyp51 [8]. Among these drugs, VT-1598 was granted orphan drug status for treating coccidioidomycosis [8]. Other novel drugs related to Histoplasma are olorofim, fosmanogepix, and nikkomycin Z [8].

Corticosteroids

Corticosteroids are suggested in patients with acute distress syndrome in addition to fungal antifungal therapy [18]. Antifungal treatment for many cases of acute Histoplasmosis can last 12 weeks when dissemination is not present [18]. Patients with chronic pulmonary Histoplasmosis must get treated to avoid the degradation of lung tissues [18]. Treatment helps decrease the rate of deaths, the disappearance of fungus in sputum, and the decrease in pulmonary infiltrates in two-thirds of cases [18]. In patients who are experiencing hypoxemia or respiratory distress, adjunctive treatment with methylprednisolone (0.5-1.0 mg/kg/day) for 1 to 2 weeks may be considered. Alternatively, IV methylprednisolone can be used for a few days, followed by a transition to oral prednisone at a dosage of 60 mg per day for one week and then a gradual tapering of the dosage over the next 1 to 2 weeks.

Treatment Regimen Monitoring

Histoplasma antigen in urine is a good test for disseminated disease, since blood antigen test is less specific. The titer indicates antigen burden and should demonstrate a response to treatment as well as relapse. For disseminated disease, the antigen should be measured at baseline, two weeks, one month, and every three months for six months after treatment has stopped. A decline in antigen should be seen two to twelve weeks after initiation of therapy [9-11].

Special Populations: Treatment in Patients Diagnosed with Human-Immunodeficiency Virus (HIV)

Induction Therapy

Disseminated Histoplasmosis is a severe infection that progresses quickly and poses a life-threatening risk to individuals living with HIV. Immediate treatment with antifungal medication is crucial. The standard treatment for this infection is deoxycholate amphotericin B, which has a good success rate but can cause significant toxicity, including infusion-related problems, electrolyte imbalances, anemia, and renal failure. The preferred treatment for treating severe or moderately severe Histoplasmosis among people living with HIV is an induction phase of liposomal amphotericin B at a dose of 3.0 mg/kg for two weeks [19]. This recommendation is conditional and based on very low certainty evidence. For mild to moderate Histoplasmosis infection, the recommendation is itraconazole 200 mg two times per day following a loading dose of 200 mg administered three times per day for three days. However, this recommendation is conditional and is based on evidence with very low certainty. Induction therapy should last for two weeks, and the duration of treatment can be reduced based on clinical evaluation of the patient's response to the medication, as amphotericin B can cause renal toxicity. If the central nervous system is affected, the duration of induction therapy may need to be extended, or the dosage may need to be increased [19].

Maintenance Therapy

Individuals living with HIV who have undergone successful induction therapy for disseminated Histoplasmosis are at high risk of relapse, with rates as high as 90% if they do not receive maintenance therapy. Relapse typically occurs within 6-18 months after the cessation of induction therapy, and reinfection is possible in areas with high rates of Histoplasmosis [19]. Therefore, antifungal maintenance therapy is necessary to effectively suppress any remaining infection and prevent relapse. Although direct randomized comparisons are lacking, itraconazole is a more effective maintenance therapy than fluconazole, with treatment success rates of 75% and 40%, respectively [19]. Usually, itraconazole treatment involves a loading dose of 200 mg thrice daily for three days, followed by 200 mg twice daily to achieve steady-state itraconazole concentrations more rapidly. However, the required efficacy and duration of such regimens for individuals with central nervous system involvement are less clear [19].

There is no established ideal duration for maintenance therapy, and it should be determined based on clinical judgment. Some national guidelines recommend lifelong maintenance antifungal therapy, and relapses are often associated with poor adherence to therapy, low levels of itraconazole, or central nervous system infection. The Infectious Diseases Society of America guidelines recommend maintenance therapy with azoles for one year [19].

Timing of Antiretroviral Therapy Initiation

Antiretroviral therapy (ART) is preferably initiated before patients infected with HIV become immunocompromised and reverses the immune defect [1]. Thus, lowering the changes of Histoplasmosis to develop [1]. Reports have shown that antiretroviral therapy alone has had improvements in HIV patients with untreated Histoplasmosis [1].

Therefore, antiretroviral therapy should not be postponed for individuals diagnosed with disseminated Histoplasmosis who are receiving antifungal therapy. This recommendation is conditional and based on very-low-certainty evidence [19]. The recommendation to not postpone ART is based on weighing the morbidity and mortality from another opportunistic infection that could occur with delayed initiation of antiretroviral therapy against the incidence of immune reconstitution inflammatory syndrome. Immune reconstitution inflammatory syndrome is not commonly seen among people with disseminated Histoplasmosis after the initiation of antiretroviral therapy, with the overall incidence occurring at about 0.74 cases per 1,000 person-years among people living with HIV [19].

Special Populations: Treatment in Immunocompromised Solid Organ Transplant Patients

Immunocompromised patients, especially solid organ transplant recipients, are at a heightened risk for Histoplasmosis due to the ability of the disease to persist in macrophages and disseminate to other parts of the body [20]. However, despite this increased risk, the occurrence of post-transplant Histoplasmosis is relatively infrequent, with an estimated incidence of less than 1% in endemic areas [20]. According to the TRANSNET study, which involved several transplant centers in endemic areas, the prevalence of Histoplasmosis among solid organ transplant recipients was only 0.14% over the study period, with a 12-month cumulative incidence rate of 0.1% [20]. The disease is primarily transmitted via inhalation through a pulmonary route, either through primary infection or reactivation of a previous infection due to immunosuppression [20]. Donor-derived infections transmitted through the allograft are rare, occurring in 1 out of 10,000 transplants, and there are no reports of human-to-human transmission [20].

The selection of antifungal therapy and duration of treatment in solid organ transplant (SOT) patients depends on various factors, such as disease severity, immune status of the patient, and potential drug interactions with other medications [20]. The classification of mild, moderate, and severe disease is subjective and mainly relies on clinical evaluation based on factors such as hospitalization requirement, respiratory status, hemodynamic stability, extent of infection, and ability to take oral medication [20]. Itraconazole monotherapy (200 mg twice daily for at least 12 months) is an effective treatment option for mild to moderate infection. For moderately severe and severe infection, initial therapy with amphotericin is recommended, but the choice of amphotericin formulation is based on availability, cost, and the risk of nephrotoxicity, as there are no randomized studies comparing their efficacy in organ transplant recipients [20]. The duration of amphotericin therapy should be 1-2 weeks or until infection stabilization, followed by step-down therapy with itraconazole (200 mg twice daily) to complete a minimum 12-month total treatment course. A concomitant reduction in immunosuppression, especially with calcineurin inhibitors, is crucial to reduce the risk of relapse [20].

The more recent azole agents such as voriconazole, posaconazole, and isavuconazole have shown activity against H. capsulatum *in vitro* [20]. Although clinical efficacy data for these agents are limited to small case reports and series, the available evidence increasingly supports their effectiveness. However, these findings are not enough to establish new treatment guidelines. Fluconazole is currently recommended as the second-line azole for Histoplasmosis, but it has a high relapse rate in immunocompromised patients who are not HIV-infected [20]. Therefore, the newer generation azoles offer alternative treatments for patients who are intolerant or unresponsive to the first-line agents, amphotericin B and itraconazole, and they may eventually become first-line agents with broader clinical experience [20].

It is important for clinicians to be aware of the potential drug interactions between itraconazole and calcineurin inhibitors, commonly used in the immunosuppressive regimens of solid organ transplant patients [7]. Itraconazole is a potent inhibitor of the cytochrome P450 3A4 isoenzyme system, which can lead to significant increases in blood levels of calcineurin inhibitors [7]. Therefore, close monitoring of calcineurin inhibitor levels is necessary. Due to variability in the pharmacokinetics and absorption of azoles, therapeutic monitoring of serum drug levels is strongly recommended to optimize therapy once steady state has been reached [20]. A serum concentration of at least 1.0 μg/mL of random itraconazole and its hydroxy-itraconazole metabolite is recommended for clinical efficacy [20]. Although the newer generation azoles have more reliable absorption, therapeutic drug monitoring is also strongly recommended for their use [20].

Primary and Secondary Prophylaxis

It is not recommended to administer primary prophylaxis for Histoplasmosis in post-transplant patients due to the low risk of the disease [11]. More than 500 patients who underwent immunosuppressive therapy for solid organ or bone marrow transplantation in an area with a high prevalence of Histoplasmosis did not develop the disease after an average follow-up of 16 months [11]. Nevertheless, transplant recipients should be advised to avoid exposure to high-risk environments [20]. Patients who have previously recovered from Histoplasmosis within two years before starting immunosuppression may be considered for secondary prophylaxis with itraconazole 200 mg daily [20]. Voriconazole, posaconazole, and isavuconazole are also potentially effective for prophylaxis. The optimal duration of secondary prophylaxis after transplantation is unknown. Solid organ transplant recipients who have had previous histoplasmosis infection should undergo regular Histoplasma antigen enzyme immunoassay (EIA) monitoring during periods of extensive immunosuppression to detect relapse [20]. The management of incidental H. capsulatum detected in explanted organs or donor tissues is not clearly established. This scenario is more common in lung transplant recipients, and antifungal prophylaxis may be considered based on the experience of a single center [20].

Histoplasmosis Secondary to Immunosuppressive Therapy

If a patient develops Histoplasmosis because of tumor necrosis factor α inhibitor therapy, antifungal treatment is necessary, and discontinuation of the tumor necrosis factor α blocker is required during this therapy [9]. Once there is a positive clinical response to treatment, pharmacological immunosuppression may be reinstated, provided that the individual receives antifungal treatment for approximately 12 months and tests negative for Histoplasma species antigen [9].

Duration of Treatment

The duration of treatment for histoplasmosis infections depends on the severity of the infection and the patient's underlying health conditions. The length of treatment can vary from several weeks to several months. Generally, antifungal therapy should last at least 12 months, regardless of disease severity [8].

For acute pulmonary Histoplasmosis, treatment lasts at a minimum of 4 to 6 weeks, while chronic pulmonary Histoplasmosis (CPH) may require longer treatment, lasting 12 to 24 months or longer [11]. Disseminated histoplasmosis and histoplasmosis meningitis are usually treated with antifungal medications for at least 12 months [11], sometimes longer depending on the patient's response to treatment. For patients needing continuous immunosuppression or after a relapse, indefinite therapy may be an option, especially with CNS involvement [8].

It is important to complete the entire course of treatment even if the symptoms improve, to ensure complete eradication of the fungus and prevent relapse. Follow-up monitoring, including repeat imaging and laboratory tests, may also be necessary to ensure the infection is fully treated [11].

Complication

Histoplasmosis severe infections may cause severe complications if not treated, especially in people with weakened immune systems or chronic lung disease [11]. CPH, a progressive lung infection, can develop in individuals with Histoplasmosis for many years. Its symptoms include chronic cough, shortness of breath, fatigue, and weight loss. Disseminated Histoplasmosis is another potential complication where the infection spreads from the lungs to other parts of the body, leading to fever, chills, night sweats, weight loss, and organ failure [11]. Acute respiratory distress syndrome (ARDS), a severe lung injury that can be life-threatening, can occur in response to Histoplasmosis, leading to mechanical ventilation [11]. Histoplasmosis can also cause pericarditis, leading to chest pain, difficulty breathing, and heart failure. Histoplasmosis can also lead to meningitis, an inflammation of the membranes surrounding the brain and spinal cord, which can be life-threatening and cause symptoms such as fever, headache, nausea, and confusion [11].

Conclusion

In developing countries, *Histoplasma capsulatum* is the prevalent cause of endemic mycosis. While it is a benign and asymptomatic disease for those with a healthy immune system, it poses a significant risk of opportunistic infection in immunocompromised individuals. Due to its expanding geographical spread and varied clinical manifestations, healthcare providers should consider Histoplasmosis a potential diagnosis in appropriate clinical scenarios. Laboratory tests have advanced to enable rapid detection and monitoring, and a broader range of antifungal therapies is now available. Diligent surveillance for active infection and targeted post-transplant antifungal prophylaxis can significantly reduce the risk of severe infection in the most vulnerable.

References

[1] Bahr N. C., Antinori S., Wheat L. J., Sarosi G. A. Histoplasmosis infections worldwide: thinking outside of the Ohio River valley. *Current tropical medicine reports*. 2015;2:70-80.

[2] Benedict K., McCracken S., Signs K., Malia Ireland, Victoria Amburgey, Jose Antonio Serrano, Natalie Christophe, Suzanne Gibbons-Burgener, Sara Hallyburton, Kimberly A. Warren, Alison Keyser Metobo, Racheal Odom, Matthew R. Groenewold, Brendan R. Jackson. Enhanced surveillance for histoplasmosis - 9 states, 2018-2019. Paper presented at: *Open Forum Infectious Diseases* 2020.

[3] Benedict K., Toda M., Jackson B. R. Revising conventional wisdom about histoplasmosis in the United States. Paper presented at: Open Forum Infectious Diseases2021.

[4] Ashraf N., Kubat R. C., Poplin V., Antoine A. Adenis, David W. Denning, Laura Wright, Orion McCotter, Ilan S. Schwartz, Brendan R. Jackson, Tom Chiller, Nathan C. Bahr. Re-drawing the maps for endemic mycoses. *Mycopathologia*. 2020;185:843-865.

[5] Arauz A. B., Papineni P. Histoplasmosis. *Infect Dis Clin North Am*. 2021;35(2):471-491.

[6] CDC. *Histoplasmosis.* 2013; https://www.cdc.gov/fungal/histoplasmosis. Accessed March 6, 2023.

[7] Cuellar-Rodriguez J., Avery R., Lard M., M. Budev, S. M. Gordon, N. K. Shrestha, D. van Duin, M. Oethinger, S. D. Mawhorter. Histoplasmosis in solid organ transplant recipients: 10 years of experience at a large transplant center in an endemic area. *Clinical Infectious Diseases.* 2009;49(5):710-716.

[8] Saullo J. L., Miller R. A. Updates on Histoplasmosis in Solid Organ Transplantation. *Current Fungal Infection Reports.* 2022:1-14.

[9] Thompson G. R., Le T., Chindamporn A., Carol A Kauffman, Ana Alastruey-Izquierdo, Neil M. Ampel, David R. Andes, Darius Armstrong-James, Olusola Ayanlowo, John W. Baddley, Bridget M. Barker, Leila Lopes Bezerra, Maria J Buitrago, Leili Chamani-Tabriz, Jasper F. W. Chan, Methee Chayakulkeeree, Oliver A Cornely, Cao Cunwei, Jean-Pierre Gangneux, Nelesh P. Govender, Ferry Hagen, Mohammad T. Hedayati, Tobias M. Hohl, Grégory Jouvion, Chris Kenyon, Christopher C. Kibbler, Nikolai Klimko, David C. M. Kong, Robert Krause, Low Lee Lee, Graeme Meintjes, Marisa H. Miceli, Peter-Michael Rath, Andrej Spec, Flavio Queiroz-Telles, Ebrahim Variava, Paul E. Verweij, Ilan S. Schwartz, Alessandro C Pasqualotto. Global guideline for the diagnosis and management of the endemic mycoses: An initiative of the European Confederation of Medical Mycology in cooperation with the International Society for Human and Animal Mycology. *The Lancet Infectious Diseases.* 2021;21(12):e364-e374.

[10] Benson C. A., Kaplan J. E., Masur H., Pau A., Holmes K. K. Treating opportunistic infections among HIV-infected adults and adolescents: recommendations from CDC, the National Institutes of Health, and the HIV Medicine Association/*Infectious Diseases Society of America*. 2004.

[11] Wheat L. J., Freifeld A. G., Kleiman M. B., John W. Baddley, David S. McKinsey, James E. Loyd, Carol A. Kauffman; Infectious Diseases Society of America. Clinical practice guidelines for the management of patients with histoplasmosis: 2007 update by the Infectious Diseases Society of America. *Clinical Infectious Diseases.* 2007:807-825.

[12] Ashley E. S. D., Lewis R., Lewis J. S., Martin C., Andes D. Pharmacology of systemic antifungal agents. *Clinical infectious diseases.* 2006;43(Supplement_1):S28-S39.

[13] PriCara. *Sporanox Prescribing Information*. 2001; https://www.accessdata.fda.gov/drugsatfda_docs/label/2009/020083s040s041s044lbl.pdf. Accessed March 6, 2023.

[14] Pfizer. *Diflucan Prescribing Information.* 2022; https://labeling.pfizer.com/ShowLabeling.aspx?format=PDF&id=575. Accessed March 6, 2023.

[15] Merck. *Noxafil Package Insert.* 2022; https://www.merck.com/product/usa/pi_circulars/n/noxafil/noxafil_pi.pdf. Accessed March 6, 2023.

[16] *Pfizer. Vfend Prescribing Information.* 2022; https://labeling.pfizer.com/showlabeling.aspx?id=618. Accessed March 6, 2023.

[17] National Institutes of Health; Centers for Disease Control and Prevention; HIV Medicine Association of the Infectious Diseases Society of America Panel on Guidelines for the Prevention and Treatment of Opportunistic Infections in Adults

and Adolescents with HIV— A Working Group of the Office of AIDS Research Advisory Council (OARAC). Guidelines for the Prevention and Treatment of Opportunistic Infections in Adults and Adolescents with HIV. [Updated 2023 Jun 14]. In: *ClinicalInfo.HIV.gov [Internet].* Rockville (MD): US Department of Health and Human Services; 2002.

[18] Azar M. M., Loyd J. L., Relich R. F., Wheat L. J., Hage C. A. Current concepts in the epidemiology, diagnosis, and management of histoplasmosis syndromes. Paper presented at: *Seminars in Respiratory and Critical Care Medicine 2020.*

[19] Organization W. H. *Guidelines for diagnosing and managing disseminated histoplasmosis among people living with HIV.* 2020.

[20] Miller R., Assi M., Practice AIDCo. Endemic fungal infections in solid organ transplant recipients - Guidelines from the American Society of Transplantation Infectious Diseases Community of Practice. *Clinical Transplantation.* 2019;33(9):e13553.

Chapter 15

Histoplasmosis in Pregnancy

Simmy Lahori[1]
Rahul Kashyap[2,3]
and Salim Surani[4,5,*]

[1]Visiting Research Fellow, Department of Radiology, Mayo Clinic, Rochester, Minnesota, USA
[2]Department of Research, WellSpan Health, York, Pennsylvania, USA;
[3]Department of Anesthesiology and Critical Care Medicine, Rochester, Minnesota, USA
[4]Adjunct Clinical Professor, Department of Medicine & Pharmacology, Texas A&M University, USA
[5]Research Collaborator, Department of Anaesthesiology, Mayo Clinic, Rochester, Minnesota, USA

Abstract

Histoplasmosis, caused by Histoplasmosis capsulatum, is a common endemic mycosis infection that is usually asymptomatic but can result in severe disease. The severity of the condition depends on the cell-mediated immunity of the host, which is reduced in pregnancy. The transplacental transmission of the infection to the offspring is still inconclusive in humans. Culture, fungal stains, serological tests for antibodies, and antigen detection can help make the diagnosis. Apart from avoiding azoles in the first trimester of pregnancy, the other recommendations for treating histoplasmosis are like those in the non-pregnant patients.

Keywords: histoplasmosis, pregnancy, transplacental transmission, amphotericin b, cell-mediated immunity

---

* Correspondence Author' Email: srsurani@hotmail.com.

In: Histoplasmosis
Editors: Salim Surani, Syed Anjum Khan and Reena Shah
ISBN: 979-8-89113-129-3

Introduction

Histoplasmosis is the most prevalent endemic fungal infection in the United States [1]. Most of the infections are asymptomatic or self-limited. However, it can affect the pulmonary system causing mild symptoms, or can cause severe and progressive disseminated infection [2]. Pregnancy increases the risk of disseminated fungal infections such as coccidioidomycosis, African histoplasmosis, blastomycosis, and cryptococcosis. Pregnancy leads to a state of suppression of cell-mediated immunity (CMI), causing the dissemination of these infections. This has played a big role of CMI in curtailing H. capsulatum infections. There has been limited information on managing less common fungal infections such as Histoplasmosis, which can be challenging for clinicians to provide evidence-based guidance while assessing risks and benefits [3].

Epidemiology

Histoplasmosis is the most common endemic fungal infection in the United States, with the Ohio and Mississippi River Valleys as the highly endemic regions [4]. As histoplasmosis is usually asymptomatic in pregnancy, in September 1954, a policy of taking routine chest X-rays during pregnancy was instituted in the Catherine Booth Hospital. They took approx. 3500 chest films of pregnant patients since then. This case demonstrated a solitary pulmonary lesion with the halo in the right lung along with extensive calcification in the mediastinal lymph nodes, which was found incidentally [5].

Risk Factors

Maternal immunosuppression or immunodeficiency with confirmed histoplasmosis diagnoses can be considered a risk factor for transmission of the disease to the newborn [6]. Infection during the previous pregnancy could be a risk factor for getting infected next time. It is thought that the fungus may remain dormant in the bone and is reactivated by the immunological effects of pregnancy. There may also be some superadded reinfection with H. duboisii [7]. There is no evidence that states that histoplasmosis is more severe during the time of pregnancy or causes dissemination to the fetus [8]. The other risk factors are similar to the ones in immunocompetent individuals that have been mentioned in the previous chapters.

Transmission

Transplacental transmission in H. capsulatum has been described by Schwarz et al., in mice by inoculation both before and after the onset of pregnancy. Inoculation before pregnancy showed no evidence of H. capsulatum in any of the subsequent offspring. Inoculation after pregnancy demonstrated the fungus in the placenta but not in the offspring. Hence, it would be best to state that no direct evidence of fetal transplacental transmission was found [5]. In previous studies, transplacental transmission has been described in horses [9]. In the case of fungal dissemination, there are chances of transplacental transmission [10].

Clinical Features

Symptomatic histoplasmosis is a rare event during pregnancy. Histoplasmosis should be kept as a differential in pregnant patients presenting with fever and non-specific pulmonary findings. There has been some association between histoplasmosis and severe anemia causing complications which could be because of folic acid deficiency or osteomyelitis of the manubrium sterni due to H. duboisii.

The extent of the disease can be determined by the number of conidia inhaled, the immune responsiveness of the host, and the integrity of the respiratory tract infection. The most benign form is acute pulmonary infections which could be asymptomatic or influenza-like illnesses. It can also be a life-threatening progressive disseminated infection that affects the immunocompromised, leading to high morbidity and mortality [11].

Brief Pathology

There has been an increase in suppressor T-lymphocyte function, and the CD4 cell function is down-regulated [12] while the lymphocyte stimulation is diminished [13]. Interferon-gamma and interleukin (IL) 2 are decreased during pregnancy. In addition, the placenta produces IL-4, IL-5, IL-6, and IL-10.

These changes contribute to the downregulation of Type 1 T-helper cell-associated immunity, and Type 2 T-helper cell-associated immunity is upregulated [14, 15]. A case series described by Whitt et al., showed that in addition to pregnancy, having diabetes mellitus or HIV could have adverse effects on the cell-mediated immunity [10].

Diagnosis

The gold standard way of diagnosing histoplasmosis is histopathology or cytopathology of the specimen and identifying the fungus [16]. Histopathologically, the specimen demonstrates a granulomatous response that can be necrotizing or non-necrotizing. Microscopy reveals ovoid, narrow-based budding yeast present within the tissues that are often phagocytosed within macrophages. The sensitivity of Histoplasmosis in the urine is approx. 91.8% [17]. Other soft clues for the diagnosis of histoplasmosis are elevated serum alkaline phosphatase, lactate dehydrogenase, ferritin levels, or the presence of hepatosplenomegaly and/or presence of mediastinal or hilar adenopathy on imaging [16].

Treatment

The treatment of Histoplasmosis in pregnancy differs from that in others. Azoles considered teratogenic are avoided during pregnancy. Amphotericin is considered the treatment of choice and is considered safe [8]. It is classified as a pregnancy risk category B drug [18]. A case has been reported in which the pregnant patient was treated in the outpatient clinic with thrice-weekly liposomal amphotericin B step-down therapy for a period of 6 weeks [19]. Patients should be monitored clinically for infusion-related reactions during and after each administration. Infusion-related reactions of thrombophlebitis can be seen. Administration of ibuprofen 30 minutes prior to amphotericin B reduced the rate of occurrence of chills to half, from 87% to 49% [17]. Nephrotoxicity is another major complicated side effect of Amphotericin B. It can be prevented by using lower doses of the drug and avoiding concurrent therapy with other nephrotoxins, such as aminoglycoside or cyclosporine [20]. The administration of N-acetylcysteine has shown to be protective against amphotericin-induced nephrotoxicity in animals by preserving the GFR and reducing apoptosis of renal tubular cells. However, its protective role in humans is inconclusive [21]. Liposomal amphotericin B is considered less nephrotoxic than the amphotericin B lipid complex [22].

Systemic azoles are considered teratogenic in animals as well as in humans. Ketoconazole has been shown to be teratogenic and embryotoxic at high doses (800 mg/kg/day) in animals [23], while Fluconazole is fetotoxic and teratogenic in rats causing craniofacial and rib abnormalities [24]. Similarly, Itraconazole is embryotoxic and teratogenic in rodents, especially in the first trimester [25]. Meperidine can also be used to reduce the amphotericin B-induced chills and rigors. However, it is avoided for premedication because of its potential side effects. Except for avoiding azoles, all the recommendations for the treatment of histoplasmosis in pregnancy remain as those of nonpregnant patients [4]. Treatment of histoplasmosis among immunocompetent, immunocompromised and pregnant patients is shown in Table 1.

Table 1. Medical management in immunocompetent, immunocompromised and pregnant patients

Immunocompetent (4)	Immunocompromised (4)	Pregnant (4)
Mild to Moderate Symptoms < 4: None Symptoms > 4 weeks: Itraconazole load, then 200 mg once or twice daily for 6 to 12 weeks.	Without CNS infection Mild to Moderate symptoms: Itraconazole)200 mg twice daily for at least 12 months	Amphotericin B 3 to 5 mg/kg once a day for 4-6 weeks. The deoxycholate formulation of Amphotericin B (0.7 to 1.0 mg/kg daily) can be given to reduce nephrotoxicity.
	Moderately severe to severe: Itraconazole (200 mg twice daily for at least 12 months	
Moderate to Severe: Liposomal Amphotericin B 3 mg/kg/day or Amphotericin B lipid complex 5 mg/kg/day IV or	CNS Histoplasmosis: Liposomal Amphotericin B (5mg/kg daily for four to six weeks) followed by Itraconazole (200 mg two to three times daily for at least 12 months).	Newborns infected with histoplasmosis are treated with Amphotericin B deoxycholate (1.0 mg/kg daily for 4 weeks)

Prevention

Pregnant patients should be advised to avoid places such as soil where the birds roost or visit buildings that have been demolished and not to explore caves to reduce the chances of getting the infection [26].

Conclusion

There are limited cases that demonstrate the presentation of histoplasmosis in pregnant patients. Antifungal prophylaxis is not recommended for at-risk populations. However, measures to minimize environmental exposure can reduce the risk of procuring infection.

References

[1] Chu J H, Feudtner C, Heydon K, Walsh T J, Zaoutis TE. Hospitalizations for endemic mycoses: a population-based national study. *Clin. Infect. Dis.* 2006;42(6):822-5.

[2] Kauffman C A. Histoplasmosis: a Clinical and Laboratory Update. *Clinical Microbiology Reviews.* 2007;20(1):115-32.

[3] Gould A P, Winders H R, Stover K R, Bookstaver P B, Griffin B, Bland C M, Eiland L S, Murray M. Less common bacterial, fungal and viral infections: review of management in the pregnant patient. *Drugs Context.* 2021;10.

[4] Wheat L J, Freifeld A G, Kleiman M B, Baddley J W, McKinsey D S, Loyd J E, Kauffman C A; Infectious Diseases Society of America. Clinical practice guidelines for the management of patients with histoplasmosis: 2007 update by the Infectious Diseases Society of America. *Clin. Infect. Dis.* 2007;45(7):807-25.

[5] SABIN M. Histoplasmosis in Pregnancy. *Obstetrics & Gynecology* 1959;13(2).

[6] Carlucci J G, Halasa N, Creech C B, Dulek D E, Gómez-Duarte O G, Nelson G E, Talbot H K, Scalise M L, Scott P L, Mahadevan U, Beaulieu D B. Vertical Transmission of Histoplasmosis Associated With Anti-Tumor Necrosis Factor Therapy. *Journal of the Pediatric Infectious Diseases Society.* 2016;5(2):e9-e12.

[7] Ajabor L N, Lucas A O, Lawson E A, Seriki O. African histoplasmosis complicating pregnancy. *Transactions of the Royal Society of Tropical Medicine and Hygiene.* 1971;65(5):650-60.

[8] Wheat J, Sarosi G, McKinsey D, Hamill R, Bradsher R, Johnson P, Loyd J, Kauffman C. Practice Guidelines for the Management of Patients with Histoplasmosis. *Clinical Infectious Diseases.* 2000;30(4):688-95.

[9] Rezabek G B, Donahue J M, Giles R C, Petrites-Murphy M B, Poonacha K B, Rooney J R, B J Smith, T W Swerczek, R R Tramontin. Histoplasmosis in horses. *J. Comp. Pathol.* 1993;109(1):47-55.

[10] Whitt S P, Koch G A, Fender B, Ratnasamy N, Everett E D. Histoplasmosis in Pregnancy: Case Series and Report of Transplacental Transmission. *Archives of Internal Medicine.* 2004;164(4):454-8.

[11] Tobón A M, Gómez B L. Pulmonary Histoplasmosis. *Mycopathologia.* 2021;186(5):697-705.

[12] Hirahara F, Gorai I, Tanaka K, Matsuzaki Y, Sumiyoshi Y, Shiojima Y. Cellular immunity in pregnancy: subpopulations of T lymphocytes bearing Fc receptors for IgG and IgM in pregnant women. *Clin. Exp. Immunol.* 1980;41(2):353-7.

[13] Sabahi F, Rola-Plesczcynski M, O'Connell S, Frenkel LD. Qualitative and quantitative analysis of T lymphocytes during normal human pregnancy. *Am. J. Reprod. Immunol.* 1995;33(5):381-93.

[14] Formby B. Immunologic response in pregnancy. Its role in endocrine disorders of pregnancy and influence on the course of maternal autoimmune diseases. *Endocrinol. Metab. Clin. North Am.* 1995;24(1):187-205.

[15] Krasnow J S, Tollerud D J, Naus G, DeLoia J A. Endometrial Th2 cytokine expression throughout the menstrual cycle and early pregnancy. *Hum. Reprod.* 1996;11(8):1747-54.

[16] Azar M M, Loyd J L, Relich R F, Wheat LJ, Hage C A. Current Concepts in the Epidemiology, Diagnosis, and Management of Histoplasmosis Syndromes. *Semin. Respir. Crit. Care Med.* 2020;41(1):13-30.

[17] Gigliotti F, Shenep J L, Lott L, Thornton D. Induction of prostaglandin synthesis as the mechanism responsible for the chills and fever produced by infusing amphotericin B. *J. Infect Dis.* 1987;156(5):784-9.

[18] Pilmis B, Jullien V, Sobel J, Lecuit M, Lortholary O, Charlier C. Antifungal drugs during pregnancy: an updated review. *Journal of Antimicrobial Chemotherapy.* 2014;70(1):14-22.

[19] Lewis P O, Khan I, Patel P. Successful stepdown treatment of pulmonary histoplasmosis with thrice-weekly liposomal amphotericin B in a hospital-associated, outpatient infusion centre: A case report. *J. Clin. Pharm. Ther.* 2018;43(2):269-72.

[20] Bates D W, Su L, Yu D T, Chertow G M, Seger D L, Gomes D R, Platt R. Correlates of acute renal failure in patients receiving parenteral amphotericin B. *Kidney Int.* 2001;60(4):1452-9.

[21] Karimzadeh I, Khalili H, Sagheb MM, Farsaei S. A double-blinded, placebo-controlled, multicenter clinical trial of N-acetylcysteine for preventing amphotericin B-induced nephrotoxicity. *Expert Opin. Drug Metab. Toxicol.* 2015;11(9):1345-55.

[22] Wingard J R, White M H, Anaissie E, Raffalli J, Goodman J, Arrieta A. A randomized, double-blind comparative trial evaluating the safety of liposomal amphotericin B versus amphotericin B lipid complex in the empirical treatment of febrile neutropenia. L Amph/ABLC Collaborative Study Group. *Clin. Infect. Dis.* 2000;31(5):1155-63.

[23] Briggs G G. Drugs in pregnancy and lactation: a reference guide to fetal and neonatal risk for PDA. Sumner J. Yaffe RKF, editor: Lippincott Williams & Wilkins, Philadelphia, 2006; 2006.

[24] Tiboni G M. Second branchial arch anomalies induced by Fluconazole, a bis-triazole antifungal agent, in cultured mouse embryos. *Res. Commun. Chem. Pathol. Pharmacol*. 1993;79(3):381-4.

[25] De Santis M, Di Gianantonio E, Cesari E, Ambrosini G, Straface G, Clementi M. First-Trimester Itraconazole Exposure and Pregnancy Outcome. *Drug Safety*. 2009;32(3):239-44.

[26] Patient education: Histoplasmosis (The Basics) [Available from: https://www.uptodate.com/contents/histoplasmosis-the-basics?search=histoplasmosis%20treatment&topicRef=2451&source=see_link#H629377858.

Chapter 16

Differential Diagnosis of Histoplasmosis

John Paul Aparece[1]
Sung Whoy[2]
Wailea Faye[3]
Gude Geethanjali[4]
Lisa Centeno[5]
Shika M Jain[6]
Sydney Boike[7]
Hasnain Saifee Bawaadam[8]
Sindu Mukesh[9]
Ibtisam Rauf[10]
Claudia Castillo Zambrano[11]
Mohamad El Labban[12]
Aysun Tekin[13]
Salim Surani[14]
and Nitesh Kumar Jain[15,*]

[1]Department of Medicine, Texas Tech University El Paso, Texas, USA.
[2]Department of Medicine, Cha Cebu Institute of Medicine, Philippines
[3]Department of Medicine, Salva Cebu Institute of Medicine, Philippines
[4]Department of Histopathology, Postgraduate Institute of Medical Education and Research, Chandigarh, India
[5]Department of medicine, University of Santo Tomas Faculty of Medicine and Surgery, Manila, Philippines

---

[*] Correspondence Author's Email: jain.nitesh@mayo.edu.

In: Histoplasmosis
Editors: Salim Surani, Syed Anjum Khan and Reena Shah
ISBN: 979-8-89113-129-3

[6]Department of Medicine, MVJ Medical College and Research Hospital, Karnataka, India
[7]Department of Medicine, University of Minnesota, Minneapolis, Minnesota, USA
[8]Department of Pulmonary & Critical Care Medicine, Aurora Medical Center, Kenosha, Wisconsin, USA
[9]Liaquat University of Medical and Health Sciences, Jamshoro, Pakistan
[10]Department of Medicine, St. George's University School of Medicine, St. George, Grenada
[11]Department of Medicine, Mayo Clinic, Rochester, Minnesota, USA
[12]Department of Internal Medicine, Mayo Clinic Health System, Mankato, Minnesota, USA
[13]Department of Medicine, Mayo Clinic, Rochester, Minnesota,USA
[14]Department of Medicine and Pharmacology, Texas A&M University, College Station, Texas, USA
[15]Department of Critical Care Medicine, Mayo Clinic Health System, Mankato, Minnesota, USA

Abstract

Histoplasmosis is an endemic fungal disease that is found in almost all major continents. It can affect many organs such as the skin, bones, joints, respiratory system, pericardial disease, gastrointestinal tract and disseminated disease. Host immunological status and the dose of infecting inoculum are important factors that determine whether disease will manifest clinically; otherwise often the disease is asymptomatic. Due to the fungus being dimorphic and clinical manifestation involves multiple organs, there is a wide array of differential diagnosis when considering this disease as diagnosis. Our current chapter reviews many of these differential diagnoses when considering histoplasmosis and various microbiological, pathological, clinical, and radiological considerations that may help in making the right diagnosis.

Keywords: histoplasmosis, blastomycosis, coccidioidomycosis, histoplasmosis capsulatum, histoplasma duboisii, cryptococcus, disseminated histoplasmosis

Introduction

Histoplasmosis is a highly endemic fungal infection in the North American continent [1]. It is primarily found in the Ohio and Mississippi river valleys, as well as other parts of the globe, such as Mexico, Central and South America,

Africa, and Asia. Although geographic distribution should be considered in formulating a differential diagnosis for mycoses, histoplasmosis has been increasingly found outside its normal geographical distribution, especially from emigrants or travelers from endemic areas [1]. Histoplasmosis presentation can be varied from asymptomatic infection to a progressive disseminated and life-threatening illness. The severity of the fungal infection can be correlated based on immunity, exposure, and even the underlying lung architecture of an individual [1]. Due to the varying clinical presentation of histoplasmosis, it can resemble many other disease entities [2]. Low levels of exposure in healthy individuals often result in asymptomatic or mild and self-limited infection [2, 3]. Radiologic and serologic findings in asymptomatic individuals are usually negative; however, some individuals may develop pulmonary lesions that can turn into calcified adenopathy and granulomas that may resemble other granulomatous diseases [3]. Symptomatic acute and subacute pulmonary histoplasmosis may present with a flu-like illness and have a fever, cough, headache, malaise, myalgia, abdominal pain, arthralgia, dyspnea, and hemoptysis 1-4 weeks after exposure [4].

The clinical manifestation of histoplasmosis is varied, and it can present with a wide variety of differential diagnosis, such as infectious, inflammatory, and even malignant conditions [3, 4]. Therefore, it is imperative to have it as a differential diagnosis and consider the different histoplasmosis syndromes and epidemiological factors when treating these patients.

This differential diagnosis spans across a wide spectrum of clinico-radiological and pathological-microbiological realms. We aim to describe this wide-ranging differential from the perspective of making a clinico-pathological-radiological diagnosis of Histoplasma capsulatum.

Microbiological Differential Diagnosis

In Africa, particularly in the central and western parts, Histoplasma duboisii is endemic. It is morphologically similar to Histoplasma capsulatum, but H.duboisii has a larger yeast form. Histoplasma duboisii rarely shows pulmonary manifestation and has two main forms of presentation. One is the localized form involving the superficial skin, subcutaneous tissue, and bone. The other is the diffuse disseminated form. Deeper subcutaneous granulomas or osteomyelitis with overlying superficial skin involvement is also seen in H. duboisii. The morphological picture of Histoplasma is similar in both epithelioid granulomatous and giant cell response. Laboratory methods used to diagnose H. duboisii also involve growth on standard culture medium. However, its yeast cells range from 8 to 15 μm in diameter, with hourglass or figure of 8 type budding similar to yeast cells of Blastomyces dermatitidis, where budding is broad-based. On culture, tuberculate macroconidia differentiate H. duboisii from B.dermatitidis. Sometimes the organism is arranged in chains. H.duboisii and B.dermatitidis cannot be differentiated with fungal-specific stains such as periodic acid-Schiff or Grocott-Gomori methenamine silver but does aid in visualizing yeast cells (Figure 1).

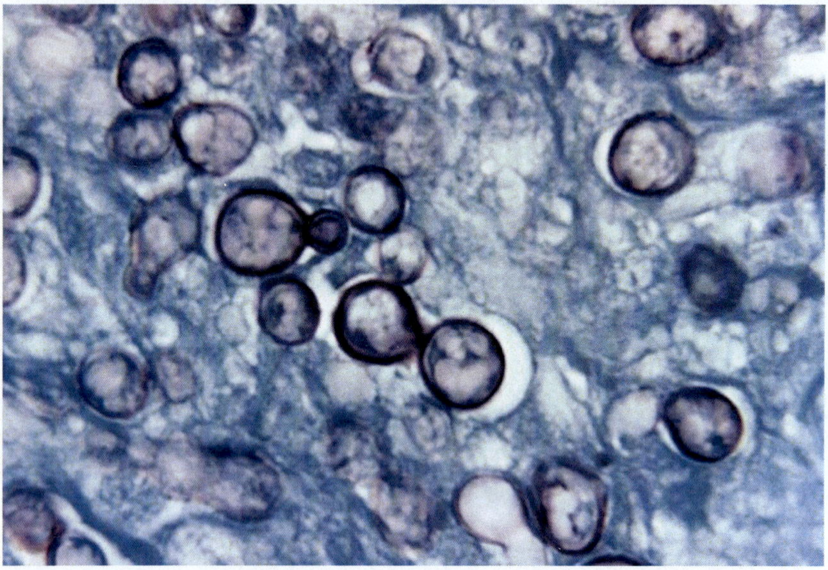

Figure 1. Tissue sample with fungal-specific strain such as Methenamine silver from a patient with a case of histoplasmosis secondary to *Histoplasma capsulatum* var. *duboisii, showing* typical yeast cells, with some undergoing replication by budding, similar to Blastomyces (Spurce: Center for disease control.ID#4221; https://phil.cdc.gov/details.aspx?pid=4221).

Although confirmation of Histoplasma infection by molecular identification is a rapid and reliable method, it has no role in differentiating the species of Histoplasma. Thus, its use will likely be terminated by the manufacturer. Antigen testing in urine and serum, originally developed for H. capsulatum, can be used in patients with *H. duboisii,*due to cross reactivity, although distinguishing between both species is not possible. Thus, the only reliable method for differentiating the Histoplasma species involves DNA sequence analysis. Moreover, patients who are immunocompromised are likely to have false negative results in the early phase of the disease.

Emergomyces: Emergomyces are dimorphic fungi that predominantly affect immunocompromised patients on several continents. Infection occurs similar to other dimorphic fungi, with inhalation of the conidia, and with changes in temperature is converted to a yeast-like form, subsequently spreading to extrapulmonary sites. While incubated in fungal media such as Sabouraud agar or potato dextrose agar, colonies of *Emergomyces* species are initially glabrous, powdery then become raised, and furrowed. In 3 weeks, the diameter reaches up to 3.5 cm. Microscopically, yeast phase is marked by colonies and mold form appears as slender conidiophores that arise from hyphae and form "floret"of short secondary conidiophores with single small subspherical conidia. As the species of emergomyces and Histoplasma cross-react, a negative urine antigen test cannot exclude the diagnosis (Figure 2).

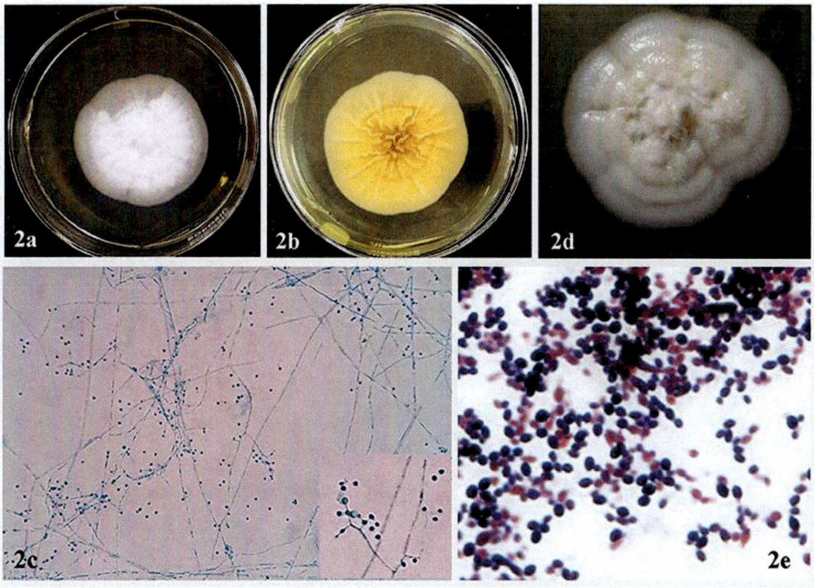

Figure 2. Mycelial form of Ergomyces- Yellowish white to tan initially glabrous colony becoming powdery and furrowed. 2C shows hyphae at right angles and form florets of short conidiophores. Courtesy of open-source article [5].

Patients with Es. africanus infection present with widely distributed skin lesions, such as papules, plaques, nodules, or ulcers. Pulmonary involvement is also seen and can present as consolidation, effusion, reticulonodular disease in diffuse pattern and/or lymphadenopathy. Other sites of involvement include gastrointestinal tract, liver, lymph nodes, and bone marrow.

Cryptococcus: Cryptococcus neoformans and *gattii* cause opportunistic infections in immunocompromised and immunocompetent patients, respectively. *C. neoformans* has a widespread distribution, readily found in soil and bird droppings, whereas *C. gattii*: has a predilection for eucalyptus trees with a tropical/subtropical distribution. Southeast parts of the U.S., Asia, Southern America, Africa, Vancouver, and British Columbia are known to be endemic. After inhalation of encapsulated yeast found in pigeon droppings, its pathogenic mechanism includes antiphagocytic and poorly immunogenic sugar capsule which acts as a major virulence factor. Its invasiveness is increased by glucuronoxylomannan (GXM), phenol oxidase, and production of various enzymes. The virulence factor inhibits phagocytosis by alveolar macrophages and inflammatory cell recruitment and migration. A chronic inflammation and pyogranulomatous response can be present.

Microscopically yeasts appear pleomorphic and variable in size, ranging from 2-20 microns. Mucinous capsule that appears bright red with mucicarmine stain surrounds yeasts with thin cell walls, and narrow-necked budding is present (as seen on Gram stain). Morphologic mimickers include *Histoplasma capsulatum* (smaller unencapsulated forms) and *Blastomyces* (unencapsulated with chronic lesions). On canavanine glycine bromothymol blue (CGB) media, *C. gattii* produces deep blue colonies. The sugar capsule contributes to the creamy, butyrous, mucoid growth on medium, and colonies appear brown on birdseed agar due to melanin production. Positive stains include methenamine silver, Fontana-Masson, and Indian Ink (rarely used in clinical practice). For bronchoalveolar lavage, pleural and cerebrospinal fluid, the Cryptococcal Antigen Lateral Flow assay, an immunochromatographic assay that qualitatively and semiquantitatively detects the capsular polysaccharide antigens of *Cryptococcus* species complex, with unchanged or increased antigen titer levers (Titer > 1:8).

CNS and pulmonary disease can manifest in both immunocompetent and immunocompromised patients, with cutaneous lesions (including pustules, papules, superficial granulomas, and cellulitis) often affecting the latter group.

Blastomyces: Blastomyces are dimorphic fungi prevalent in the soil in the Southeastern United States and Canada, Mexico, Africa, India, and the Middle East. Inhalation of the soil containing microconidia initiates infection, and pulmonary disease can present as consolidative pneumonia, ARDS, or apical nodules that resemble carcinoma. There is a mixed acute and granulomatous inflammation. Skin lesions can occur secondary to pulmonary blastomycosis. Grossly, lesions resemble tuberculosis, and yeasts are easily seen on H&E, taking the form of large budding yeasts (10-15 microns) with refractile walls and broad-based buds.

Coccidioidomycosis, is a dimorphic fungus that contains two species, namely Coccidioides immitis and Coccidioides posadasii, found in Central and Southern California and latter outside California. It is commonly known as Valley fever or San Joaquin Valley fever. Both species have similar clinical courses and microscopic morphology. It is a primary lung infection wherein lower respiratory tract symptoms resemble bacterial pneumonia (pulmonary coccidioidomycosis). Extrapulmonary sites include joints, bones, and meninges. Dissemination is present in 1-5% of cases, mainly in immunocompromised patients. Desert rheumatism or coccidioidomycosis includes the combination of fever, arthralgia, and erythema nodosum. But most individuals infected are minimally symptomatic or asymptomatic. The symptoms include cough, fever, dyspnea, and pleuritic chest pain. Patients with chronic infection can have a cavity-forming mass lesion.

In chronic infection, a mass lesion that is well circumscribed with central cavitation is formed, and a fungus ball mycetoma has been found in up to 28% of these cases. Within the cavitary lesion, one may find fibrosis with chronic inflammation and palisading fibroblasts, as well as occasional multinucleated giant cells. The wall of the central cavity is lined with squamous metaplastic cells, and hyphal elements can sometimes be identified. The surrounding lung parenchyma exhibits organizing pneumonia with chronic bronchiolitis and lymphoid hyperplasia. If blood vessel lesions are present, they take the form of arteritis with fibrinoid necrosis and rupture, thrombus, and mural inflammation.

Arthroconidia (3-5 microns) found in soil are inhaled when they are aerosolized, forming a specialized spherule in the lung. This rupture releases new endospores that develop into new spherules that disseminate hematogenously. Larger spores (20-200 microns) have thick walls, and granular basophilic endospores (2-4 microns) can be present, whereas patients with diabetes mellitus can have thin, septate hyphae where granular basophilic endospores may or may not be present. A necrotizing granulomatous inflammation (often with suppuration), with eosinophilic infiltration is present. GMS and PAS are positive stains, whereas mucicarmine is a negative stain. On cytologic examination of bronchoalveolar lavage, acute inflammation accompanies varying forms of spherules, and immature, smaller, empty, or fractured ones poorly absorb stains.

Although real time PCR assays and in situ hybridization specific for coccidioides are helpful for identifying different types of specimens, diagnosis by histology, culture or serology is the mainstay to identify fungal organisms. As the pathogen can cause severe infection, laboratory technicians should be aware of the diagnosis. While it has varying plate morphologies on standard fungal culture, a lactophenol cotton blue stain has been used to show septated hyphae with alternating barrel-shaped arthroconidia. Positive serology for anticoccidioidal IgG, IgM, and sometimes eosinophilia on complete blood count (found in 27%), are indicative of disease.

Clinico-Radiological Considerations

Pulmonary Infection: Since acute symptomatic histoplasmosis presents commonly as Pneumonia, it must be distinguished from the more common causes of pneumonia, including viral, community-acquired bacterial, and atypical pneumonia such as Legionella and Chlamydia pneumonia [3, 4]. Due to the vast differentials in patients who present with pulmonary symptoms, imaging of the thorax such as x-rays and Computed tomography(CT) scans are initially obtained, which shows infiltrates that are diffuse interstitial or reticulonodular in pattern, as well as hilar or mediastinal lymphadenopathy[3].Further diagnostic workups such as Histoplasma antigen (bronchoalveolar lavage (BAL) fluid, serum, or urine), BAL fluid cytopathology, fungal serology such as Galactomannan testing, and Histoplasma IgG and IgM serology may be warranted [1].

Chronic pulmonary histoplasmosis usually occurs in older patients with past medical history of structural lung disease or smoking and presents with cough, night sweats, low-grade fever, and weight loss [3]. This may present similarly to mycobacterial infections such as tuberculosis and fungal infections such as blastomycosis and coccidioidomycosis [1]. Chest imaging may demonstrate upper lobe cavities with granuloma formation, fibrosis, and pleural thickening [1, 2, 5, 6]. Granulomas are non-specific findings, and it is important to consider granulomatous lung diseases such as sarcoidosis as they may also present similarly[7]. Granulomatous diseases involving the lung are a category of diseases with varied manifestations and can be both infectious and noninfectious in origin; it is associated with granuloma formation like histoplasmosis. Differential diagnoses can include infectious causes such as mycobacteria, fungal infections including Histoplasma, aspiration pneumonia, syphilis, leprosy, and parasitic infections. Noninfectious causes of granulomatous lung disease include inflammatory disorders such as sarcoidosis, exposures and toxins, vasculitis, and autoimmune diseases such as rheumatoid nodules, malignancy, Pulmonary Langerhans cells histiocytosis, and Granulomatous–lymphocytic interstitial lung disease [7]. Fungal cultures of BAL fluid and Histoplasma IgG and IgM serology may also be useful in differentiating chronic pulmonary or cavitary histoplasmosis from other causes [1].

Integumental and Bony Lesions

Histoplasma capsulatum var. capsulatum (Hcc) or Histoplasma capsulatum var. duboisii (Hcd) are commonly found in the African continent. It is also known as Classical or African Histoplasmosis. A comparison of the two phenotypes is tabulated in Table1 [8].

Table 1. Differentiating features between classical and african histoplasmosis. [Adapted from open-source article] [8]

Characteristic Feature	Classical Histoplasmosis	African Histoplasmosis
Size of Cell (Microns)	3-5	7-15
Cell wall width	Thin	Thick
Most common geographical location in Africa	Northern and southern Africa	Central and West Africa.
Route of transmission	Inhalation of spores	Direct inoculation of skin and inhalation.
HIV association	Common	Uncommon
Most common sites	Pulmonary, bone marrow and Reticulo endothelial system, adrenals.	Integument, lymph node and internal viscera.
Treatment	Anti-infective chemotherapy	Surgery and anti-infective chemotherapy.

Both the species of Histoplasma such as H.Capsulatum and H. duboisii, enter the body through the inhalation route but direct penetration through skin has been proposed for the latter [8]. Commonly involved sites include skin, subcutaneous tissue, lymph nodes and bones. Two main skin lesions have been described in Africa; lesions that are localized with no systemic manifestation or widespread disease involving bone and or internal viscus [8]. The circumference of skin lesions can vary from 5 to 80 mm [8]. These skin lesions can have different morphologies, such as papules, nodules, ulcers, eczema, psoriasiform, or circinate lesions [8]. Therefore, these lesions can have a broad differential diagnosis, as enumerated in Table 2. [8]. In addition, tuberculosis is an important differential diagnosis [1, 8].

Table 2. Differential diagnosis of histoplasmosis skin lesions. [Adapted from open-source article [8]]

Integumental lesions (Type)	Differential diagnosis
Papules and nodules	Molluscum Contagiosum, Bromoderma, Kaposi sarcoma, Sarcoidosis, Common warts, Sporotrichosis, Leishmaniasis, Cryptococcosis, Emergo mycosis.
Infiltrated plaques	Lichen planus, Eczema, Psoriasis, Emergo mycosis.
Ulcer	Basal cell ca, cutaneous TB, Buruli ulcer, Sporotrichosis, Leishmaniasis, Cryptococcosis, Emergo mycosis.
Circinate lesions	Tinea corporis, Granuloma annulare.
Multiple granulomas	Malignant tumor, Blastomyces infection, Mycetoma.
Abscess	Bacterial infection, Helminthic abscess, foreign body, Lipoma, chromoblastomycosis and cryptococcosis.
Bony lesions	
Sinuses	Mycetoma, TB and bacterial bone infection, Actinomyces infection.
Giant granuloma	Blastomycosis, Chronic osteomyelitis, malignant tumor.

While older skin lesions heal, simultaneously newer lesions develop [8]. Like in tuberculosis, older lesions may evolve into large cold suppurative lesions, while singular lesions may spontaneously resolve. Lymph node involvement can be local or disseminated involving, the groin, neck, and axilla commonly [8]. When internal viscera are involved, malignancy is a consideration and may require more extensive work up which often can be invasive [8].

Malignancy

In patients with a history of residing in endemic regions, pulmonary nodules are commonly seen in imaging such as x-rays and Computed tomography(CT) scans. Histoplasmosis is one of the common fungal infections mimicking malignancy of the lung. In patients presenting with certain features such as lymphadenopathy or nodules, malignancy is often the primary concern, particularly in the appropriate epidemiological setting [9]. Although clinical features are often inconclusive due to the varied manifestation of both these conditions, certain features, including involvement of the anterior mediastinum, lymphopenia, or cervical lymph nodes, suggest malignancy to be more likely than histoplasmosis [10, 11].

Among the spectrum of malignancy presenting with solitary nodules, primary lung cancer, carcinoid tumors, and solitary lung metastasis may present with nodules like that of histoplasmosis. CT imaging findings suggesting malignancy include a stippled or eccentric calcification pattern, spiculated border, doubling of growth rate, and a lower density (< 185 Hounsfield units) [3]. Differentiating the nodules from malignancy may be difficult for these patients, requiring biopsy. Evidence suggests a decreased radionuclide uptake on PET scans in histoplasmosis-associated nodules compared to malignancy [6].

Mediastinal histoplasmosis syndromes can also present as a mass and cause complications that must be differentiated from malignancy and infection. Mediastinal adenitis occurs in young patients less than 20 years old. It may present as a homogenous mass on chest CT obstructing the airway, esophagus, and other vascular structures[6]. Mediastinal granulomas occur in all ages and present as a heterogenous mass in chest CT. It causes obstruction, fistula formation, bacterial superinfection, and pain [6]. Fibrosing mediastinitis typically occurs in 20-30-year-olds and is a late complication obstructing the airway, esophagus, and vascular structures [6]. Histoplasma serology may help diagnose mediastinal histoplasmosis syndromes in these patients [6]. Histoplasma may present with mediastinal lymphadenopathy, often caused by a hematologic malignancy such as lymphoma. Often, imaging and biopsy are required to differentiate between those conditions as both may present with non-specific symptoms [12]. Some features, such as location in the middle mediastinum and elevation of anti-Histoplasma titer, suggest that histoplasmosis is more likely [3]. Endobronchial histoplasmosis may rarely present with a fixed, obstructing endobronchial lesion clinically associated with hemoptysis and dyspnea, presenting similarly to primary bronchogenic carcinoma [13].

Disseminated and Miscellaneous Considerations

Immunocompromised patients presenting with constitutional and respiratory symptoms for 1-2 weeks may have Progressive disseminated Histoplasmosis (PDH). The radiologic examination would show diffuse reticulonodular and interstitial lung infiltrates[6].. 80% of cases of PDH clinically present as fever of unknown origin with constitutional symptoms resembling disseminated tuberculosis infection. From the lungs, the fungus can disseminate to virtually any system in the body [14].

PDH may form lesions in different areas, including the tongue, buccal mucosa, larynx, lip, and genitalia. Such lesions are often confused with squamous cell carcinoma or other malignancy [14]. Bronchoalveolar lavage, Histoplasma antigen, cytopathology and cultures, including both blood and bone marrow, may be necessary to diagnose these patients [6]. Outside malignancy, clinical and laboratory features resemble other granulomatous infections like tuberculosis or other fungal infections, including cryptococcosis and blastomycoses [14]. Gastrointestinal histoplasmosis is a rare manifestation of Histoplasma infection [15]. In PDH involving the GI tract, lymphoid tissue from the mouth to the anus may be involved, with the terminal ileum being the most common due to Peyer patches [16]. GI symptoms can be non-specific, such as abdominal pain or diarrhea, or site-specific, in the form of an obstructing or fungating mass, oropharyngeal and anorectal ulcers, GI bleeding, or clinical signs of bowel obstruction [15, 17]. The wide range of symptoms resembles appendicitis, inflammatory bowel disease, malignancy, and other diseases of the GI tract [17, 18]. Central nervous system (CNS) involvement is another rare manifestation of Histoplasmosis infection. Intracerebral Histoplasma may cause mass effects and resemble brain tumors or brain abscesses in CT scans, showing ring enhancement with contrast. PDH involving the CNS may present with subacute signs and symptoms, including headaches, altered mental status, focal neurologic deficits, cognitive deficits, and seizures, which may be due to other causes in the spectrum of CNS infections in the immunocompromised patient, such as progressive multifocal leukoencephalopathy, cryptococcal meningoencephalitis, toxoplasma encephalitis, tuberculous meningitis, cytomegalovirus encephalitis, and varicella-zoster virus meningitis [19-21].

Histoplasmosis may also present as inflammatory syndromes usually found with subacute pulmonary histoplasmosis. Rheumatologic manifestations such as arthritis and arthralgias, associated with erythema nodosum, can also be found in 5-10% of acute infections [1]. Rheumatologic manifestations are more common in the female sex and must be differentiated from other rheumatologic conditions [22]. Chest pain and pericarditis can develop due to the inflammatory response to the infection; risk factors for pericarditis include healthy, young patients, male sex, and the African race; it is important to distinguish from other causes of chest pain [1, 22].

Although pathophysiology is still unknown, another manifestation of histoplasmosis is the presumed ocular histoplasmosis syndrome (POHS) presents with atrophic chorioretinal scars, peripapillary atrophy, and the absence of vitreous inflammation. POHS can be asymptomatic until choroidal neovascularization develops [23]. Multiple differential diagnoses can include other causes of chorioretinitis, autoimmune conditions such as sarcoidosis, Behcet syndrome, Vogt-Koyanagi-Harada syndrome, and infections such as toxoplasmosis, toxocariasis, and rubella [1, 23].

Conclusion

The clinical manifestation of histoplasmosis is varied, and it can present similarly to other infectious, inflammatory, and even malignant conditions. Thus, it is essential to have it as a differential diagnosis and consider the different histoplasmosis syndromes and epidemiological factors when treating these patients.

References

[1] Loscalzo J, Fauci A, Kasper D, Hauser S, Longo D, Jameson JL: Preface. Harrison's Principles of Internal Medicine, 21e. McGraw-Hill Education, New York, NY; 2022.

[2] Azar M M, Loyd J L, Relich R F, Wheat L J, Hage C A: Current Concepts in the Epidemiology, Diagnosis, and Management of Histoplasmosis Syndromes. *Semin. Respir. Cri.t Care Med. 2020*, 41:013-030. 10.1055/s-0039-1698429.

[3] Wheat L J, Conces D, Allen S D, Blue-Hnidy D, Loyd J: Pulmonary histoplasmosis syndromes: recognition, diagnosis, and management. *Semin. Respir. Crit. Care Med.* 2004, 25:129-144. 10.1055/s-2004-824898.

[4] Update on emerging infections: News from the Centers for Disease Control and Prevention. Annals of Emergency Medicine. 2003, 42:110-112. https://doi.org/10.1067/mem.2003.318.

[5] Samaddar A, Sharma A: Emergomycosis, an Emerging Systemic Mycosis in Immunocompromised Patients: Current Trends and Future Prospects. *Frontiers in Medicine.* 2021, 8. 10.3389/fmed.2021.670731.

[6] Azar M M, Hage C A: Clinical Perspectives in the Diagnosis and Management of Histoplasmosis. *Clin. Chest. Med.* 2017, 38:403-415. 10.1016/j.ccm.2017.04.004.

[7] Ohshimo S, Guzman J, Costabel U, Bonella F: Differential diagnosis of granulomatous lung disease: clues and pitfalls. *European Respiratory Review*. 2017, 26:170012. 10.1183/16000617.0012-2017.

[8] Ocansey B K, Kosmidis C, Agyei M, Dorkenoo A M, Ayanlowo O O, Oladele R O, Darre T, Denning D W: Histoplasmosis in Africa: Current perspectives, knowledge

gaps, and research priorities. *PLoS Negl. Trop. Dis.* 2022, 16:e0010111. 10.1371/journal.pntd.0010111.

[9] Gazzoni F F, Severo L C, Marchiori E, Irion K L, Guimarães M D, Godoy M C, Sartori A P G, Hochhegger B: Fungal diseases mimicking primary lung cancer: radiologic–pathologic correlation. *Mycoses.* 2014, 57:197-208. https://doi.org/10.1111/myc.12150.

[10] Dall Bello A G, Severo C B, Guazzelli L S, Oliveira F M, Hochhegger B, Severo L C: Histoplasmosis mimicking primary lung cancer or pulmonary metastases. *J. Bras. Pneumol.* 2013, 39:63-68. 10.1590/s1806-37132013000100009.

[11] Naeem F, Metzger M L, Arnold S R, Adderson E E: Distinguishing Benign Mediastinal Masses from Malignancy in a Histoplasmosis-Endemic Region. *The Journal of Pediatrics. 2015*, 167:409-415. https://doi.org/10.1016/j.jpeds. 2015.04.066.

[12] McGraw E P, Kane J M, Kleiman M B, Scherer L R: Cervical abscess and mediastinal adenopathy: an unusual presentation of childhood histoplasmosis. *Pediatr. Radiol.* 2002, 32:862-864. 10.1007/s00247-002-0808-2.

[13] Ross P, Jr., Magro CM, King MA: Endobronchial histoplasmosis: a masquerade of primary endobronchial neoplasia--a clinical study of four cases. Ann Thorac Surg. 2004, 78:277-281. 10.1016/j.athoracsur.2003.12.045.

[14] Donegan JO, Wood MD: Histoplasmosis of the larynx. *The Laryngoscope.* 1984, 94:206-209. https://doi.org/10.1288/00005537-198402000-00011.

[15] Mullick S S, Mody D R, Schwartz M R: Cytology of gastrointestinal histoplasmosis. A report of two cases with differential diagnosis and diagnostic pitfalls. *Acta Cytol.* 1996, 40:989-994. 10.1159/000334015.

[16] 16. Cappell MS, Mandell W, Grimes MM, Neu HC: Gastrointestinal histoplasmosis. Digestive Diseases and Sciences. 1988, 33:353-360. 10.1007/BF01535762.

[17] Kahi C J, Wheat L J, Allen S D, Sarosi G A: Gastrointestinal Histoplasmosis. *Official journal of the American College of Gastroenterology* | ACG. 2005, 100:220-231.

[18] Koot R A, van Uum S H, Naber A H, Meis J F: [Generalized histoplasmosis due to endogenous reactivation of a latent infection in an HIV-seronegative man]. *Ned. Tijdschr. Geneeskd.* 1995, 139:1454-1456.

[19] Epelboin L, Dione A, Serris A, Blanchet D, Bidaud B, Walter G, Abboud P, Mosnier E, Gaillet M, Michaud C, Couppié P, Demar M, Nacher M, Djossou F, Adenis A: Histoplasmosis of the Central Nervous System: A Case Series between 1990 and 2019 in French Guiana. *The American Journal of Tropical Medicine and Hygiene.* 2021, 105:125-129. 10.4269/ajtmh.20-1486.

[20] Sheybani F, van de Beek D, Brouwer MC: Suspected Central Nervous System Infections in HIV-Infected Adults. *Frontiers in Neurology.* 2021, 12. 10.3389/fneur.2021.741884.

[21] Nyalakonda H, Albuerne M, Suazo Hernandez L P, Sarria J C: Central Nervous System Histoplasmosis in Acquired Immunodeficiency Syndrome. *The American Journal of the Medical Sciences.* 2016, 351:177-186. https://doi.org/10.1016/j.amjms.2015.11.016.

[22] Bahr N C, Antinori S, Wheat L J, Sarosi G A: Histoplasmosis Infections Worldwide: Thinking Outside of the Ohio River Valley. *Current Tropical Medicine Reports.* 2015, 2:70-80. 10.1007/s40475-015-0044-0.

[23] Oliver A, Ciulla TA, Comer G M: New and classic insights into presumed ocular histoplasmosis syndrome and its treatment. Current Opinion in Ophthalmology. 2005, 16:160-165. 10.1097/01.icu.0000161228.21797.d9.

Chapter 17

Histoplasmosis-Induced Hemophagocytic Syndrome

Noura Attallah[1]
Ibtisam Rauf[2]
Abbas B. Jama[1]
Esraa Hassan[1]
Syed Anjum Khan[1]
and Mohamad El Labban[3]
[1]Critical Care Medicine Department,
Mayo Clinic Health System, Mankato, Minnesota, USA
[2]Medicine Department, St. George's School of Medicine,
University Centre Grenada, West Indies, Grenada, USA
[3]Internal Medicine Department,
Mayo Clinic Health System, Mankato, Minnesota, USA

Abstract

This chapter provides an overview of hemophagocytic lymphohistiocytosis (HLH) specifically HLH secondary to histoplasmosis. It starts with an introduction that defines HLH and disseminates histoplasmosis. This is followed by discussion of the pathophysiology behind HLH and the mechanism through which histoplasmosis can induce HLH. The diagnostic criteria of HLH in addition to scoring algorithms to diagnose secondary HLH are then reviewed in depth. Finally, treatment and prognosis compendium are discussed at the end of the chapter.

In: Histoplasmosis
Editors: Salim Surani, Syed Anjum Khan and Reena Shah
ISBN: 979-8-89113-129-3

Keywords: hemophagocytic lymphohistiocytosis, secondary hemophagocytic lymphohistiocytosis, histoplasmosis, disseminated histoplasmosis, histoplasmosis-induced hemophagocytic lymphohistiocytosis

Introduction

Hemophagocytic lymphohistiocytosis (HLH) is defined as a severe hyperinflammatory syndrome driven by immune cells' abnormal activation that is now more recognized across all age groups. Histoplasmosis is the most prevalent endemic mycotic infection in the United States [1]. H. capsulatum var. capsulatum is endemic in the regions of Ohio and the Mississippi River [2]. Disseminated histoplasmosis is defined as a severe widespread extrapulmonary infection. Immunocompromised or elderly patients are at increased risk.

Pathophysiology of HLH

The pathogenesis of HLH is due to dysregulation and uncontrolled immunological activation. The HLH pathophysiology is not entirely explained; it is postulated that the reason behind the hyperinflammatory immune response is a disruption in the negative feedback mechanisms [3, 4]. The result is excessive secretion of pro-inflammatory cytokines as tumor necrosis factor α (TNFα), interferon γ, and interleukins (1, 4, 6, 8, 10, and 18) 8 causing a possibly fatal "cytokine storm" [4]. In secondary HLH, the immune system cannot limit the stimulatory effects of multiple triggers. Cell-mediated immunity is the primary immune response involved in the defense against histoplasmosis. After natural killer cells recognize the histoplasma antigen, cytokines activate macrophages to kill the fungus [4].

Types of HLH

HLH is classified as familial (primary) or acquired (secondary). Familial HLH is the primary subtype in children, whereas secondary HLH is more recognized in adolescents and adults. Infections are still the most common triggering factor of HLH [5, 6]. Primary familial hemophagocytic lymphohistiocytosis (FHL), with an incidence of 1:50,000 live births, is the predominant autosomal recessive type [7]. Infection-triggered is the most common subtype in secondary HLH. EBV, CMV, and HIV remain the leading culprits. Other infectious triggers include bacteria (e.g., mycobacteria and spirochaetes) and fungi (e.g., histoplasmosis). The majority of HLH cases linked to histoplasmosis were in patients with disseminated histoplasmosis. The most prevalent immunodeficiency causing HLH still is HIV [8]; however, there is increasing evidence of HLH occurring in other etiologies of immunosuppression (e.g., chronic steroid use, transplant patients) [2].

Diagnosis

HLH is a potentially fatal disease. Prompt recognition and treatment are crucial for better outcomes. The clinical presentations of HLH and acute disseminated histoplasmosis frequently overlap, making the diagnosis much more challenging. Fever, fatigue, cytopenia, and splenomegaly can be caused by either condition in the setting of immunocompromised patients. Because of that reason, a high level of suspicion is warranted to diagnose HLH in cases with histoplasmosis dissemination.

Diagnostic Criteria of HLH

The HLH-2004 diagnostic criteria:

If either criterion 1 or criterion 2 below is fulfilled, the HLH diagnosis can be confirmed.

(1) A molecular diagnosis of HLH [7] (common mutations detection such as mutations in the perforin gene (*PRF*) [9], *UNC13D* [10], or *STX1* [11].
(2) HLH Diagnostic criteria are established (at least five out of the eight criteria below) [7].

(A) Preliminary diagnostic criteria:
 1. High Temperature.

2. Splenomegaly.
3. Hypertriglyceridemia and/or hypofibrinogenemia:
   Fibrinogen level ≤ 1.5 g/L.

   Fasting triglycerides level ≥ 3.0 mmol/L (i.e., ≥ 265 mg/dl).

   Hemophagocytosis present in the spleen or lymph nodes or bone marrow (Figure 1).

4. Cytopenias (in two or more of 3 peripheral blood lineages):
   Hemoglobin < 90 g/L (in infants < 4 weeks: hemoglobin < 100 g/L).

   Neutrophils $< 1.0 \times 10^9$/L.

   Platelets $< 100 \times 10^9$/L.

5. Exclusion of malignancy.

(B) New diagnostic criteria:
1. Low or absent activity of Natural Killer cells [12].
2. Ferritin ≥ 500 μg/L [13].
3. Soluble CD25 ≥ 2,400 U/ml [14].

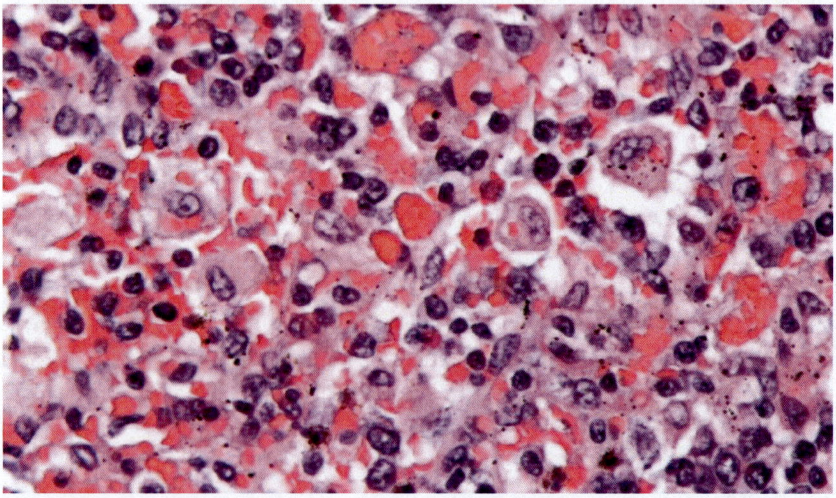

Figure 1. Hemophagocytic Syndrome (H&E Stain) Nephron, CC BY-SA 3.0 <https://creativecommons.org/licenses/by-sa/3.0>, via Wikimedia Commons.

In addition, there is also Hscore and Delphi study scoring algorithms which is shown in Table 1.

Diagnostic Methods of Histoplasmosis [6]

1. A lung or lymph node specimen can be collected for histopathology and serology tests to determine the diagnosis.
2. Fungal culture using multiple sputum bronchoalveolar lavage (BAL) samples.
3. Antigen detection in the blood, urine, or BAL samples of infected individuals.
4. by utilizing enzyme immunoassay (EIA).
5. Serology by performing complement fixation, enzyme immunoassay, and immunodiffusion.
6. Polymerase chain reaction (PCR).

Table 1. Available Scoring algorithms used for the secondary HLH diagnosis

HScore [15]	Delphi study [16]
History of immunosuppression	History of Immunosuppression
High temperature	High Temperature
Hepatosplenomegaly	Hepatosplenomegaly
Increased Ferritin	Increased Ferritin
Cytopenia	Cytopenia
Hemophagocytosis	Hemophagocytosis
High Triglycerides	High LDH
High SGOT/ALT	
Low fibrin	

Treatment of HLH

The goal of treating HLH is to remove any possible trigger to the overreactive immune system. If a neoplasm or infection is detected, treatment targeted to that condition should immediately begin. For histoplasmosis-associated HLH syndrome, antifungal treatment consisting of amphotericin B formulation or

Azole has been shown to decrease mortality in histoplasmosis-associated HLH [17].

The HLH-94 Treatment Protocol for the Pediatric Population [6]

Infants, toddlers, and children up to 18 are treated with the HLH-94 pediatric treatment protocol. The regimen consists of an induction phase, an 8-week chemotherapy course with etoposide and dexamethasone, followed by a remission phase. A bone marrow transplant is eventually required to reach a cure. Patients with familial HLH and persistent secondary HLH were more likely to proceed with BMT after the induction phase. On the other hand, patients with secondary HLH with partial or complete remission can be treated intermittently with HLH-94 protocol in case of relapse. Prophylactic antimicrobial therapy, including antifungals, antibiotics, and antivirals, is required during periods of immunosuppression.

Adult Treatment Protocol [18]

In adults, acquired/secondary HLH is more prevalent, and treatment is directed to the underlying trigger (infection, malignancy, immune disorders, or drug interactions). Common chemotherapy regimens include CHOP (cyclophosphamide, doxorubicin, vincristine, and prednisone) corticosteroid, etoposide, methylprednisolone, or IVIG. Alternative therapies, including chemotherapy with ruxolitinib, doxorubicin, emapalumab, alemtuzumab, and plasma exchange, have proven efficacy in treating refractory/relapsed (r/r) HLH. If clinical improvement is observed, we believe immunosuppressive medication can be weaned.

Prognosis

About 198 patients with HLH had follow-up data available with diverse durations of monitoring. One hundred and three (52%) of children with HIH died due to severe infection due to pancytopenia, disseminated intravascular coagulation, or multi-organ failure. Infection Associated Hemophagocytic

Syndrome (IAHS) caused by bacterial infections had a reasonable recovery rate; EB virus infection associated-HLH had the poorest prognosis [19]. Based on a recent report, 27 patients of HLH related to progressive disseminated histoplasmosis (PDH) have been documented, with a 38% fatality rate [20].

Conclusion

This book chapter provides a much-needed review of HLH and more specifically histoplasmosis induced HLH. The latter is due to a dysregulated immunological activation secondary to histoplasma. A criterion must be met before establishing the diagnosis and the treatment is directed towards both HLH and the trigger in cases of secondary HLH such as disseminated histoplasmosis.

References

[1] Chu J H, Feudtner C, Heydon K, Walsh T J, Zaoutis T E. Hospitalizations for endemic mycoses: a population-based national study. *Clinical Infectious Diseases*. 2006;42(6):822-5.

[2] Assi M, Martin S, Wheat L J, Hage C, Freifeld A, Avery R, Baddley J W, Vergidis P, Miller R, Andes D, Young J A, Hammoud K, Huprikar S, McKinsey D, Myint T, Garcia-Diaz J, Esguerra E, Kwak E J, Morris M, Mullane K M, Prakash V, Burdette S D, Sandid M, Dickter J, Ostrander D, Antoun S A, Kaul D R. Histoplasmosis after solid organ transplant. *Clinical infectious diseases*. 2013;57(11):1542-9.

[3] Al-Samkari H, Berliner N. *Hemophagocytic lymphohistiocytosis*. Annual review of pathology: mechanisms of disease. 2018;13:27-49.

[4] Townsend J L, Shanbhag S, Hancock J, Bowman K, Nijhawan A E, editors. Histoplasmosis-induced hemophagocytic syndrome: a case series and review of the literature. *Open forum infectious diseases*; 2015: Oxford University Press.

[5] McClain K L, Eckstein O. Clinical features and diagnosis of hemophagocytic lymphohistiocytosis. *UpToDate*, Waltham, MA, USA; 2018.

[6] La Rosée P, Horne A, Hines M, von Bahr Greenwood T, Machowicz R, Berliner N, Birndt S, Gil-Herrera J, Girschikofsky M, Jordan M B, Kumar A, van Laar J A M, Lachmann G, Nichols K E, Ramanan A V, Wang Y, Wang Z, Janka G, Henter J I. Recommendations for the management of hemophagocytic lymphohistiocytosis in adults. *Blood*. 2019;133(23):2465-77.

[7] Henter J I, Elinder G, Ost A. Diagnostic guidelines for hemophagocytic lymphohistiocytosis. The FHL Study Group of the Histiocyte Society. *Semin. Oncol.* 1991;18(1):29-33.

[8] Jabr Re, El Atrouni W, Male H J, Hammoud K A. Histoplasmosis-associated hemophagocytic lymphohistiocytosis: a review of the literature. *The Canadian Journal of Infectious Diseases & Medical Microbiology= Journal Canadien des Maladies Infectieuses et de la Microbiologie Médicale*. 2019;2019.

[9] Stepp S E, Dufourcq-Lagelouse R, Le Deist F, Bhawan S, Certain S, Mathew P A, Henter J I, Bennett M, Fischer A, de Saint Basile G, Kumar V. Perforin gene defects in familial hemophagocytic lymphohistiocytosis. *Science*. 1999;286(5446):1957-9.

[10] Feldmann J, Callebaut I, Raposo G, Certain S, Bacq D, Dumont C, Lambert N, Ouachée-Chardin M, Chedeville G, Tamary H, Minard-Colin V, Vilmer E, Blanche S, Le Deist F, Fischer A, de Saint Basile G. Munc13-4 is essential for cytolytic granules fusion and is mutated in a form of familial hemophagocytic lymphohistiocytosis (FHL3). *Cell*. 2003;115(4):461-73.

[11] Zur Stadt U, Schmidt S, Kasper B, Beutel K, Diler A S, Henter J I, Kabisch H, Schneppenheim R, Nürnberg P, Janka G, Hennies H C. Linkage of familial hemophagocytic lymphohistiocytosis (FHL) type-4 to chromosome 6q24 and identification of mutations in syntaxin 11. *Human molecular genetics*. 2005;14(6):827-34.

[12] Perez N, Virelizier J-L, Arenzana-Seisdedos F, Fischer A, Griscelli C. Impaired natural killer activity in lymphohistiocytosis syndrome. *The Journal of pediatrics*. 1984;104(4):569-73.

[13] Esumi N, Ikushima S, Todo S, Imashuku S. Hyperferritinemia in malignant histiocytosis, virus-associated hemophagocytic syndrome and familial erythrophagocytic lymphohistiocytosis. A survey of pediatric cases. *Acta Paediatr. Scand*. 1989;78(2):268-70.

[14] Komp D M, McNamara J, Buckley P. *Elevated soluble interleukin-2 receptor in childhood hemophagocytic histiocytic syndromes*. 1989.

[15] Fardet L, Galicier L, Lambotte O, Marzac C, Aumont C, Chahwan D, Coppo P, Hejblum G. Development and validation of the HScore, a score for the diagnosis of reactive hemophagocytic syndrome. *Arthritis & Rheumatology*. 2014;66(9):2613-20.

[16] Hejblum G, Lambotte O, Galicier L, Coppo P, Marzac C, Aumont C, Fardet L. A web-based delphi study for eliciting helpful criteria in the positive diagnosis of hemophagocytic syndrome in adult patients. *PloS one*. 2014;9(4):e94024.

[17] Risdall R J, McKenna R W, Nesbit M E, Krivit W, Balfour H H Jr, Simmons R L, Brunning R D. Virus-associated hemophagocytic syndrome A benign histiocytic proliferation distinct from malignant histiocytosis. *Cancer*. 1979;44(3):993-1002.

[18] Schram A M, Berliner N. How I treat hemophagocytic lymphohistiocytosis in the adult patient. Blood, *The Journal of the American Society of Hematology*. 2015;125(19):2908-14.

[19] Janka G, Imashuku S, Elinder G, Schneider M, Henter J-I. Infection-and malignancy-associated hemophagocytic syndromes: secondary hemophagocytic lymphohistiocytosis. *Hematology/oncology clinics of North America*. 1998;12(2): 435-44.

[20] Henter J I, Elinder G, Söder O, Öst Å. Incidence in Sweden and clinical features of familial hemophagocytic lymphohistiocytosis. *Acta Paediatrica.* 1991;80(4):428-35.

About the Authors

Salim R. Surani, MD, MPH, MSHM, FACP, FCCP, FAASM, FCCM

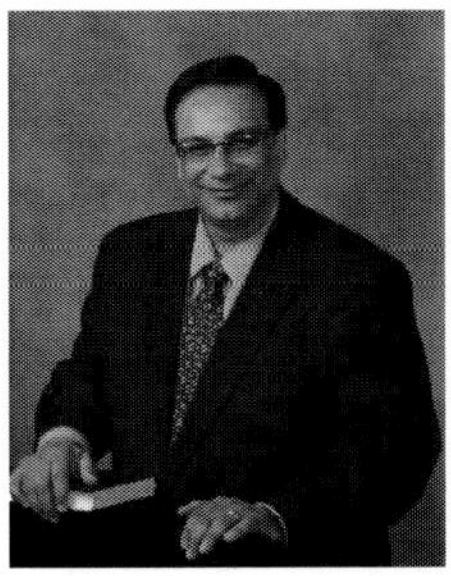

Dr. Salim Surani serves as Adjunct Clinical Professor of Medicine, Department of Pulmonary, Critical Care & Sleep Medicine at Texas A&M University, as well as Clinical Professor of Pharmacology at Texas A&M University Kingsville. In addition, he serves as the voluntary Professor at the University of Houston and the Research Collaborator at Mayo Clinic, Minnesota. He has served as the program director for Pulmonary Fellowship Program at Bay Area Medical Center, Corpus Christi. He has done his fellowship in Pulmonary Medicine at Baylor College of Medicine, Houston, Texas. Dr. Surani has done his master's in public health & Epidemiology from Yale University and master's in health management from the University of Texas, Dallas. Dr. Surani also serves as a board trustee for THE CHEST Foundation and on numerous national and international committees. He is serving as editor in chief, editorial board member, and reviewer for several peer-review journal. Dr. Surani has authored more than 300 articles in the peer review journals and has written 50 book chapters. He has established himself as a Master Clinician who has trained significant numbers of practicing primary care, internal medicine, and emergency physicians in the Coastal Bend region in the USA. He has served as an independent grant reviewer for the Government of Australia, the Government of Singapore, and the European Nation via Rannis.

During the pandemic, Dr. Surani has been involved in taking care of critically ill patients with COVID and has been relentlessly involved in educating the community locally and medical community globally during his role as the resident medical expert in KIII TV Coastal bend, as well as educator and academician globally.

Dr. Surani serves as a resident health expert, first edition in Kiii TV (affiliate of ABC News). Dr. Surani is highly regarded among his peers and is very well respected as a mentor, clinician, and humanitarian

Dr. Syed Anjum Khan

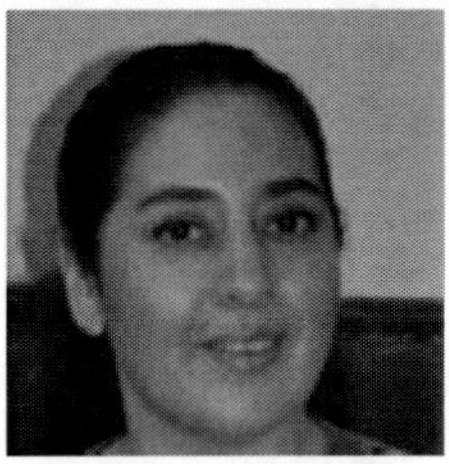

Dr. Syed Anjum Khan has been involved in patient care, education, and curriculum development for Critical Care education for more than two decades. She serves as the regional chair of critical care division for Southwest Minnesota Mayo Clinic Health system from 2007-present. She also serves as the member of specialty critical care council committee member for the Southwest Minnesota Mayo Clinic Health system for past 10 years. She also serves as a member of Mayo Enterprise Critical care specialty council and a Member of Mayo Enterprise Critical care practice committee for past several years. She played an instrumental role in taking care of critically ill covid patients during the COVID-19 pandemic and was the site investigator for the Discovery virus trial which was a collaboration between Society of Critical Care Medicine and mayo clinic. Exceptional educator, researcher, mentor, and very well reputed critical care physician. She brings a diverse expertise for editing this book on Respiratory insufficiency.

Professor Reena Shah

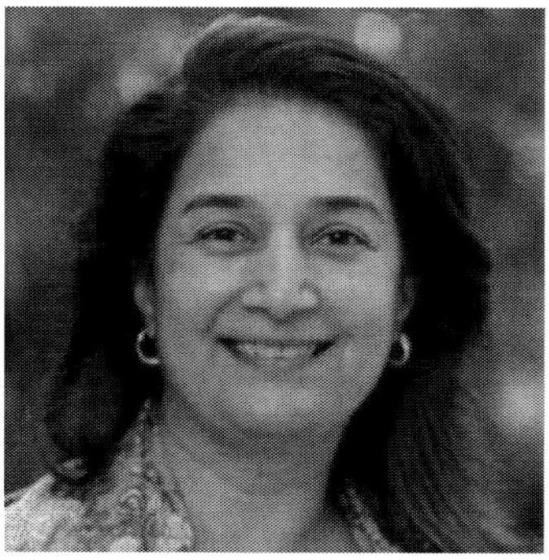

Professor Reena Shah is a Consultant Physician, Section Head of Infectious Diseases and the Fellowship Director for Infectious Disease Fellowship Program at Aga Khan University Hospital. She has recently been appointed head of department of Medicine.

She received her MBBS degree from the University of Southampton (UK) in 1996 and her MRCP from the Royal College of Physicians London in 2000. She obtained a Diploma in Infectious Diseases from the University of London, UK in 2008 as well as completed Diploma in Tropical Medicine and Infectious Diseases from the London School of Tropical Medicine and Hygiene (UK) in 2009. She also holds a Masters in Infectious Diseases from the University of London since 2008. She obtained Fellowship of the Royal College of Physicians Edinburgh (FRCPE) in 2014 and Fellowship of the Royal College of Physicians London (FRCP) London in 2018.

She is currently leading the hospital in COVID-19 response as Head of Infectious Diseases and a frontline worker. She has also been involved in the development of the national case management guidelines in Kenya. With her new appointment she oversees all the section in internal medicine which includes cardiology, pulmonology, gastro, neuro, ICU among others.

Index

A

E

F

G

H

I

R

S

T

U

V